STRUCTURAL APPROACHES IN PUBLIC HEALTH

That health has many social determinants is well established and a myriad range of structural factors – social, cultural, political, economic, and environmental – are now known to impact on population well-being. Public health practice has started exploring and responding to a range of health-related challenges from a structural paradigm, including individual and population vulnerability to infection with HIV and AIDS, injury prevention, obesity, and smoking cessation.

Recognizing the inadequacy of public health responses that focus solely on individual behaviour change to improve population health outcomes, this text promotes a more holistic approach. Discussing the structural factors related to health and well-being that are both within and outside an individual's control, it explores what form structural approaches can take, the underlying theory of structure as a risk factor and the local realities, environments, and priorities that public health practitioners need to take into consideration. Anchored in empirical evidence, the book provides case studies of innovative and influential interventions – from the 100% Condom Use Programme, to urban planning, injury prevention, and the provision of adequate clean drinking water and sanitation systems – and concludes with a section on implementing and evaluating structural public health programmes.

This comprehensive text brings together a selection of internationally recognized authors to provide an overview for students and practitioners working in or concerned with public health around the globe.

Marni Sommer is Assistant Professor of Sociomedical Sciences, and Director of the Global Health Track for the Department of Sociomedical Sciences, at Columbia University's Mailman School of Public Health, USA. She is the Executive Editor of the journal *Global Public Health*.

Richard Parker is Professor of Sociomedical Sciences and Anthropology, and Director of the Center for the Study of Culture, Politics, and Health at Columbia University, USA. He is Editor-in-Chief of the journal *Global Public Health*.

STRUCTURAL APPROACHES IN PUBLIC HEALTH

Edited by
Marni Sommer and Richard Parker

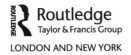

Routledge
Taylor & Francis Group

LONDON AND NEW YORK

First published 2013
by Routledge
2 Park Square, Milton Park, Abingdon, Oxon, OX14 4RN

Simultaneously published in the USA and Canada
by Routledge
711 Third Avenue, New York, NY 10017

Routledge is an imprint of the Taylor & Francis Group, an informa business

British Library Cataloguing in Publication Data
A catalogue record for this book is available from the British Library

Library of Congress Cataloging in Publication Data
Structural approaches in public health / edited by Marni Sommer, Richard Parker.
    p. ; cm.
    Includes bibliographical references.
    I. Sommer, Marni. II. Parker, Richard G. (Richard Guy), 1956–
    [DNLM: 1. Public Health. 2. Social Medicine. 3. Health Policy.
    4. Social Environment. 5. World Health. WA 31]
    362.1--dc23   2012039032

ISBN: 978-0-415-50085-2 (hbk)
ISBN: 978-0-415-50086-9 (pbk)
ISBN: 978-0-203-55829-4 (ebk)

Typeset in Bembo
by Bookcraft Ltd, Stroud, Gloucestershire

DEDICATED TO THE MEMORY OF
ALAN BERKMAN

CONTENTS

WITHDRAWN

CONTENTS

CONTENTS

LIST OF ILLUSTRATIONS

Figures

Tables

ACKNOWLEDGEMENTS

The editors would particularly like to thank Margaret Bradley who greatly assisted in preparing the manuscripts for publication, and Alana Kolundzija at the Mailman School of Public Health, Columbia University, who liaised with contributors and assisted with related administrative support. We would also like to acknowledge the ongoing institutional support of the Center for the Study of Culture, Politics, and Health, based in the Department of Sociomedical Sciences at Columbia University's Mailman School of Public Health.

NOTES ON CONTRIBUTORS

Peter Aggleton is Professor of Education and Health at the National Centre in HIV Social Research, Faculty of Arts and Social Sciences, University of New South Wales, Australia. He has authored and edited numerous books in the fields of sexuality, health and human rights, and is the Editor-in-Chief of the international peer-reviewed journals *Culture, Health and Sexuality*, and *Sex Education*. His most recent book (edited jointly with Richard Parker) is the *Routledge Handbook of Sexuality, Health and Rights* (2010).

Clare Barrington is an Assistant Professor in the Department of Health Behavior and Health Education at the University of North Carolina at Chapel Hill Gillings School of Global Public Health, USA. Dr Barrington's research examines social and structural influences on health and health behaviours, in particular HIV/AIDS. She has been working on community-based research in the Dominican Republic since 1996, and has projects examining HIV vulnerability among Mexican migrant men in North Carolina and men who have sex with men and transgender persons in Central America.

Ruth Bell is a Senior Research Fellow in the Department of Epidemiology and Public Health at University College London (UCL), England, UK. She was a member of the UCL-based secretariat of the World Health Organization (WHO) Commission on Social Determinants of Health (CSDH) and the Marmot Review team in England. Her interests are in global health and health equity, in particular the processes whereby public health knowledge is translated into policy action to tackle health inequalities within and between countries.

Christopher Buckley is a Research Professor in the School of Chemical Engineering and head of the Pollution Research Group (PRG) at the University of KwaZulu-Natal, South Africa. He has conducted research in water and effluent management at the University of Natal (now University of KwaZulu-Natal) since 1976. Current research interests centre on urban and industrial water management in a developing country context with core funding for the municipal component of this activity obtained from eThekwini Municipality (Water and Sanitation Unit) in Durban. He coordinates the research and development activities for BORDA, a German NGO in the field of basic needs services for the poor in Asia and Africa, and was awarded a Reinvent the Toilet Challenge grant from the Bill and Melinda Gates Foundation.

Deborah A. Cohen is a researcher in the area of the built environment and health, and is the co-author of *Prescription for a Healthy Nation: A New Approach to Improving our Lives by Fixing our Everyday World*, published by Beacon Press. She is currently a senior natural scientist at the RAND Corporation, USA. For more than a decade her research studies have focused on the role of the built environment in physical activity and dietary behaviours. She has conducted multiple environmental assessments over the past 15 years, developing tools to study neighbourhood design, physical indicators of collective efficacy, billboards, alcohol outlets and in-store marketing strategies, and parks.

Jonathan Cohen is the Deputy Director of the Open Society Foundations' (OSF) Public Health Program (PHP), USA, and oversees the PHP's work with respect to Roma Health and the Campaign to Stop Torture in Health Care. He was previously the PHP's Senior Human Rights Advisor and founding director of its Law and Health Initiative. In 2011, he was appointed co-chair of the Joint United Nations Programme on HIV/AIDS (UNAIDS) Reference Group on HIV and Human Rights. He previously served as a law clerk at the Supreme Court of Canada and as co-Editor-in-Chief of the *University of Toronto Faculty of Law Review*.

James Colgrove is an Associate Professor in the Center for the History and Ethics of Public Health at Columbia University's Mailman School of Public Health, USA. His research examines the relationship between individual rights and the collective well-being, and the social, political, and legal processes through which public health policies have been mediated in American history. His most recent book is *Epidemic City: The Politics of Public Health in New York* (Russell Sage Foundation, 2011).

Jason Corburn is an Associate Professor jointly appointed in the School of Public Health and the Department of City and Regional Planning at the University of California, Berkeley, USA. He is author of *Toward the Healthy City: People, Places and the Politics of Urban Planning* (2009) and *Street Science: Community Knowledge and Environmental Health Justice* (2005), both published by the MIT Press. He is on the editorial boards of the *Journal of Urban Health* and the *Journal of Planning, Education and Research*.

Heather Doyle directs the Sexual Health and Rights Project at the Open Society Foundation (OSF) in New York, USA, a global human rights and health funding and advocacy project. Her focus areas include minority health equity, sexual rights, and community-based health. Her current project promotes the health and health-related rights of sex workers and sexual and gender minorities in Eastern Europe, Central Asia, sub-Saharan Africa, and Southeast Asia. Prior to joining OSF, Heather worked extensively throughout Eastern Europe, the Balkans, and Africa designing, implementing and evaluating maternal and child health projects and HIV prevention and treatment initiatives.

Andrew Ellner is Co-Director of the Center for Primary Care and Director of the Program in Global Primary Care and Social Change, at Harvard Medical School, USA. He is also an Associate Physician in the Division of Global Health Equity at Brigham and Women's Hospital and Assistant Medical Director of the Phyllis Jen Center for Primary Care. He previously served as the Clinical Policy Director of the Clinton HIV/AIDS Initiative's Rural Initiative and managed the Academic Consortium of the World Health Organization's (WHO) Maximizing Positive Synergies initiative. His work focuses on studying and improving health systems for vulnerable populations.

Amy Fairchild is a Professor of Sociomedical Sciences (SMS) at Columbia University Mailman School of Public Health, USA, and served as Chair of the Department of SMS from 2008 to 2012. She is a historian researching the broad social forces that produce disease and shape public health policy and a public health policy analyst focused on dilemmas in the ethics and politics of contemporary debates. Dr Fairchild's book, *Science at the Borders* (Johns Hopkins University Press, 2003) is a revisionist history uncovering the ways that the machinery of processing unskilled immigrant labourers at the United States' borders in the early 1900s helped to define inclusion into industrial citizenship, the state, and social power. Her book *Searching Eyes: Privacy, the State and Disease Surveillance in America*, co-authored with Ronald Bayer and James Colgrove (University of California Press/Milbank Books on Health and the Public, 2007), focuses on policy challenges that arise when it becomes necessary to report the names of individuals with disease.

Paul Farmer is a founding director of Partners In Health (PIH), an international non-profit organization that provides direct health care services, and has undertaken research and advocacy activities on behalf of those who are sick and living in poverty. He is the Kolokotrones University Professor and Chair of the Department of Global Health and Social Medicine at Harvard Medical School; Chief of the Division of Global Health Equity at Brigham and Women's Hospital; and the United Nations Deputy Special Envoy for Haiti, under Special Envoy Bill Clinton. Dr Farmer has written extensively on health, human rights, and the consequences of social inequality. His books include *Haiti after the Earthquake*; *Partner to the Poor: A Paul Farmer Reader*; *Pathologies of Power: Health, Human Rights, and the New War on the Poor*; *The Uses of Haiti*; *Infections and Inequalities: The Modern Plagues*; and *AIDS and Accusation: Haiti and the Geography of Blame*.

Peter Goldblatt is a Deputy Director of the Institute of Health Equity at University College London (UCL) and an Honorary Professor in the Department of Epidemiology and Population Health. He was seconded from the Office of National Statistics (ONS) to UCL for the duration of the Strategic Review of Health Inequalities in England post–2010 (the Marmot Review). He headed the World Health Organization (WHO) UK Collaborating Centre on Disease Classification within ONS from 1999–2004. Prior to joining ONS, he worked at the Home Office on re-offending statistics and development of a crime reduction strategy; the Department of Health on demographic advice, developing an information strategy for hospital and community health services and statistics on local authority social services for children and families; the Office of Population Censuses and Surveys on longitudinal and vital statistics; City University on a Medical Research Council (MRC) programme on differentials in mortality; and Manchester University on perceptions of risk.

Lori Heise is a Senior Lecturer at the London School of Hygiene and Tropical Medicine, England, UK, and Chief Executive of STRIVE, a research and action consortium dedicated to expanding the evidence base on structural drivers and

HIV. She is founding Director of two NGOs: the Center for Health and Gender Equity (CHANGE) and the Global Campaign for Microbicides, a civil society effort dedicated to expanding research into new methods of HIV prevention, especially for women.

Adnan A. Hyder is an Associate Professor in the Department of International Health, Bloomberg School of Public Health, Johns Hopkins University, USA. He is Director of the International Injury Research Unit (IIRU), a leading centre on injury research and training for the developing world, and a World Health Organization (WHO) Collaborating Centre for Injuries, Violence and Accident Prevention. He is also Director of the Bloomberg School of Public Health's PhD Program in Health Systems, and Associate Director for Global Bioethics of the Johns Hopkins Berman Institute of Bioethics. Dr Hyder directs the global Road Safety in 10 Countries (RS–10) Project supported by Bloomberg Philanthropies, is the current Chairman of the global Road Traffic Injuries Research Network, and a member of the International Organizing Committee of the World Conferences on Injury Prevention and Safety Promotion.

Smarajit Jana is the Principal of the Sonagachi Research and Training Institute. Dr Jana served as the National Programme Advisor at the National AIDS Control Organization for the Government of India from 2007 to 2009, as the Assistant Country Director at CARE India from August 2003 to March 2006, and as the CARE Regional HIV Advisor overseeing 15 countries in the Asia region. He initiated the Sonagachi Project in Kolkata, India, an organization run by sex workers called the Durbar Mahila Samanwaya Committee, which represents 65,000 male, female and transgender sex workers.

Thomas Kerr is the Co-Director of the Urban Health Research Initiative at the British Columbia Centre for Excellence in HIV/AIDS, an Associate Professor in the Department of Medicine at the University of British Columbia, and a Michael Smith Foundation for Health Research Scholar, Canada. Dr Kerr was the co-recipient of the inaugural Population and Public Health Research Milestones Initiative award for his contribution to developing Canada's research base for harm reduction and health equity approaches to HIV prevention and control. Dr Kerr was also the co-recipient of the Alfred R. Lindesmith Award for Achievement in the Field of Scholarship.

Deanna Kerrigan is an Associate Professor of Health, Behavior, and Society and International Health at the Bloomberg School of Public Health, Johns Hopkins University, USA. Her research focuses on the social and structural factors affecting the health and well-being of marginalized populations. Dr Kerrigan currently directs a global HIV prevention research project entitled Research to Prevention (R2P), which conducts applied research in 18 countries aimed at improving the quality and effectiveness of HIV prevention programming and policies.

Rod Knight is a doctoral student at the University of British Columbia's Interdisciplinary Studies Graduate Program within the School of Population and Public Health, Canada. He was a co-founder of the University of British Columbia's CampOUT! programme, a camp for lesbian, gay, bisexual, transgender, and allied youth ages 15 to 21, and served as the inaugural Camp Director. Rod is also the Executive and Academic Coordinator of the Canadian Institutes of Health Research

(CIHR)-funded Population Health Intervention Research Network (PHIRNET), a pan-Canadian strategic training network in population health intervention research.

Scott Lee is a doctoral student in Health Policy and Management at Harvard Medical School and Harvard Business School, USA. His research interests lie in improving the delivery of primary health care both in the United States and in developing countries. He is the President of Common Hope for Health, an NGO that provides technical assistance to grassroots health initiatives in developing countries.

Jeffrey Craig Lunnen is a Research Program Coordinator at the International Injury Research Unit (IIRU) at the Bloomberg School of Public Health, Johns Hopkins University, USA. He is responsible with Dr Hyder for coordinating the monitoring, evaluation, and reporting activities for the Bloomberg Philanthropies-funded Road Safety in 10 Countries Project (RS–10). In 2011, Jeffrey served as a consultant for the Pan American Health Organization (PAHO) and prepared a case study of the growing burden of motorcycle injuries in Guyana.

Neil Macleod has been Head of Water and Sanitation at the eThekwini Municipality since 1992, responsible for ensuring the provision of water and sanitation services to the 3.8 million people living in South Africa's Durban Metropolitan region. He has more than 39 years of experience in the water and sanitation sector and has served on the board of directors of the Municipal Infrastructure Investment Unit, Johannesburg Water, and Umgeni Water. He is a registered professional engineer and holds an MBA degree. He serves on steering committees for the Water Research Commission, and is currently Chairman of BPD Water and Sanitation, a UK-based organization.

Tatyana Margolin is a Program Officer at the Open Society Foundation's (OSF) Public Health Program, where she focuses on the Law and Health Initiative and the International Harm Reduction Development Program. She oversees a diverse portfolio of grantees working to improve the lives of injecting drug users through legal aid, legal empowerment, and strategic litigation in East Africa and Eastern Europe. She also leads the PHP's efforts to improve health outcomes in pre-trial detention settings. Tatyana was previously a foreign law clerk at the Supreme Court of Israel, and a staff attorney at the Women's Law Project.

Michael Marmot is Director of the International Institute for Society and Health and the Medical Research Council (MRC) Research Professor of Epidemiology and Public Health at University College London (UCL), England, UK. He chaired the Commission on Social Determinants of Health (CSDH) set up by the World Health Organization (WHO), as well as the Strategic Review of Health Inequalities in England Post 2010 (Marmot Review). He was a member of the Royal Commission on Environmental Pollution for six years, and served as President of the British Medical Association (BMA) from 2010 to 2011. In 2000, he was knighted by Her Majesty the Queen, for services to epidemiology and the understanding of health inequalities. Professor Marmot is a Foreign Associate Member of the Institute of Medicine, and a former Vice President of the Academia Europaea. He was Chair of the CSDH, which was established by the WHO in 2005, and produced the report entitled *Closing the Gap in a Generation* in August 2008.

Mary Byrne McDonnell is Executive Director of the Social Science Research Council (SSRC) in New York City, USA. As director of the SSRC's Vietnam programme, she has worked since 1986 with national and international partners to strengthen individual and institutional capacity in research design and implementation in Vietnam. She has been involved in working with the United Nations Development Programme (UNDP) and the Vietnamese government to assess the impact of Doi Moi (reforms) and social change. She serves on the board of directors at the School of Social Development and Public Policy at Beijing Normal University. She is currently co-editing *The Handbook of Research Management* (Sage, forthcoming).

Alyson Metzger is Managing Editor of the Social Science Research Council (SSRC), USA, where she oversees publications and contributes to internal and external communications. Before joining the SSRC, she worked for many years as a commercial writer and editor for both private and public clients; as an academic editor and copy-editor; and as a film and video producer and production coordinator. She has served as editor for a number of digital and print publications and the online essay forum *10 Years after September 11*.

Luis Moreno is a sociologist with 25 years of HIV research experience, particularly among female sex workers in the Dominican Republic. He was previously the head of the research and evaluation unit at the Centro de Orientación e Investigación Integral and is currently a programmatic advisor for HIV prevention programming in the Dominican Republic supported by the Global Fund to Fight AIDS, TB and Malaria (GFATM).

Peter Muennig is an Associate Professor at the Columbia University Mailman School of Public Health, USA. He co-founded the Burmese Refugee Project, an NGO in northern Thailand. His primary area of research interest is in the evaluation of the health effects of major social policies, such as early childhood interventions, lead control, housing, and community enhancements. He and his work have appeared on NPR, CNN, MSNBC and in major print media sources such as the *New York Times*, the *Washington Post*, and *Slate*.

Kevin O'Reilly is a Scientist in the Department of HIV/AIDS at the World Health Organization (WHO) focusing on prevention of sexual transmission of HIV. He is a medical anthropologist and epidemiologist with extensive experience designing multi-site community demonstration projects for HIV prevention in the United States. He has worked on HIV prevention in more than 30 developing countries and as a result is keenly aware of the gap between the current needs for programme direction in countries and the need for better application of research results. Dr O'Reilly received his PhD in Medical Anthropology at the University of Connecticut. In 1981, he served as an Epidemiology Intelligence Service (EIS) Officer at the Centers for Disease Control and Prevention (CDC) and was a key figure in HIV prevention research there for more than a decade.

Christine Pace is a primary care physician and Addiction Medicine Fellow at Boston Medical Center in Boston, MA, USA. Her clinical work and research are focused on the integration of addiction treatment and prevention services with primary care, and on improving care for women with addiction, particularly during and after pregnancy.

Richard Parker is Professor of Sociomedical Sciences (SMS) and Anthropology and Director of the Center for the Study of Culture, Politics, and Health in the Mailman School of Public Health at Columbia University, USA, where he also served as Chair of the Department of SMS from 2001 to 2008. He is the Editor-in-Chief of *Global Public Health*, co-editor of *The Routledge Handbook of Global Public Health*, as well as author of *Bodies, Pleasures, and Passions: Sexual Culture in Contemporary Brazil* (1991; 2nd edition, 2009) and *Beneath the Equator: Cultures of Desire, Male Homosexuality, and Emerging Gay Communities in Brazil* (1999). Dr Parker is also the Director and President of ABIA, the Brazilian Interdisciplinary AIDS Association, and has been active in advocacy work in the fields of HIV and AIDS, sexual rights, and globalization in Latin America and other regions.

Paul Pronyk is a physician and public health researcher with faculty appointments at the Mailman School of Public Health and the School of International Affairs at Columbia University, as well as at the School of Public Health at the University of the Witwatersrand (South Africa). Dr Pronyk has worked extensively in sub-Saharan Africa, researching a range of issues including clinical and structural interventions for HIV/AIDS; child health and nutrition; tuberculosis epidemiology and prevention; gender-based violence; the health and social impacts of economic development programmes; social capital; health systems development; and public health ethics.

Wiwat Rojanapithayakorn is the Representative of the World Health Organization (WHO) in Mongolia. He has been working with the WHO since 2002, serving in the capacities of medical officer of WHO Mongolia (2002–2004) and HIV/AIDS team leader of WHO China (2005–2008). Previously he was the team leader of the Joint United Nations Programme on HIV/AIDS (UNAIDS) Southeast Asia and Pacific Inter-country Team, and worked in the Ministry of Public Health of Thailand for 23 years. He has authored or co-authored more than 100 publications in English and Thai, and was editor or chief editor of over ten public health journals. In 1989, Dr Rojanapithayakorn established the 100% Condom Use Programme, and in 2010, he received the Prince Mahidol Award in Public Health.

Elisa Roma is based at the London School of Hygiene and Tropical Medicine, England, UK, working for the Sanitation and Hygiene Applied Research for Equity (SHARE) consortium. She has over five years' experience in the sanitation and hygiene sector, during which she been involved in the theoretical and applied social science research on sustainability of water and sanitation and appropriate hygiene behaviour in low-income countries. Dr Roma's doctoral research explored the role of socio-economic and behavioural determinants of adoption of water and sanitation technologies and policies in South Africa and Indonesia. From November 2010 until February 2011, Dr Roma worked as a research fellow at the University of KwaZulu-Natal, where she was principal researcher on several projects funded by Unilever and the Bill and Melinda Gates Foundation.

David Rosner is the Ronald H. Lauterstein Professor of Sociomedical Sciences (SMS) at Columbia University Mailman School of Public Health and Professor of History at Columbia University Graduate School of Arts and Sciences, USA. His research focuses on the intersection of public health and social history and the politics of occupational disease and industrial pollution. In 2010, he was elected to the National

Academy of Sciences' Institute of Medicine. He has been a Guggenheim Fellow, a recipient of a Robert Wood Johnson Investigator Award, a National Endowment for the Humanities Fellow and a Josiah Macy Fellow. Dr Rosner is an author of many books on occupational disease, epidemics and public health. His latest work, *The Best of Intentions* (University of California Press/Milbank Fund, 2012), details the recent conflicts at Johns Hopkins over studies of children placed in homes with low level lead exposure and what it says about public health research.

Jonathan M. Samet is Professor and Flora L. Thornton Chair for the Department of Preventive Medicine at the Keck School of Medicine at the University of Southern California (USC) and Director of the USC Institute for Global Health, USA. His research has focused on the health risks of inhaled pollutants. He currently chairs the Clean Air Scientific Advisory Committee of the US Environmental Protection Agency (EPA) and the Food and Drug Administration's (FDA) Tobacco Products Scientific Advisory Committee. He was appointed to the National Cancer Advisory Board in 2011. Dr Samet received the Surgeon General's Medallion in 1990 and 2006, the 2004 Prince Mahidol Award for Global Health, and the 2006 Public Service Award of the American Thoracic Society.

Jennifer Schaefer is a research officer at the Center for Global Health and Economic Development, Columbia University, USA. She coordinates performance monitoring and quarterly reporting for the Millennium Villages Project. Her particular interests are infectious disease and vital events surveillance, and the use of mobile and electronic health applications in resource-poor settings, with a focus on paediatric and newborn care.

Kate Shannon is the Director of the Gender and Sexual Health Initiative at the British Columbia Centre for Excellence in HIV/AIDS, Assistant Professor in the Department of Medicine, and Associate Faculty in the School of Population and Public Health at the University of British Columbia, Canada. She leads a large research programme on the social and structural determinants shaping sexual health and HIV/STI prevention and care for marginalized populations in Canada and sub-Saharan Africa. She is the Associate Editor of the *International Journal of Drug Policy* and is working with the World Health Organization (WHO) on the development of international guidelines and best practices for violence and HIV/STI prevention among sex workers and clients. She was awarded the Canadian Institutes of Health Research (CIHR) Peter Lougheed Award in 2010.

Jean Shoveller is a Professor at the University of British Columbia's School of Population and Public Health in Vancouver, Canada. She is a leading researcher focusing on the social contexts of youth health inequities, with a particular emphasis on sexual health. She currently holds a Senior Scholar Award from the Michael Smith Foundation for Health Research and a Canadian Institutes of Health Research (CIHR) Applied Public Health Chair in Improving Youth Sexual Health.

Marie-Andrée Somers is senior statistician at the Center for Global Health and Economic Development at Columbia University, USA, where she is primarily involved in the evaluation of the Millennium Villages Project in Africa. She has conducted programme and policy evaluations for several organizations including the US Department of Education, Statistics Canada, United Nations Education, Scientific and Cultural Organization (UNESCO), and the Organisation for Economic Co-operation and Development (OECD).

Marni Sommer is Assistant Professor of Sociomedical Sciences (SMS) and Director of the SMS Global Health Track at the Mailman School of Public Health at Columbia University, USA. Her particular areas of expertise include participatory research with adolescents, understanding and promoting healthy transitions to adulthood, and the intersection of public health with education, gender, and sexual health. She is a member of the hygiene working group for the Joint Monitoring Programme (JMP), is the Executive editor of *The Routledge Handbook of Global Public Health*.

Richard Steen has worked as a public health clinician in designing, implementing and evaluating interventions and operations research in the areas of STI control and HIV prevention since 1989. He has developed guidelines for the World Health Organization (WHO) including *Sexually Transmitted and Other Reproductive Tract Infections: A Guide for Essential Practice*; *The HIV/AIDS and Sex Work Toolkit*; and the *South-East Asia Regional Strategy for Prevention and Control of STIs*. In collaboration with the WHO, Erasmus University MC, Rotterdam, and the University of the Witswatersrand, Johannesburg, he is currently working on guideline development, implementation support, and modelling related to targeted STI control and HIV prevention interventions for sex workers and their clients.

Celina Su is currently an Associate Professor of Political Science at the City University of New York (CUNY) and a Visiting Scholar at the New York University (NYU) Wagner Graduate School of Public Service, USA. Her publications include *Streetwise for Book Smarts: Grassroots Organizing and Education Reform in the Bronx* (Cornell University Press, 2009) and *Our Schools Suck: Young People Talk Back to a Segregated Nation on the Failures of Urban Education* (co-authored with Gaston Alonso, Noel Anderson, and Jeanne Theoharis, New York University Press, 2009). She is co-founding Executive Director of the Burmese Refugee Project. Su's honours include the Berlin Prize and the Whiting Award for Excellence in Teaching.

Michael Sweat is Professor and Director of the Family Services Research Center in the Department of Psychiatry and Behavioral Sciences at the Medical University of South Carolina, USA. He previously worked as the Director of the Behavioral Research Unit for Family Health International (FHI), conducting HIV-related prevention studies in developing countries in Africa, Latin America, and Asia. Some of his current studies include a community-randomized trial examining large-scale HIV testing and counselling in rural Tanzania, and a systematic review and meta-analysis project being conducted in collaboration with the WHO and Johns Hopkins University.

Dallas Swendeman is Assistant Professor-in-Residence at the University of California Los Angeles (UCLA) David Geffen School of Medicine, Department of Psychiatry and Biobehavioral Sciences, Center for Community Health, and the Center for HIV Identification, Prevention, and Treatment Services, USA. His graduate studies focused on multi-level theory, intervention, and research methods applied to the Durbar/Sonagachi community-led structural HIV intervention in India, and resulted in a 10-year and ongoing mixed-methods research collaboration with the Durbar/Sonagachi project. Dr Swendeman is a member of the University of California Global Health Institute's Center of Expertise in Women's Health and Empowerment.

Jonathan L. Weigel is a PhD candidate in Political Economy and Government at Harvard, and a research assistant to Dr Paul Farmer in the Department of Global Health and Social Medicine at Harvard Medical School, USA. His research interests include the political economy of development, foreign aid effectiveness, and integrated public–private approaches to health system strengthening.

Heather L. Wipfli is an Assistant Professor in the Department of Preventive Medicine at the University of Southern California (USC) Keck School of Medicine and in the Department of International Relations at the USC Dana and David Dornsife College of Letters, Arts and Sciences, USA. She is also the Associate Director of the USC Institute for Global Health. Her research focuses on global health politics and the development of innovative forms of global health governance. Prior to joining USC, Dr Wipfli directed research and training for the Institute for Global Tobacco Control at the Johns Hopkins Bloomberg School of Public Health and also worked as a technical officer at the World Health Organization headquarters in Geneva on the development of the Framework Convention on Tobacco Control.

Daniel Wolfe is the Director of the Open Society Foundation's (OSF) International Harm Reduction Development (IHRD) programme, USA. He is a core member of the United Nations (UN) Reference Group on HIV and Injecting Drug Use and the former director of communications at GMHC, the first AIDS NGO in the USA. He is co-author of a working paper commissioned by the HIV/AIDS Task Force of the Millennium Project of the UN to examine the effects of UN and national illicit drug policies on the spread of HIV, and is the author of multiple books, chapters, and articles in popular and peer-reviewed publications.

1

INTRODUCTION

Structural approaches in public health

Marni Sommer and Richard Parker

The field of public health in the early twenty-first century has seen a resurgence of interest in what can be described as 'structural approaches' (Blankenship *et al.* 2000). In relation to topics as diverse as HIV/AIDS and other newly emerging or re-emerging infectious diseases, injury and violence prevention, and the growing global incidence of chronic or non-communicable diseases, increasing attention has focused on the structural factors – social, cultural, political, economic, and environmental – that shape and constrain individual, community, and societal health outcomes. This emphasis on structural factors that make both individuals and the communities to which they belong vulnerable to negative health outcomes has also led to a growing focus on structural and environmental interventions in public health – interventions that seek to alter the context within which health and illness are produced and reproduced (Blankenship *et al.* 2006; Gupta *et al.* 2008; Parker *et al.* 2000; Sweat and Denison 1995).

The growing use of structural approaches in contemporary public health is not an entirely novel phenomenon. On the contrary, the history of public health offers a wide range of case examples in which practitioners and policymakers, often for moral, economic, or social (rather than health-related) reasons, have implemented structural interventions aimed at changing the social conditions in which people live (Porter 1997). In the nineteenth and early twentieth centuries, for example, reformers in the United States, Europe, and other industrializing nations focused on the problematic conditions of populations living in increasingly crowded urban environments. Advocating for the need to address people's working and living conditions, often from the perspective of wanting to reduce the risks of perceived immoral behaviour posed by unsanitary surroundings, significant efforts were made to implement structural interventions such as improved water supplies and laws on tenement housing. Such efforts, implemented through effective interdisciplinary action, which at times impinged on the civil liberties of selected populations, had an enormous influence on population health outcomes, and in particular on the rates of infectious disease (Rosen 1993; Rosner and Markowitz 1985; Schmid *et al.* 1995). These types of interdisciplinary approaches diminished in the early twentieth century, however, with the rise of the germ theory of disease, a turn by public health clinicians and practitioners toward the laboratory, and a focus on the individual and his or her behaviour as the key to reducing health-related risks (Tomes 1998).

Over the course of the twentieth century, more individualistic and behavioural approaches came to dominate both theory and practice in relation to health promotion and disease prevention and were applied to almost all major public health challenges (Matarazzo 1980). The outcomes of such approaches were often disappointing. Efforts to improve population health, ranging from health education on diet and exercise, to guidance on wearing condoms at every sexual encounter, driving more safely, and avoiding injuries in the home or work environment, were all found to be limited in their effectiveness given the numerous influences shaping, and constraining, individual behaviour and choice. Such influences emerged from the structural realities affecting people's lives and the social forces, or the social drivers, influencing the distribution of health and illness (Auerbach *et al.* 2011). For example, the toxic food environment of high-income countries, now spreading to low- and middle-income countries, combined with the change in everyday activity levels and the physiology of automatic eating behaviour, has prevented many individuals from maintaining a healthy weight. The social, economic, and gendered realities of people's lives in numerous contexts prevented the use of condoms with every sexual encounter. Inadequate road construction and insufficient traffic safety legislation and enforcement made safe driving a reality far removed from individual control. Injuries in a range of settings, including in the home or resulting from the use of unsafe equipment in the workplace, were unavoidable as long as the infrastructure within which they occurred remained unchanged. While individual behaviour and agency play an important role in protecting and maintaining a person's health, many of the priority public health interventions that focus on the individual alone, with little to no attention to the structural and environmental influences shaping their lives, proved to be insufficient to accomplish the stated public health goals of reducing morbidity and mortality. Such individually focused interventions nonetheless continued to dominate the public health arena for much of the twentieth century.

Recognizing the limitations of mainstream health education and behavioural prevention programmes, in the past two decades attention began to shift to structural approaches and interventions as an important alternative to concentrating on individual health behaviours (Blankenship *et al.* 2000). This renewed interest in structural and contextual factors that shape health-related risks and vulnerability to disease has been especially strong in work focusing on HIV and AIDS, where the relatively limited success of health education and behavioural interventions has led researchers and policymakers to explore alternative strategies, ranging from community mobilization activities to reduce the spread of HIV, to the use of anti-discrimination legislation and similar policies aimed at protecting those already living with HIV (Blankenship *et al.* 2006; Gupta *et al.* 2008; Parker *et al.* 2000; Sweat and Denison 1995). Increasingly, there has been a growing trend toward focusing on structural and environmental factors not only in research and programmes focusing on HIV and AIDS, but across a wide range of topical areas and in countries and communities around the world. Examples include the impact of improved accessibility to clean water to combat diarrhoeal disease; the mandated use of seat belts and motorcycle helmets aimed at reducing traffic injuries; the banning of tobacco use; and the prohibition of certain kinds of foods and beverages known to cause cancer or obesity-related chronic diseases (Brownson *et al.* 2006; Katz 2009; Schmid *et al.* 1995). Indeed, by the early twenty-first century, many leading figures in public health policy and practice had returned to focusing attention on confronting and changing the structural and environmental factors in the everyday world around us that pose major health risks – and on promoting public health policies aimed at creating a healthier environment (Farley and Cohen 2005).

As important and widespread as the renewed uptake of such structural and environmental approaches has been, it is still limited and fraught with controversy about the extent to which policymakers and public health experts have the right to protect people from the consequences of their own behavioural choices (Bayer *et al.* 2006). In addition to the important ethical debates generated by this turn to structural and environmental approaches and interventions, another key factor limiting their uptake in many settings has been a relative lack of consensus concerning the definition of what constitutes *structure* together with a range of differing theoretical frameworks that exist for conceptualizing structural factors (Blankenship *et al.* 2000). While researchers trained in the social sciences and those trained in public health or behavioural medicine may use the same terminology, they frequently mean very different things when they describe the workings of structure (Parker *et al.* 2000).

In much of the social science research on structural factors that impact health, primary emphasis has focused on the role of social inequality in structuring health-related vulnerabilities. Medical anthropologists or medical sociologists are more likely to frame the discussion of structural factors in relation to aspects of political economy and emphasize how broad macro-economic processes and social structural inequalities such as class, race or ethnicity, and gender shape the vulnerability of different groups to a range of health conditions. They have thus tended to focus on the negative health impact of what they frequently describe as 'structural violence' (Farmer 2002, 2004; Parker 2002) and explore the ways in which multiple and intersecting forms of inequality create a kind of synergy – quite literally producing what have been described as 'syndemics' that affect poor and marginalized populations (Singer and Clare 2003). This focus, in turn, has led many researchers working at the interface of social science and public health to emphasize the need for broad social and economic transformations in order to truly change negative health outcomes (Farmer 2005), and to focus on intervention approaches aimed at community mobilization and collective empowerment as key to promoting population health (Laverack and Labonte 2000; Parker 1996; Wallerstein 1992).

In contrast, public health and health behavioural researchers, while sensitive to the importance of social structural inequalities, are more likely to conceptualize structural and environmental factors as aspects of health policy and institutional programmes and practices that influence the context in which health behaviours take place. Indeed, perhaps because of the lack of consensus concerning its meaning, they are less likely to use the term 'structure', and instead frequently speak in terms of 'environmental and policy approaches' (Brownson *et al.* 2006; Schmid *et al.* 1995). Even when they do use the language of structure and structural interventions, they downplay the social science focus on macro-economic structures (that are seen as only minimally subject to transformation), placing greater emphasis on policy changes that might influence more 'proximal' aspects of the context and environment in which health behaviours take place, rather than 'distal' factors such as the broader structures of social inequalities (Krieger 2001).

In spite of these important differences, both in relation to terminology and in relation to conceptualization, there has nonetheless been a growing approximation in recent years between social science and public health approaches to issues of inequality as well as to interventions aimed at responding to their negative health impact. This is perhaps especially evident in the increasingly widespread uptake in public health of frameworks focusing on the 'social determinants' of health (Marmot and Wilkinson 1999) and the 'fundamental causes' of disease (Link and Phelan 1995). In emphasizing the social and economic conditions that shape health outcomes – and that have maintained health disparities over time – such approaches have provided an important point of convergence for both public health and social science thinking on the relationship between social inequality and health. They have also focused new attention on factors such as prestige and power as central to understanding differential health outcomes, and helped the field move beyond notions of proximal and distal causes of health disparities in examining processes through which power differentials operate in producing health and disease (Krieger 2008). Through the work of the World Health Organization's (WHO) Commission on the Social Determinants of Health (CSDH) (CSDH 2008), and the extensive activities that this Commission's work has stimulated at the country level around the globe, extensive new space has opened for social science and public health research on the structural dimensions of health globally in the early twenty-first century. Perhaps never before has so much attention focused on these issues – nor have conditions been so favourable for seeking to address the health impact of social inequalities through the design and implementation of structural and environmental interventions.

In spite of these positive recent developments, many challenges continue to confront work on these issues. Just as differing notions of what structure is and how it operates has made the analysis of structural factors and the design of interventions more difficult, measuring the effectiveness of structural interventions has also raised major challenges. In contrast to individually or even culturally focused interventions that are evaluated in terms of individual behavioural changes, structural or environmental interventions are evaluated in terms of social transformations, such as community mobilization or social movement empowerment. Measuring change at this scale involves a whole new set of considerations that the field has only begun to understand and confront (Bonell et al. 2006).

It is in relation to these important challenges that the current volume on Structural Approaches in Public Health seeks to make a key contribution. The chapters brought together here aim to map out the ways in which the notion of structure has been conceptualized in relation to health, both over time and across a range of different disciplinary perspectives. They also explore how structural interventions have been conceived and implemented in various contexts to address different topics related to population health. Finally, they explore some of the important challenges that must be addressed in seeking to assess the impact of structural interventions in practice. Taken together, they make a case for the central importance of structural approaches in confronting the most pressing practical challenges in the field of public health today, and point the way forward in relation to the continued refinement of these approaches in the future. In the discussion to follow, we will briefly summarize the contents of the chapters that have been included in each of the three major sections of this volume and present our vision of how to further develop this field of work.

Defining structural factors

As mentioned above, one of the key challenges to the broader adoption of structural approaches has been the relative lack of consensus on precisely what so-called 'structural approaches' actually entail. While diversity in conceptual frameworks can be highly productive, in this case, it has been an impediment to more fruitful discussion and debate. One of the major obstacles has been the perception that different scholars and scientists are talking about the same thing when, in fact, their intended meanings are quite different. It is thus useful to look at some of the different ways in which definitions of structure have been articulated in various disciplinary and even epistemological traditions.

The chapters in the first section of *Structural Approaches in Public Health* do exactly that. They explore a number of the different ways in which notions of structure and structural factors affecting health outcomes have been conceptualized, both historically, as well as from different disciplinary and epistemological perspectives. These chapters examine the similarities and differences in existing definitions of structural factors in an effort to highlight areas of definitional understanding and consensus among the leading experts within the field. The section also includes chapters on structure as a risk factor, structural violence as a local and global challenge, and descriptions of theoretical approaches as applied to structural and environmental approaches.

The first chapter in this section, Chapter 2, 'The history of structural approaches in public health', by James Colgrove, Amy Fairchild, and David Rosner, provides a rich overview of the historical evolution of structural approaches within public health. It begins with a discussion of interventions framed in the nineteenth century as ecological and environmental approaches, highlighting the dramatic impact such approaches had on improving the health of the poor. Such interventions prefigured the modern conception of structural approaches. The authors then describe the shift in the field toward more individual-focused interventions as attention to bacteriology grew and public health transitioned toward exploring non-communicable diseases. The latter led to a shift away from efforts aimed at the social and environmental context as an important factor influencing population health. The chapter ends with a description of the more recent return of public health to its historical roots, with a renewed emphasis in the field to utilizing structural approaches, a trend that has been growing steadily over the last few decades.

Following this historical overview, in Chapter 3, 'Social inequalities and public health', Ruth Bell, Peter Goldblatt, and Michael Marmot focus on the social determinants of health inequalities and describe the importance and contributions of the WHO Commission on the Social Determinants of Health (CSDH 2008). Work on the social determinants of health constitutes one of the most important contemporary attempts to revive the historical tradition described in the previous chapter by Colgrove and his colleagues. As summarized in this chapter by Bell, Goldblatt, and Marmot, the work of the WHO Commission identified various social (or structural) factors which led to differential exposures, risks, vulnerabilities and assets among different groups within a given population, all determined by the distribution of power, money, and resources within that society. Through an extensive presentation of global data, the authors demonstrate how even when overall health indicators improve for a country or region, health inequities may remain when the lowest income quintiles have less improvement than the wealthier quintiles. Also presented is the causal framework that shapes our understanding of persistent health inequities and the range of factors contributing to this causal pathway across the life course. Such factors include early childhood development, gender equity, fair financing, universal health care, and the built environment, among others. The chapter concludes with a discussion of how action on the social determinants of health is now occurring in countries around the world.

In Chapter 4, 'Embracing complexity: toward platforms for integrated health and social service delivery', Andrew Ellner, Christine Pace, Scott Lee, Jonathan L. Weigel, and Paul Farmer describe the challenges that face clinicians and public health practitioners who aim to address the health risks experienced by individuals as a result of structural inequalities. They emphasize how social determinants of health become forms of structural violence and how clinicians routinely encounter such collective forces embodied in the lives of their individual patients. In presenting the intertwining nature of social phenomena and illness within an individual, the authors suggest that traditional definitions of 'communicable' and 'non-communicable' disease are problematic when social determinants, such as stress, economic status, place in the social hierarchy, exposure to trauma, and other factors may be enhancing the spread of illnesses traditionally labelled as non-communicable. They argue that only a truly 'biosocial' approach, one that integrates interventions aimed at both human biology and social conditions, can allow for an improved understanding and response to improving health outcomes. As a specific example, the authors discuss how health service delivery systems could be transformed to account for the social determinants of health.

The fifth chapter, 'Ideological barriers to structural interventions: toward a model of values-based interventions', by Michael Sweat and Kevin O'Reilly, moves from the impact of structural factors in the clinic to the level of social policy. It explores the possible reasons behind perceived political barriers to past and present widespread acceptance of structural approaches. The authors argue that although structural approaches to public health challenges are not new, a growing market-centric ideology that promotes individual and corporate interests over a more equitable society, along with limited existing theories defining the role of structural approaches as mechanisms for social change, impede their effective implementation. They also compare differing views on the use of state power and its application to the issue of equality in different countries, with some countries preferring to restrict state power while others permit its broader use in addressing inequalities. As this comparative perspective makes clear, structural interventions are more widely accepted in contexts where the leading ideology is more centrist, that is, focused on equality and engendering values of enhanced agency.

In Chapter 6, the final chapter in this section of the volume, 'Getting the balance right: agency and structure in HIV prevention', Peter Aggleton, Jean Shoveller, Kate Shannon, Thomas Kerr, and Rod Knight move from the level of broad social policies to exploring the evolution of structural approaches as they have been applied to HIV prevention. They trace the history of interventions in response to HIV and AIDS as it has moved from initial individual-focused approaches to those addressing the large-scale structural factors influencing people's lives and shaping their vulnerability to HIV. They discuss how social responses to the epidemic have paralleled existing social inequalities within populations, including those shaped by gender, age, class, race, and sexuality. They also emphasize the responses of solidarity that have arisen within communities responding to the epidemic. They present three case studies (on sex work, injecting drug use, and young people and sexuality) that highlight these trends and stress the importance of a multidimensional approach to HIV, one that incorporates social structure and individual agency as well as efforts happening both globally and locally.

Taken together, the chapters in this section explore definitions of structure in different contexts: in the history of public health, in the literature on contemporary social determinants of health, at the level of the clinic and the interface between clinical care and public health programmes, at the level of policy and the state, and in relation to specific policies and programmes that target structure while promoting individual agency. Our goal is not to forge a single, unified theory of structure, but rather to deepen our understanding of the range of different meanings that have been associated with structural approaches in public health and the challenges we face in seeking to apply structure as an analytical frame in diverse contexts. This collection of chapters calls for more detailed description and analysis of the design and implementation of different structural interventions, as explored in the next section of this book.

Designing and implementing structural interventions

The second section of *Structural Approaches in Public Health* examines past and present structural interventions in public health to emphasize the more practical aspects of this work, that is, how programmes are developed and implemented. The early chapters included in this section analyze water and sanitation and urban planning, among the key areas in which structural interventions were first developed in public health, followed by HIV and AIDS and illegal drug use, topics which have been especially important in stimulating a revival of interest in structural approaches. The later chapters focus on issues such as chronic and non-communicable disease and injury prevention, which are increasingly being addressed through the design and implementation of structural interventions.

In Chapter 7, 'Integrating water and sanitation interventions for health: a case study from eThekwini Municipality', Elisa Roma, Neil Macleod, and Christopher Buckley describe an approach aimed at providing safe and affordable water and sanitation to over three million people living within the rural, peri-urban, and urban areas of eThekwini Municipality in Durban, South Africa. They highlight the various challenges that impede the population's access to adequate and appropriate water and sanitation sources, including those that are environmental as well as those found within the social and economic context of the municipality. The chapter subsequently provides a comprehensive description of the multiple interventions that were implemented and evaluated, such as a waterless sanitation system provided to rural households outside the sewerage system, related educational activities, and water and sanitation facilities provided to densely populated informal settlements. The authors emphasize the importance of holistic approaches to the water and sanitation challenges facing populations in low-income settings, along with the thorough evaluation of such efforts to assure the most appropriate, effective, and affordable approaches are being utilized.

In Chapter 8, 'City planning as a structural determinant of health: toward healthy urban governance in the century of the city', Jason Corburn discusses how and why the fields of city planning and public health have separated over the last century, in turn contributing to the existence and perpetuation of social inequities. He makes a strong case for how city planning thus constitutes yet another structural determinant of health affecting populations in urban environments. Prior to and following this period of separation, the fields of city planning and public health also had moments of overlap and collaboration. From the shared and separate histories of these two fields, we are offered key lessons and other important insights for further reconnecting the two through improved urban governance.

In Chapter 9, 'The 100% Condom Use Programme: a structural intervention to prevent HIV and sexually transmitted infections in Asia', Wiwat Rojanapithayakorn and Richard Steen reflect on the success of the 100% Condom Use Programme (CUP) in Thailand, which dramatically reduced the incidence of HIV in selected populations across the country. They then critically assess various attempts to adapt the 100% CUP to other countries, including Cambodia, China, and Mongolia, highlighting the challenges that can arise in modifying effective structural approaches to new and different contextual settings. The authors describe how the efforts to adapt the 100% CUP to new countries have contributed to a deeper understanding of the structural factors involved in sex work, the most effective approaches to utilize in addressing HIV risk, and the continual need for flexibility given the unique conditions of each new setting. The chapter concludes with a return to the Thailand case study to show how particular strategies, such as changing the power balance within condom negotiation and the *de facto* decriminalization of sex work to allow sex workers more autonomy in adopting risk reduction strategies, were key to the programme's success.

The tenth chapter, 'The Sonagachi/Durbar Programme: a prototype of a community-led structural intervention for HIV prevention', by Dallas Swendeman and Smarajit Jana, describes the development and evolution of a very successful community-led structural intervention (CLSI) in India. The programme began as a conventional HIV and sexually transmitted infection (STI) intervention that took a clinical, individualistic approach to prevent and treat HIV and other STIs among sex workers. Over almost 20 years, it expanded into a much broader social mobilization of sex workers in Kolkata that sought to address the range of structural factors that contributed to their sense of vulnerability, including financial constraints to saving money, harassment by the police, inadequate educational institutions for their children, and stigma and discrimination. From this overview, we learn what aspects are essential for a CLSI to succeed, information that is critical for other marginalized groups seeking to replicate this success.

In Chapter 11, 'Breaking the links: legal and paralegal assistance to reduce health risks of police and pre-trial detention of sex workers and people who use drugs', Daniel Wolfe, Jonathan Cohen, Heather Doyle, and Tatyana Margolin emphasize the growing evidence suggesting that routine and sometimes abusive law enforcement practices may contribute to an increased risk of infection with HIV among targeted populations, particularly sex workers and people who use drugs. While previous research has documented how incarceration serves as a structural determinant of HIV risk, the authors argue that a much wider range of police and law enforcement-related activities contribute to and augment risk. They focus on the critical role of harm reduction approaches in reaching populations at high risk, with important case examples from Kenya, Indonesia, and the Ukraine. Through the guiding framework and cases presented, the authors highlight how pre-detention aspects of the legal processing and detention systems both place such populations at greater risk of infection with HIV and STIs, while simultaneously being targets for effective structural intervention.

In the twelfth chapter, 'Structured environments and dietary-related chronic diseases', Deborah A. Cohen argues that, while policy and regulation have served in the effort to prevent infectious disease, injury, and toxic exposure, such approaches are absent in the case of chronic disease. The focus on individual behaviour as the cause of chronic disease, including the view that obesity arises from personal failures and a lack of individual willpower, has hindered a broader understanding of the structural and contextual factors influencing dietary behaviours. The chapter presents an overview of the multiple influences, both biophysical and social, that shape population food intake. For example, the food industry creates desire for its products through the use of marketing strategies that tap into 'eyegaze', a neural pathway response in consumers. This is compounded by retailers' relentless efforts to encourage increased consumption of relatively low-cost, high calorie foods, and people's limited cognitive capacity to refrain from overeating. Cohen concludes that excess exposure to food, rather than individual knowledge or behaviour, must be the target of regulatory intervention if the epidemic of overweight, obesity, and chronic disease are to be effectively controlled.

In the final chapter in this section of the volume, Chapter 13, 'Structural approaches for unintentional injury prevention', Adnan A. Hyder and Jeffrey C. Lunnen focus on global morbidity and mortality from preventable injuries. As is true in other fields, injury prevention and control has shifted its focus from individual-level interventions to interventions that are more structural in nature. The structural approaches have proven to be more effective; however, they are not without challenges, especially when applied to low-income countries. Hyder and Lunnen describe these challenges. They argue that an interdisciplinary approach to injury prevention and control, one that draws from education, law, engineering, transportation, and public health, is ideal. Through the use of case examples from around the world, they show us how an interdisciplinary model can be applied and what core components are essential for preventing different types of injuries in different contexts.

By providing us with a clear view of the wide range of different topical areas – water and sanitation, urban planning and environmental health systems, HIV and AIDS, sex work and injecting drug use, obesity and other dietary-related health conditions, and injury prevention – these chapters provide deeper understanding of the breadth of different contexts in which structural approaches and interventions can be employed, as well as the diverse challenges that must be confronted both in the design and the implementation of such programmes. They highlight the extent to which addressing structural issues demands long-term, ongoing public health action as well as the positive outcomes that such action can frequently produce. They also underline the complexity of evaluating structural intervention approaches, particularly given how different these programmes tend to be when compared with more individualistic and behavioural public health programmes. The difficulties associated with evaluation are the focus for the next section of this book.

Evaluating structural interventions

The third and final section of *Structural Approaches in Public Health* focuses on the challenge of evaluating the impact of structural interventions. It discusses existing and recommended methodologies for evaluating structural approaches and identifies gaps in the broader understanding of effective mechanisms for evaluating structural approaches. Part 3 begins with an overarching presentation of how to evaluate structural interventions and continues with examples of intervention programmes that have effectively incorporated evaluation into the implementation design, such as the structural intervention addressing HIV vulnerability in the Dominican Republic, the banning of tobacco in bars and public spaces in New York City, the effectiveness of a helmet law implemented in Vietnam, and other structural approaches around the world.

In Chapter 14, 'Evaluating structural interventions in public health: challenges, options and global best practice', Paul Pronyk, Jennifer Schaefer, Marie-Andrée Somers, and Lori Heise discuss the many challenges inherent in the effort to evaluate structural approaches in various contexts around the world, while also providing detailed guidance on methodologies and approaches that can be utilized in such efforts. They describe the importance of various aspects of evaluating structural interventions, such as the role of context, sampling, the use of mixed methods, and short- versus long-term measures. The chapter provides guidance on the major evaluation approaches that can be utilized, such as impact assessment, implementation research and economic evaluation, and how to overcome barriers associated with their use. The authors provide three useful case study examples of effective evaluations that were conducted in very different contexts. The chapter concludes by emphasizing the importance of increasing efforts to conduct high-quality evaluations of structural interventions in order to improve resource allocation and public health impact.

In the fifteenth chapter, 'Developing and evaluating structural-environmental interventions to reduce HIV risk among female sex workers and their sexual partners in the Dominican Republic', Deanna Kerrigan, Clare Barrington, and Luis Moreno provide an in-depth overview of the adaptation of the 100% Condom Use Programme in Thailand to the context and realities of female sex workers living in the Dominican Republic. They describe the formative research that was conducted in the Dominican Republic prior to the implementation of the intervention, the key components of the research design for the structural-environmental intervention that was ultimately implemented, and the methods and indicators used to capture and evaluate the influence of both individual and structural-environmental factors. The chapter provides a useful example of an effective evaluation that measured both process and impact outcomes, the findings from which provide important insights for future such HIV interventions and evaluations.

In Chapter 16, 'Helmet Day! Structural intervention and strategic learning in Vietnam', Mary Byrne McDonnell and Alyson Metzger present the successful case of the Vietnam helmet policy intervention that combined strong political will and a coalescing of funding, vision, and leadership to shift the Vietnamese population toward a very high usage of helmets on motorcycles and bicycles. This was a structural solution to an undeniably structural problem. As Vietnam's economy grew, more people relied upon motorcycles for commuting purposes, thus leading to an unexpected increase in morbidity and mortality from road accidents. The authors describe the careful process of stakeholder building utilized to effect the legislation, enforcement, and public awareness needed to change the social norm around helmet wearing in the Vietnamese context, and the evaluation methodology utilized to measure its success.

In Chapter 17, 'Ending the tobacco epidemic: from the genetic to the global level', Jonathan M. Samet and Heather L. Wipfli trace the history of the tobacco epidemic and efforts to control it. They utilize a life course perspective in presenting the various factors that may influence tobacco uptake and addiction, along with providing opportunities for public health intervention. The chapter highlights the successful structural interventions utilized to reduce tobacco consumption in high-income countries and current efforts to adapt these approaches to low- and middle-income countries where global and local tobacco companies are now focusing their markets and advertising. The authors also provide an overview of the global strategy known as the World Health

Organization's Framework Convention on Tobacco Control (FCTC), its ratification and implementation in countries around the world, and suggestions of directions for future global tobacco control post-implementation of the FCTC. The chapter concludes by discussing the tobacco industry's efforts to thwart tobacco control interventions and by emphasizing the importance of local and global surveillance for effective tobacco control.

Finally, in Chapter 18, 'Social policy interventions and health', Celina Su and Peter Muennig explore the use of social policy interventions outside the health care system. They review a range of approaches, including conditional cash transfers to enhance school attendance, changes to the built environment, and improved administration and governance, all of which have been shown in various contexts around the world to positively impact health outcomes. The chapter includes details on various evaluation measures developed and utilized to capture the impact of the different interventions. It also highlights challenges that were encountered in implementation. The authors emphasize the importance of not attempting to generalize the social policy success of selected interventions in one setting to another given the many local contextual factors that play a role in a given intervention's effectiveness. The chapter concludes by highlighting the need for structural approaches that combine various levels of intervention, while also pointing to the inherent complexity of such approaches, the need for continual critique and improvement, and the length of time needed to observe improved health outcomes.

By looking at the very different challenges entailed in evaluating structural approaches and interventions in highly varied contexts – condom use in the context of sex work, motorcycle helmets in a rapidly changing society undergoing an economic boom, tobacco control through health diplomacy on a truly global scale, and social policy interventions aimed at impacting health outcomes by addressing social inequalities – these chapters alert us to the diverse solutions that must be sought to assess the impact of such programmes. In addition, they highlight the role of context, the need to develop rigorous standards for evaluation, and the importance of using the limitations of traditional evaluation strategies as a platform for designing novel approaches more suited to evaluation at a structural level. The chapters illustrate how the field of structural approaches, including their evaluation, has evolved and will continue to evolve in the future.

The future of structural approaches in public health

The various chapters that make up *Structural Approaches in Public Health* provide a broad overview of what we see as the 'state of the art' in this field of work. They provide us with a clear sense of how structural factors are being addressed in the analysis of the most pressing problems that face us in public health today, how to confront these problems using structural interventions and programmes, and how to evaluate the effect of such interventions. Without a crystal ball, it would be impossible to fully predict how this field is likely to evolve in the future. But the richness of the material collected here, together with our analysis above of the trends characterizing this line of work, suggest a number of likely developments. We would like to end this 'Introduction' by briefly commenting on some developments that we think are most crucial: in particular, the continued importance of structural approaches in responding to health problems driven by social inequalities; the growing importance of such approaches in confronting the new health challenges associated with ongoing processes of globalization; and the fundamental need for long-term commitment to such approaches as central to public health over the foreseeable future.

To the extent that significant – and frequently growing – inequalities characterize all societies and play a preponderant role in patterning the most important health problems, we are convinced that the importance of structural approaches in public health will continue to grow in the future. The range of factors that structure inequality in societies around the world today – including economic exclusion, racial and ethnic discrimination, gender power differentials, sexual stigma and discrimination, age-related power inequalities, and so on – continue to function with ruthless efficiency. While biomedical and behavioural approaches to health promotion offer important benefits in relation to many different health problems, they have been proven to have limited efficacy in relation to the challenges driven by such inequalities. Structural approaches will continue to offer us our most effective alternative in response to such health inequalities for the foreseeable future.

We are also convinced that the ongoing globalization of the world during these first decades of the twenty-first century guarantees the continued importance of the kinds of structural problems that this volume seeks to highlight. The present time has marked a disintegration of old binaries, such as first world and third world, developed and developing countries, and core and periphery. The world has become more integrated and interactive than ever before in human history. A key feature of this transformation is a kind of 'epidemiological transition', in which the health problems that were seen to be most associated with poverty and underdevelopment (such as newly emerging and re-emerging infectious diseases) have become serious challenges for what are thought to be the rich countries of the industrialized North, just as those most associated with wealthy settings (such as the increased incidence in chronic diseases) have become growing challenges in the emerging and rapidly growing countries of the global South. Structural factors are at the heart of each of these complex and rapid social and epidemiological changes taking place. We will adequately confront these changing health problems only by recognizing this and committing ourselves to the kinds of structural programmes and interventions that are described in this volume. In a globalized world – a world in which the most important health challenges are also global – structural approaches will continue to be centrally important to the policies and programmes of public health for the future.

Finally, we think that it is important to stress the importance of long-term commitment to further this kind of work. There will always be a desire to invent and deploy quick fixes (the ongoing search for a magic bullet) in order to have a major impact in solving any public health problem. As such, the implementation of rapid biomedical or behavioural solutions and interventions will continue. However, as this volume attests, many of the most profound structural factors that shape health and illness in all societies are caused by what we recognize as deep social, cultural, political, and economic structures that, by their very nature, are highly resistant to change. They would withstand even the most powerful magic bullet available. In acknowledging that fully confronting structural and environmental factors influencing health and illness thus requires more than a quick solution, there must be long-term investments of financial and human resources, broad social development strategies, and ongoing political will. Recognizing this to be true should not discourage us. On the contrary, it is only through this recognition that we will find the force and resources required to make change. It is only through a long-term commitment to developing sustainable programmes that confront the structural factors driving disease that we will overcome our greatest health challenges.

We hope that the chapters brought together here in this edited collection on *Structural Approaches in Public Health* will fill an important gap in publications in the field of public health and will be a source of both insight and inspiration for our readers. By describing the historical roots and current definitions of structural approaches and the present trends in implementation and evaluation, we want to provide readers with insight into an area of work that has captured our own attention for many years now. We hope that you find this book helpful, a useful source of reference for many years to come. We have selected and incorporated a range of contributions with a diverse readership in mind. We aim to open up our collective thinking about research, intervention, and evaluation to reflect on the successes and failures of the past, and to devise new approaches for the future.

References

Auerbach, J., Parkhurst, J., and Caceres, C. (2011) 'Addressing social drivers of HIV/AIDS for the long-term response: conceptual and methodological considerations', *Global Public Health*, 6 (Suppl. 3): S293–309.

Bayer, R., Gostin, L.O., Jennings, B., and Steinbock, B. (eds) (2006) *Public Health Ethics: Theory, Policy, and Practice*, New York: Oxford University Press.

Blankenship, K., Bray, S., and Merson, M. (2000) 'Structural interventions in public health', *AIDS*, 14 (Suppl. 1): S11–21.

Blankenship, K., Friedman, S., Dworkin, S., and Mantell, J. (2006) 'Structural interventions: concepts, challenges and opportunities for research', *Journal of Urban Health*, 83 (1): 59–72.

Bonell, C., Hargreaves, J., Strange, V., Pronyk, P., and Porter, J. (2006) 'Should structural interventions be evaluated using RCTs? The case of HIV prevention', *Social Science & Medicine*, 63 (5): 1135–42.

Brownson, R.C., Haire-Joshu, D., and Luke, D.A. (2006) 'Shaping the context of health: a review of environmental and policy approaches in the prevention of chronic diseases', *Annual Review of Public Health*, 27: 341–70.

Commission on Social Determinants of Health (CSDH) (2008) *Closing the Gap in a Generation: Health Equity through Action on the Social Determinants of Health*, Geneva: World Health Organization. Online, available at: http://whqlibdoc.who.int/publications/2008/9789241563703_eng.pdf (accessed 27 August 2012).

Farley, T. and Cohen, D.A. (2005) *Prescription for a Healthy Nation: A New Approach to Improving our Lives by Fixing our Everyday World*, Boston, MA: Beacon Press.

Farmer, P. (2002) *Infections and Inequalities: The Modern Plagues*, Berkeley: University of California Press.

Farmer, P. (2004) 'An anthropology of structural violence', *Current Anthropology*, 45 (3): 305–25.

Farmer P. (2005) *Pathologies of Power: Health, Human Rights, and the New War on the Poor*, 2nd edition, Berkeley, CA: University of California Press.

Gupta, G., Parkhurst, J., Ogden, A., Aggleton, P., and Mahal, A. (2008) 'Structural approaches in HIV prevention', *The Lancet*, 372: 764–75.

Katz, M.H. (2009) 'Structural interventions for addressing chronic health problems', *Journal of the American Medical Association*, 302 (6): 683–5.

Krieger, N. (2001) 'Theories for social epidemiology in the 21st century: an ecosocial perspective', *International Journal of Epidemiology*, 30: 668–77.

Krieger, N. (2008) 'Proximal, distal, and the politics of causation: what's level got to do with it?', *American Journal of Public Health*, 98 (2): 221–30.

Laverack, G. and Labonte, R. (2000) 'A planning framework for community empowerment goals within health promotion', *Health Policy and Planning*, 15: 255–62.

Link, B.G. and Phelan, J.C. (1995) 'Social conditions as fundamental causes of disease', *Journal of Health and Social Behavior*, 35 (extra issue): 80–94.

Marmot, M. and Wilkinson, R. (1999) *Social Determinants of Health*, New York: Oxford University Press.

Matarazzo, J.D. (1980) 'Behavioral health and behavioral medicine: frontiers for a new health psychology', *American Psychologist*, 35 (9): 807–17.

Parker, R.G. (1996) 'Empowerment, community mobilization and social change in the face of HIV/AIDS', *AIDS*, 10 (Suppl. 3): S27–31.

Parker, R.G. (2002) 'The global HIV/AIDS pandemic, structural inequalities, and the politics of international health', *American Journal of Public Health*, 93 (3): 343–6.

Parker, R.G., Easton, D., and Klein, C. (2000) 'Structural barriers and facilitators in HIV prevention: a review of international research', *AIDS*, 14 (Suppl. 1): S22–32.

Porter, R. (1997) *The Greatest Benefit to Mankind*, New York: W.W. Norton.

Rosen, G. (1993) *A History of Public Health*, Baltimore, MD: Johns Hopkins University Press.

Rosner, D. and Markowitz, G. (1985) 'The early movement for occupational safety and health, 1900–1917', in J. Leavitt and R. Numbers (eds) *Sickness and Health in America, Readings in the History of Medicine and Public Health*, 2nd edition, Madison: University of Wisconsin Press.

Schmid, T.L., Pratt, M., and Hovze, E. (1995) 'Policy as intervention: environmental and policy approaches to the prevention of cardiovascular disease', *American Journal of Public Health*, 85 (9): 1207–11.

Singer, M. and Clare, S. (2003) 'Syndemics and public health: reconceptualizing disease in bio-social context', *Medical Anthropology Quarterly*, 17 (4): 423–41.

Sweat, M. and Denison, J. (1995) 'Reducing HIV incidence in developing countries with structural and environmental interventions', *AIDS*, 9 (Suppl. A): S251–7.

Tomes, N. (1998) *The Gospel of Germs: Men, Women, and the Microbe in American Life*, Cambridge, MA: Harvard University Press.

Wallerstein, N. (1992) 'Powerlessness, empowerment, and health: implications for health promotion programs', *American Journal of Health Promotion*, 6 (3): 197–205.

Part 1

DEFINING STRUCTURAL FACTORS

2

THE HISTORY OF STRUCTURAL
APPROACHES IN PUBLIC HEALTH

James Colgrove, Amy Fairchild, and David Rosner

Structural approaches in public health have a long history. When it emerged as an organized endeavour in the nineteenth century, public health concerned itself primarily with environmental and ecological approaches: water supplies and sewer systems, laws governing tenement construction, and regulation of hazardous industries and workplaces. These efforts prefigured the modern conception of structural interventions, although the political motivations of early public health reformers were mixed and there remains debate about whether their efforts should be thought of as radical or conservative.[1] Whatever their intent, the public health innovations of the nineteenth century in Europe and in the cities of the urban northeast in the United States achieved dramatic improvements in public health by addressing fundamental living and working conditions, especially those of the poor.

In the first decades of the twentieth century, as the germ theory of disease achieved widespread popular and scientific acceptance, US public health professionals withdrew from their engagement with broad social and economic factors affecting health and adopted a more narrowly conceived, laboratory- and biology-based approach. Over the course of the twentieth century, some public health practitioners sought to reorient the field toward a greater focus on social context, but they remained in the minority.

The current emphasis on structural approaches in public health therefore represents not so much an innovation as a return to the field's earliest historical roots. This chapter will examine the antecedents of current efforts to improve health by altering broad social, political, economic, and environmental factors. It will also trace the shifting attitudes within the field of public health in the United States about whether the individual or the society is the appropriate locus for public health intervention.

European beginnings

Outbreaks of epidemic infectious diseases such as cholera and typhus in the 1830s and 1840s gave rise to the first sustained movement to improve public health. Most diseases were thought to arise from miasmas – clouds of noxious gases arising from decaying animal and vegetable matter and other forms of filth – so environmental approaches were seen as the most effective way of preventing epidemics. Efforts to create more sanitary streets, markets, homes, and workplaces were given urgency by the fear of social unrest. In the rapidly urbanizing, industrializing societies of England, France, and Germany, the squalid living conditions endured by the poor created the potential for riots, and even insurrection or revolution. Moreover, physical health was closely linked with morality and spiritual well-being, so measures to prevent sickness among the labouring classes would also improve their character and make them less prone to vice and sloth and less likely to become dependent on charity. In this way, public health reform was linked to an expansive vision of social and political stability and economic productivity (Nathanson 2007).

In England, the desire to maintain order and decrease dependency led reformers such as Edwin Chadwick, a lawyer, politician, and member of the royal commission studying the country's system of public welfare, to call for improvements in urban infrastructure (Hamlin 1999). Chadwick's *Report on the Sanitary Condition of the Labouring Population of Great Britain* (1843) remains a seminal document in the history of public health and was critical to the development of clean water supplies and sewage disposal. Over the second half of the nineteenth century, Britain created a strong, decentralized system of public health administration and passed a series of landmark laws establishing that civic hygiene was a matter of state responsibility.

In Germany, the physician Rudolf Virchow advanced a radical vision of medicine and public health at the height of the European revolutions of 1848. 'Severe and mighty political storms such as now roar over the thinking portion of Europe, shaking to the foundation all elements of the state, indicate radical changes in the prevailing conceptions of life', Virchow wrote. 'In this situation, medicine cannot alone remain untouched; it too can no longer postpone a radical reform of its field' (as cited in Rosen 1947: 676).

When the Prussian government commissioned him to investigate a disease outbreak in the rural province of Silesia, Virchow found that poverty, poor housing, and inadequate food supply lay at the root of the epidemic. In his *Report on the Typhus Epidemic in Upper Silesia*, Virchow recommended modernizing the region's political and economic institutions and creating an educational system. The report's critique of the dominant political structures proved too radical for its government sponsors, and Virchow was temporarily removed from his position, though he later returned to favour and pursued a successful career as an influential politician and legislator (Porter 1997).

Today, Virchow is best remembered for a declaration that might serve as a definition of structural interventions:

> Medicine is a social science, and politics is nothing else but medicine on a large scale. Medicine, as a social science, as the science of human beings, has the obligation to point out problems and to attempt their theoretical solution: the politician, the practical anthropologist, must find the means for their actual solution. … The physicians are the natural attorneys of the poor, and social problems fall to a large extent within their jurisdiction.
>
> (as cited in Sigerist 1941: 93–4)

Atlantic crossing

In the United States, the field of public health emerged when physicians, housing reformers, advocates for the poor, and scientists trained in new techniques of chemistry and civil engineering came together to fight problems growing out of urbanization, industrialization, and large-scale immigration. This coalition transformed the nation's economy and environment and, as a result, its health. High death rates and pestilence had long affected rich and poor communities alike. In contrast to the Colonial period, when life spans in many towns were relatively long, Americans' health had deteriorated by the mid-nineteenth century (Demos 1983; Greven 1972; Lockwood 1978). Epidemic diseases such as smallpox, cholera, typhoid, yellow fever, and intestinal diseases became powerful symbols of uncontainable social decline – and were often blamed on the immigrant poor (Fairchild *et al.* 2010).

Amid this atmosphere of alarm over the conditions of the poor, civic leaders launched expansive investigations into the social and environmental, as well as the individual, causes and consequences of disease. In Philadelphia, New York, and Boston, reformers focused on housing as a cause of the city's physical, social, and moral decline (Citizens' Association of New York 1865). American reformers explicitly drew upon models from abroad. For example, physician John Griscom's influential 1845 report *The Sanitary Condition of the Laboring Population of New York* echoed the title of Edwin Chadwick's document; similarly, Lemuel Shattuck, a statistician commissioned by the Massachusetts legislature to investigate the health of the commonwealth, patterned his *Report of the Sanitary Commission* (1850) on Chadwick's work.

The 'sanitarians' (as they were known) who led reform efforts in the nineteenth and early twentieth centuries generally saw themselves as more than technical experts trained in a specific skill. Some had come from elite merchant families and others had been educated in the ministry. Others had been militant abolitionists, allied with the growing anti-slavery movement; still others were suffragists, seeking equality for women in the workplace and in the voting booths (Rosenkrantz 1972). They defined their mission as much in moral as in secular terms and believed that illness, filth, class, and disorder were intrinsically related. Individual transgression and social decay were equally at fault for poor health.

With the turn to bacteriology that followed the discoveries of Louis Pasteur, Joseph Lister, and Robert Koch in later decades of the nineteenth century, a new faith in laboratory science emerged among physicians engaged in public health. A new model began to gain greater acceptance: germs, not miasmas, made people sick. The slums of large cities were 'breeding grounds' that were 'seeded' with bacilli waiting to infect the susceptible victim. For a period of time, however, sanitarian dictums meshed quite well with the new bacteriological discoveries (Tomes 1998). United by moral certainty regarding the need to act, sanitarians, epidemiologists, and bacteriologists, the old and new sciences of public health, were marshalled to achieve radical reform. Although the movement could and often did focus on the moral characteristics of those who succumbed to disease, it was nonetheless allied with social and labour reformers seeking to transform housing and work conditions for city dwellers in the decades at the turn of the century (Rosner and Markowitz 1985).

New housing was now required to have indoor plumbing and connections to the new water and sewer lines that were replacing wells and privies. Tenement laws were passed that mandated that all rooms in newly constructed buildings have windows opening to the outside. Restrictions on housing density and new nuisance laws began to have an effect on rates of tuberculosis and other devastating diseases (Blackmar 1995). Laws requiring the refrigeration of foodstuffs, meat-inspection laws, pure-milk laws, and regulation of the 'noxious trades' like slaughterhouses and tanneries began to be reflected in improvements in health (Fee 1987; Fee and Hammonds 1995; Schultz and McShane 1978).

In rural areas, malaria, yellow fever, and pellagra were addressed through a host of engineering and social reform efforts from the draining of swamps to the provision of better diets and work to poor sharecroppers both black and white. Perhaps most remarkable was the degree to which public health served as both an organizing and unifying concept. Throughout the country, health officials sought to control the tuberculosis bacillus, but they did so with an eye to the individual in his or her social context (Abel 1997; Fox 1975).

Within the field of industrial health, crusaders like Alice Hamilton and Florence Kelley, who were focused on the link between illness and working conditions, likewise operated within a broad network. Such reformers forged links between the settlement house, industrial reform, and labour movements. This type of alliance helped to spur factory inspection after the tragic 1911 fire at the Triangle Shirtwaist Company, which marked a turning point in the regulation of the workplace and the movement for workers' compensation laws. The understanding that working conditions were critical to health would continue to inform the efforts of the Consumers League and the International Ladies' Garment Workers' Union to attach the 'union label' to garments as a symbol of clean working conditions (and, therefore, healthy, tuberculosis-free garments) in the 1920s (Fairchild *et al.* 2010). Although she was speaking specifically of the federal government, understanding the intersection of different groups around public health issues helps to shed light on what Alice Hamilton meant when she said that the state was no more or less than 'ourselves – ourselves organized' (as cited in Viseltear 1973: 991).

The turn away from environmental approaches

If epidemics were a hallmark of the crowded, centralized cities of the East Coast during the nineteenth century, then cancers and other chronic diseases were the paradigmatic conditions that plagued cities in the twentieth century. The new century saw fundamental change in land use and transportation that improved health in many respects but created new hazards and diseases for the urban United States. Exposures to synthetic materials; air, water, and soil pollution; and the creation of a huge marketing industry that promoted toxic materials for consumer uses – such as lead paints and tobacco – led to an epidemiological revolution as infectious diseases gave way to chronic conditions. Ironically, in the wake of these social and epidemiological transformations, the public health community embraced bacteriology, with its focus on the laboratory rather than the social and environmental context, as an authoritative science that did not require any political alliances: science spoke for itself. Departments of public health shed sanitation, housing reform, and even hospital care. The interdisciplinary alliance that lent power to public health splintered, with profound consequences for the subsequent evolution of the field (Fairchild *et al.* 2010).

This fragmentation was reflected in the rise of academic public health. As Elizabeth Fee has argued, bacteriology and sanitary reform had been 'the twin pillars of public health': 'Bacteriology represented the achievements of laboratory research' while sanitary engineering represented 'the practice of providing clean water supplies and treating sewage wastes' (Fee 1987: 60). William Welch, the first dean of the Johns Hopkins

School of Hygiene and Public Health and one of the early pioneers of public health education, recognized the housing and urban reforms' contributions to health but saw them as properly located in the fields of engineering, social work, and urban planning. Public health education would centre on the laboratory (Fee 1987; Rosner and Markowitz 1973).

In 1913, Hibbert Hill, a public health official and author, wrote a provocative book entitled *The New Public Health*. In it he sought to capture the fundamental changes that had overtaken the field over the course of the previous 50 years and to present a roadmap to the future. The 'essential change' he characterized succinctly:

> The old public health was concerned with the environment; the new is concerned with the individual. The old sought the sources of infectious disease in the surroundings of man; the new finds them in man himself. The old public health … failed because it sought them … in every place and in every thing *where they were not*.
> (Hill 1913: 10; emphasis in original)

For Hill, to improve the health of the nation, one had to begin changing behaviour one person at a time. Public health had to abandon universalist environmental solutions – introducing pure water, sewage systems, street cleaning – and begin focusing on training people on how to live cleaner, more healthful lives. Bacteriology held out the hope for an 'efficient' public health. The logic of the old sanitarians' ideas ultimately led to radical reformation of the environment – tearing down filthy, air-deprived slums, improving infrastructures of entire neighbourhoods – while 'education' and the control of the actions of the infected individual merely required a focus on the renegade few (Fairchild *et al.* 2010). Treating a few thousand victims of disease was, in his analysis, far cheaper – he estimated 'one seven-hundredth the magnitude' – than improving housing for millions (Hill 1913: 17). Hill's analysis marked the beginning of a struggle to define the mandate of public health – a struggle that has consumed the field since the early years of the twentieth century. Public health professionals made more than 100 efforts, in books, journal articles, and reports, to define the 'new' public health in the decades following Hill's 1916 call for refocusing. At the heart of these efforts has been the question of whether public health, as an agent of science, can also promote fundamental social, economic, and political reforms.

The death of progressivism and the advent of the conservative political and social environment of the 1920s pushed public health into the laboratory and away from the progressive traditions that had once been central to its identity. While the Depression created new opportunities for public health, allowing for alliances with the labour movement in support of a national health plan and even local initiatives to set up community health centres for the vast number of unemployed, the growing power of medical science and narrowly defined 'efficiency' continued to push public health away from its reformist roots. In the years following the Second World War, the end of the New Deal, the rise of consensus politics of the 'affluent' consumer society, and the invention of new medical and therapeutic technologies led public health to shift its focus away from social reform in favour of 'magic bullets' as the preferred means for addressing disease.

While in the US the activities of states and localities were (and still are) the centre of public health activities, the shifting terrain of public health was evident at the national level as well. In the two decades between the beginning of the Roosevelt and the Eisenhower administrations, Congress considered five major national health proposals. The general purpose of the National Health Act of 1939 – the first attempt after the failed efforts to incorporate a national health programme in the Social Security Act of 1935 – was 'to provide for the general welfare' by providing broad support for public health and hospital and clinic construction, particularly for economically distressed areas. Significantly, the 1939 proposal contained no provisions for paying for medical care, public or private. Rather, it sought to ensure environmental reforms and economic services that spoke to older conceptions of the province of public health. The 1939 proposal thus reflected the degree to which the Roosevelt Administration, as it attempted to resurrect the national health programme sacrificed to assure passage of the Social Security Act of 1935, saw poor health not only as a problem of being able to afford care, but as one of the underlying economic structure: 'The records of dependency and relief show how frequently illness is the cause of economic breakdown' (as cited in Hirschfield 1970: 102). The Technical Committee of Roosevelt's Interdepartmental Committee to Coordinate Health and Welfare Activities consequently recommended a plan to compensate workers' wages during times of sickness as well as disability insurance, modelled on 'old age insurance'. Concluded the Committee, 'Since not only the health of the wage earner, but that of his dependents is at stake, the Committee feels that maintenance of the sick worker's purchasing power is an important part of any program for national health' (Interdepartmental Committee to Coordinate Health and Welfare Activities 1939: 25–7).

The 1939 proposal did not simply imagine that the sick should be able to purchase medical care. Florence Greenberg, representing the Citizens Committee for Adequate Medical Care at the 1939 hearings, argued that while workers needed to be able to pay for medical services, 'of equal importance is finding ways to increase economic security of the worker, the assurance of a job and income' (Interdepartmental Committee to Coordinate Health and Welfare Activities 1939: 229). The critical importance of assuring wages in the context of maintaining public health was also given voice by representatives from the National Association for the Advancement of Colored People (NAACP), though with an eye to curbing racism.

By the beginning of the Cold War, the idea of public health as a sweeping reformist enterprise was all but moribund in the United States. In the national health insurance proposals to emerge after Second World War, the idea of disability insurance was replaced by a 'pre-paid health benefit' plan for medical services. Hospital construction and clinical, not population-based, research became a national priority. At the same time, some of the sanitary activities for which health departments had been responsible, such as garbage collection, air pollution control, and noise abatement, were pulled under the aegis of other professions and government agencies (Fox 1995; Melosi 2000). It was medicine, now, that was positioned to protect the nation's health. But the rise of the hospital and hegemony of medical research were not inevitable. 'Deficiencies in basic living conditions ... are the breeding ground for disease and poor health', argued Solomon Barkin of the Textile Workers Union of America: 'No program for the improvement of the Nation's health is complete which does not have the elimination of ... deficiencies in basic living conditions ... as one of its goals' (US Senate 1946: 2617).

Biomedical science become a great leveller, allowing public health professionals to ignore social factors – such as racial segregation, poverty, inequality, and poor housing, which had been the foci of earlier public healthy reformers – and to explain disease without any of the disruptive implications of a class analysis. This was Thomas McKeown's 1950s critique of prevailing understandings of disease as a medical phenomena rather than an indicator of social relations. A Progressive Era emphasis on social welfare and urban reform became ideologically dangerous when class analysis was equated with anti-Americanism in the context of the 'affluent society' of the McCarthy era. This was also the era in which new medical technologies – antibiotics, vaccines, psychotropic medications, and a host of other clinical interventions – provided apolitical means of attacking disease without disrupting the social order (Foner 1998).

Social medicine and a new focus on structure

Ironically, it was in the face of the retrenchment of public health that a heterogeneous group of doctors, nurses, epidemiologists, and educators claimed a more enlightened, sociologically informed view than the narrow focus of biomedicine, and some of the profession's activist members sought to advance a broadly social vision of health that gave greater attention to structural forces. In the 1940s and 1950s, physicians in the United States and the United Kingdom such as McKeown, Zena Stein, and Mervyn Susser articulated a new vision for medicine itself: social medicine (Rosen 1947).

George Rosen, the eminent historian and editor of the *American Journal of Public Health*, sought to import the European social medical tradition into the US context and introduced public health practitioners to their roots in social activism, recalling the work of Virchow and Chadwick. In turn, the field of social medicine helped spawn social epidemiology as a discipline within schools of public health. But while social epidemiology began to mark academic public health, the vision remained marginal within the US context, where class politics was less pronounced than in Europe and even the most radical Progressive Era visions of social and political reforms rejected class struggle. Hence public health practitioners in the United States missed opportunities to shape the institutional landscape of health and disease (Brandt and Gardner 2000).

Profound social, cultural, and institutional changes provide the backdrop to the waning authority of public health beginning after the Second World War. The rise of medical authority went hand in hand with the ascendance of the hospital as the centre of treatment and research with the development of an array of therapeutic tools, such as antibiotics, vaccines, and biotechnologies. Power was consolidated in corporate interests and given force by a general cultural ethos of mass consumption and market-driven health care. A powerful discourse of 'personal responsibility' for health and disease placed blame on individuals and absolved corporations that marketed potentially harmful products like cigarettes or put lead paint on the walls knowing the hazards it posed to children or polluted the nation's water and air (Fairchild *et al.* 2010). An influential 1974 report by the Canadian Minister of Health, Marc Lalonde, signalled a new focus on health promotion in the industrialized democracies: it was time to focus on changing risky behaviours. In a similar vein, John Knowles, former president of the Rockefeller Foundation, argued in a widely read and discussed article, 'The solution to the problems of ill health in modern American society involves individual responsibility' (Knowles 1977: 58). Knowles set a critical tone for subsequent policy, which placed the blame for morbidity and mortality in the United States not just on personal habits but careless habits and individual indulgence in private excesses. An increasing focus on individual health promotion and disease prevention intersected with powerful social movements concerned with issues of race, gender, sexuality, and medical authority. The antiwar movement, the women's movement, and the civil rights movement all challenged public trust in expert judgements. This emphasis was given force by revelations such as in 1972 about the Tuskegee syphilis study and in 1976 by the Centers for Disease Control and Prevention's ill-fated plan to protect the nation from swine flu (Colgrove 2011). While all helped to propel a sweeping social and health policy emphasis not only on individual autonomy and rights but also on social justice, they contributed to deep fissures in the field of public health.

The historical demographer Thomas McKeown argued that fundamental social and economic changes were responsible for altering patterns of health and illness (McKeown 1979). Jack Geiger, a co-founder of Physicians for Human Rights and for decades one of the most politically active public health leaders in the United States, worked with civil rights organizations such as the Congress of Racial Equality and travelled to Mississippi to establish health centres for impoverished African Americans; Lorin Kerr, a physician with the US Public Health Service, partnered with the United Mine Workers to conduct research and advocacy that forced black lung disease in Appalachia onto the national agenda; and many in the American Public Health Association pressed for strong alliances with women's organizations, civil rights groups, and peace activists (Fairchild et al. 2010). Yet, while they may have represented the social conscience of public health, they were rarely able to change power relationships on a broader scale. Still others did not seek to define the mandate of public health as affecting social reform and, in fact, openly opposed any role outside public health 'science' in addressing health concerns of the nation. For example, the epidemiologist Kenneth Rothman and his colleagues argued that, as a science, epidemiology had no advocacy role in broad social debates: it might document the effects of poverty on health, for example, but it had no mandate to attack poverty (Rothman et al. 1998).

A return to structural approaches?

Over the course of the past century, public health officials defined their mandate ever more narrowly and shrank from political engagement with powerful interests such as corporations and businesses that created unhealthful environments. They failed to confront medical specialists interested in defining preventive interventions as clinical and, hence, as reimbursable. This critique was made perhaps most memorably in a 1970 address to the American Public Health Association by Paul Cornely. Newly elected as the group's first African American president, Cornely levelled a blistering attack on what he saw as the complacency of his profession. It had been 'a mere bystander' to profound changes in the health care system that had taken place in the 1960s; its members wasted their time on 'piddling resolutions and their wordings'. Public health, he charged, remained 'outside the power structure' (Cornely 1971: 16). Cornely's address was a clarion call for more aggressive action against a host of health problems integral to modern industrial society.

A century ago, Hermann Biggs described public health as 'autocratic' and 'radical' in nature. To be sure, such an outlook shored up authoritarian and paternalistic public health practices that, today, are often condemned by human rights activists. But at the same time it conveyed a sense of ambition and authority on the part of a host of public health actors. But this capacity for deliberate action represented more than just a resolute mindset of public health officials that allowed the field to overcome all obstacles through the force of sheer will and moral fibre: it represented real alliances with social and political groups that were struggling for a place and power in US society (Fairchild *et al.* 2010).

For many decades the field has been constrained by self-imposed limitations and, too often, has avoided collaboration with people who challenge complacency and existing power relationships. Public health became unwilling or uncertain about how to use science to challenge powerful corporate interests or profound social inequalities linked to gender, race, and class (Tomes 2008). Yet, as various institutions, organizations, and communities mobilized in the name of public health, the field was pressed to join the coalitions that had some of the radical characteristics of the late nineteenth and early twentieth centuries. Whether the field will return to its social-reformist roots and an emphasis on structural approaches remains to be seen, however.

The worldwide financial crisis of 2008, which affected the health and well-being of hundreds of millions of people in the United States and around the world, provided the chance to rethink the fundamental assumptions of a society's economic and social systems. Public health is now positioned to reclaim its place as part of an emerging worldwide reform movement. The future will present new challenges – from global warming and industrial pollution to bioterrorism and universal health care – that will bring practitioners into very dramatic confrontation with their history. The field will either accommodate to the status quo or confront political and economic structures in the name of the public's health.

Note

1   As Nathanson (2007: 247) notes, 'Public health originated as much from fear of social change – the revolutionary potential of the desperate poor huddled together in the teeming cities of the nineteenth century – as from the desire for social reform. Public health was conceived as a means to public order.' On the conservative nature of nineteenth century public health reform, see Nathanson 2007 and Hamlin 1999.

References

Abel, E.K. (1997) 'Taking the cure to the poor: patients' responses to New York City's tuberculosis program, 1894 to 1918', *American Journal of Public Health*, 87: 1808–15.

Blackmar, E. (1995) 'Accountability for public health: regulating the housing market in nineteenth-century New York City', in D. Rosner (ed.) *Hives of Sickness: Public Health and Epidemics in New York City*, New Brunswick, NJ: Rutgers University Press.

Brandt, A.M. and Gardner, M. (2000) 'Antagonism and accommodation: interpreting the relationship between public health and medicine in the United States during the 20th century', *American Journal of Public Health*, 90: 707–15.

Citizens' Association of New York (1865) Sanitary Condition of the City, Report of the Council of Hygiene and Public Health of the Citizens' Association of New York, New York: Citizens' Association of New York.

Colgrove, J. (2011) *Epidemic City: The Politics of Public Health in New York*, New York: Russell Sage Foundation.

Cornely, P. (1971) 'The hidden enemies of health and the American Public Health Association', *American Journal of Public Health*, 61: 16–17.

Demos, J. (1983) 'Notes on life in Plymouth Colony', in S.N. Katz and J.M. Murrin (eds) *Colonial America: Essays in Politics and Social Development*, 3rd edition, New York: Alfred A. Knopf.

Fairchild, A.L., Rosner, D., Colgrove, J., Bayer, R., and Fried, L.P. (2010) 'The exodus of public health: What history can tell us about the future', *American Journal of Public Health*, 100: 54–63.

Fee, E. (1987) *Disease and Discovery: A History of the Johns Hopkins School of Hygiene and Public Health, 1916–1939*, Baltimore, MD: Johns Hopkins University Press.

Fee, E. and Hammonds, E.M. (1995) 'Science, politics and the art of persuasion: promoting the new scientific medicine in New York City', in D. Rosner (ed.) *Hives of Sickness: Public Health and Epidemics in New York City*, New Brunswick, NJ: Rutgers University Press.

Foner, E. (1998) *The Story of American Freedom*, New York: W.W. Norton and Company.

Fox, D.M. (1975) 'Social policy and city politics: tuberculosis reporting in New York, 1889–1900', *Bulletin of the History of Medicine*, 49 (2): 169–72.

Fox, D.M. (1995) 'The politics of public health in New York City: contrasting styles since 1920', in D. Rosner (ed.) *Hives of Sickness: Public Health and Epidemics in New York City*, New Brunswick, NJ: Rutgers University Press.

Greven, P.F. (1972) *Four Generations: Population, Land, and Family in Colonial Andover, Massachusetts*, Ithaca, NY: Cornell University Press.

Hamlin, C. (1999) *Public Health and Social Justice in the Age of Chadwick: Britain, 1800–1854*, Cambridge: Cambridge University Press.

Hill, H. (1913) *The New Public Health*, Minneapolis, MN: Journal-Lancet Press.

Hirschfield, D.S. (1970) *The Lost Reform: The Campaign for Compulsory Health Insurance in the United States from 1932–1943*, Cambridge, MA: Harvard University Press.

Interdepartmental Committee to Coordinate Health and Welfare Activities (1939) *Toward Better National Health*, Washington, D.C.: United States Government Printing Office.

Knowles, J. (1977) 'The responsibility of the individual', in J. Knowles (ed.) *Doing Better and Feeling Worse: Health in the United States*, New York: W.W. Norton.

Lockwood, R.A. (1978) 'Birth, illness, and death in 18th-century New England', *Journal of Social History*, 12: 111–28.

McKeown, T. (1979) *The Role of Medicine: Dream, Mirage, or Nemesis?*, Princeton, NJ: Princeton University Press.

Melosi, M.V. (2000) *The Sanitary City: Urban Infrastructure in America from Colonial Times to the Present*, Baltimore, MD: Johns Hopkins University Press.

Nathanson, C. (2007) *Disease Prevention as Social Change: The State, Society, and Public Health in the United States, France, Great Britain, and Canada*, New York: Russell Sage Foundation.

Porter, R. (1997) *The Greatest Benefit to Mankind*, New York: W.W. Norton.

Rosen, G. (1947) 'What is social medicine? A genetic analysis of the concept', *Bulletin of the History of Medicine*, 21: 674–733.

Rosenkrantz, B. (1972) *Public Health and the State: Changing Views in Massachusetts, 1842–1936*, Cambridge, MA: Harvard University Press.

Rosner, D. and Markowitz, G. (1973) 'Doctors in crisis: the uses of medical education reform to establish modern professional elitism in medicine', *American Quarterly*, 25: 83–107.

Rosner, D. and Markowitz, G. (1985) 'The early movement for occupational safety and health, 1900–1917', in J. Leavitt and R. Numbers (eds) *Sickness and Health in America: Readings in the History of Medicine and Public Health*, 2nd edition, Madison: University of Wisconsin Press.

Rothman, K.J., Adami, H.-O., and Trichopoulos, D. (1998) 'Should the mission of public health include the eradication of poverty?', *The Lancet*, 5: 810–13.

Schultz, S.K. and McShane, C. (1978) 'To engineer the metropolis: sewers, sanitation, and city planning in late-nineteenth-century America', *Journal of American History*, 65: 389–411.

Sigerist, H. (1941) *Medicine and Human Welfare*, New Haven, CT: Yale University Press.

Tomes, N. (1998) *The Gospel of Germs: Men, Women, and the Microbe in American Life*, Cambridge, MA: Harvard University Press.

Tomes, N. (2008) 'Speaking for the public: the ambivalent quest of twentieth century public health', in J. Colgrove, G. Markowitz, D. Rosner (eds), *The Contested Boundaries of American Public Health*, New Brunswick, NJ: Rutgers University Press.

United States Senate (1946) *National Health Program: Hearings before the Committee on Education and Labor on S. 1606, 79th Congress, 2nd session, Part 5: 24, 25, 26, 27 June, 10 July 1946*, Washington, D.C.: Government Printing Office.

Viseltear, A.J. (1973) 'Emergence of the medical care section of the American Public Health Association, 1926–1948', *American Journal of Public Health*, 63: 986–1007.

3

SOCIAL INEQUALITIES AND PUBLIC HEALTH

Ruth Bell, Peter Goldblatt, and Michael Marmot

Introduction

A person's health is determined by a wide range of influences they experience during their lives – from the genes they inherit, and the conditions they experience during their lives from before birth to older ages. These influences are many and complex. The very different experiences lead to variation in health. To the extent that there are systematic differences in these experiences of individuals and groups related to the social conditions in which a person is born, lives, works, and dies, the resulting health differences are referred to as health inequalities. Where inequalities are avoidable by reasonable means, they are considered to be inequitable (CSDH 2008). A distinction is also made between the determinants of population health (such as the cleanliness of a water supply that affects everyone in the area supplied) and the social determinants of health inequities. The latter cover factors that impact differently on groups according to a range of social factors.

The WHO Commission on the Social Determinants of Health (CSDH) (CSDH 2008) has highlighted the many factors, including education, employment and work, health care, transport and housing, the societal stage of industrialization, urbanization, and globalization that shape health and health inequities. Most important, it has indicated how these factors lead to differential exposures to risks and different vulnerabilities and assets – all ultimately determined by the distribution of power, money, and resources in society.

Inequalities in health between and within countries

Health improvements are achievable by reasonable means. During the twentieth century, many countries have achieved major improvements in population health. Taking life expectancy as a summary measure of population health, there was a remarkable increase of 20 years in average global life expectancy since 1950 (UN 2011). Notably, however, progress in population health has been uneven across regions (Figure 3.1) and stark inequalities in health and life expectancy exist between and within countries (CSDH 2008).

When overall health improvements are achieved, it is frequently the case that health inequities remain. Figure 3.2 demonstrates trends in the social gradient in under-five mortality in Egypt according to the distribution of wealth, measured in terms of

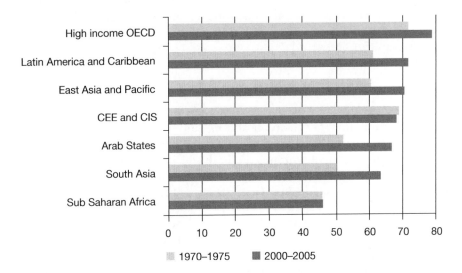

Figure 3.1 Life expectancy at birth by region, 1970–1975 and 2000–2005

Source: UNDP 2006

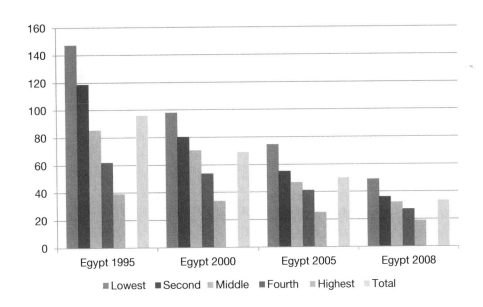

Figure 3.2 Trends in under-five mortality per 1,000 births by wealth quintile: Egypt

Source: Prepared by the authors using data from MEASURE DHS 2011

household assets. Between 1995 and 2008, the overall rate of child deaths fell by two-thirds, but the ratio of the lowest to the highest wealth quintile only fell by one-third, so while there were improvements for all, substantial inequalities remained. To reduce inequalities, it is necessary for those who are worse off to improve more quickly than those who are better off.

Social determinants of health

The explanatory framework used by the CSDH builds on previous work (Solar and Irwin 2010) and outlines how health and health inequities such as those described in Figures 3.1 and 3.2 are created. The framework (Figure 3.3) draws together both 'the social factors promoting and undermining the health of individuals and populations' and 'the social processes underlying the unequal distribution of these factors between groups occupying unequal positions in society' (Solar and Irwin 2010: 27). The term 'social determinants of health' encompasses all these factors.

Health is shaped by a person's genes and by the conditions experienced throughout life; before birth and in early life; and by the social and physical environments of daily life throughout adult life (Figure 3.4).

Factors of daily life include material conditions, such as access to nutritious food, clean water and sanitation, basic health care, safe and health-promoting living and working

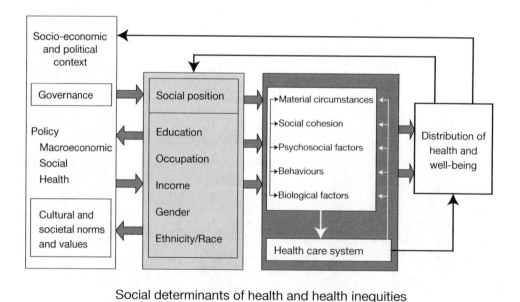

Figure 3.3 Conceptual framework of the Commission on Social Determinants of Health

Source: CSDH 2008, reproduced with permission

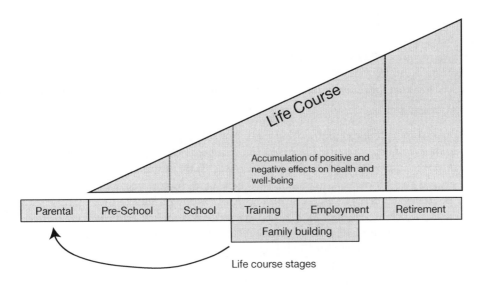

Figure 3.4 Accumulation of influences on health through the life course

Source: Marmot Review 2010

conditions, as well as psychosocial factors. Within countries the link between poverty, poor material living and working conditions, and poor health and disease is apparent. But health inequalities are also seen among groups that are not poor. For example, the Whitehall studies of British civil servants showed that, even among employed people who are not poor, there is a social gradient in mortality and morbidity that runs from the bottom to the top of society (Marmot *et al.* 1984, 1991). The search for explanations therefore includes examination of material conditions and psychosocial factors – including lack of control, social support, and social cohesion – as well as the connections between material and psychosocial factors.

Material conditions and psychosocial factors are experienced differently by groups within a social structure depending on the nature of social stratification in a society making groups more or less vulnerable to disease. Lower material living conditions and lower control experienced by disadvantaged groups in society are reflected in poorer health and lower life expectancy compared to more advantaged groups.

Behavioural choices also influence health outcomes across society. These include health-related behaviours that are risks for non-communicable disease, including smoking, harmful use of alcohol, physical inactivity, and diets that are high in saturated fats, sugar, and salt. However, individual choices that people make are shaped by the social environment they inhabit, as well as cultural norms and values. For example, smoking has been identified as a coping strategy among women in England struggling with psychological stresses associated with multiple life challenges of caring for relatives and living on low incomes (Graham 1987).

The functioning of health systems is an important influence on health and the distribution of health. Inequity in access to health care and preventive services contributes to differential health outcomes, but does not fully explain the distribution of health in society. Beyond health care, the health care system has a wider role through working with other sectors for health promotion (for example, risk reduction in lifestyles and behaviours) and ill health prevention.

The nature and level of social stratification flow from inequalities in wealth, income, and education. Differential vulnerability is also created by experiences of people in their daily lives, for example power relations between men and women and the extent to which they are balanced, and discrimination on the basis of race or ethnicity.

Social stratification within a society is driven by national socio–economic context, governance arrangements, economic and social policies, and cultural and societal norms, values and biases. These national-level factors are in turn influenced by systems of global governance, trade, aid, and international relations (CSDH 2008).

The centrality of power differentials in the causal framework leading to health inequalities led the CSDH to emphasize the role of empowerment in improving health and reducing health inequalities. The CSDH described empowerment in three dimensions operating at individual, community, and national levels – the material requirements for a decent life; psychosocial empowerment, having control over one's life; and political empowerment, having a political voice and participating in the decisions that affect lives. The notion of empowerment aligns with Amartya Sen's capability approach to human well-being, in which well-being is linked to the capabilities of people to realize various functionings or freedoms that enable people to live a life they have reason to value (Sen 1999).

The social determinants approach to health goes beyond considering how to encourage behaviour change to reduce exposure to lifestyle risks, although behaviour change will be part of what is needed. Indeed, it goes beyond what is traditionally considered to be the domain of the health sector. The social determinants of health approach applies values of social justice in every sphere of public and private sector policy. Simply put, the social determinants of health approach implies asking the question 'How does this strategy/policy/intervention affect people's lives and the ability of people to live a life they have reason to value?'

The CSDH made its recommendations across a framework that takes a life course perspective on 'the conditions in which people are born, grow, live, work and age', and examines 'the inequitable distribution of power, money and resources' (CSDH 2008: 2). The CSDH described three principles of action to tackle health inequities:

1   Improve the conditions of daily life – the circumstances in which people are born, grow, live, work, and age;
2   Tackle the inequitable distribution of power, money and resources – the structural drivers of those conditions of daily life – globally, nationally, and locally;
3   Measure the problem, evaluate action, expand the knowledge base, develop a workforce that is trained in the social determinants of health, and raise public awareness about the social determinants of health.

Within these three overarching recommendations, the CSDH arranged its full set of recommendations under the following areas for action:

Daily living conditions
   Equity from the start (early child development and education)
   Healthy places

Fair employment and decent work
Social protection
Universal health care

Power, money, and resources
Health equity in all policies, systems, and programmes
Fair financing
Market responsibility
Gender equity
Political empowerment – inclusion and voice
Good global governance

Monitoring, research, and training

The following sections use this framework to outline how social determinants affect health.

Early child development and education

The period before birth and during early childhood is the most important development phase throughout the lifespan (CSDH Early Child Development Knowledge Network 2007). Development across the interrelated domains of physical, social-emotional, and language-cognitive development strongly influences 'well-being, obesity/stunting, mental health, heart disease, competence in literacy and numeracy, criminality, and economic participation throughout life' (CSDH Early Child Development Knowledge Network 2007: 15).

Good conditions for development in early childhood set the foundations for building resilience to stressful situations faced throughout life, enabling development of self-esteem and sense of control that are fundamental to health and well-being. Brain development at critical periods in early life responds to stimuli in the social environment, such as those that arise in interactions between babies and caregivers. The quality of the psychosocial stimulation that babies and young children receive and elicit through engagement with their social and physical environment shapes the development of cognitive function and the development of habitual ways of responding to and reacting towards others. The health and nutritional status of women before, during, and after pregnancy, good nutrition and health care, and nurturing, supportive, caring, and responsive living environments for children in the early years affect their development and future life trajectory.

Interventions such as parenting support and home-based and centre-based programmes can improve children's cognitive and social-emotional development in the early years of life (Engle *et al.* 2011). Children from poorer backgrounds are less likely to attend early child development programmes (Figure 3.5). This situation contributes to widening social inequalities from which health inequities flow.

To the extent that good conditions for early child development vary across a continuum of social advantage and disadvantage, approaches that improve the conditions for development before birth and in early life proportionately according to need are a promising way to improve health and reduce health inequities.

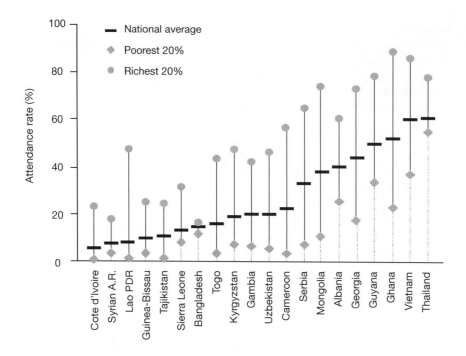

Figure 3.5 Percentage of 3- and 4-year-olds attending early learning programmes by family household wealth (2005–2007)

Source: Nonoyama-Tarumi and Ota 2010, reproduced with permission

Healthy places

Both the built environment and the social environment in which people live affect health in multiple ways. The world population became predominantly urban in 2008 and it is predicted that by 2030 around 60 per cent of the world's population will live in urban areas (Population Reference Bureau 2007). There are several correlates of urbanization that impact health and health inequities. Over one billion people worldwide live in overcrowded slum areas with poor and inadequate access to vital services such as water and sanitation. At the same time, concentration of resources in urban areas can contribute to rural underdevelopment and poverty. Urbanization is associated with increased consumption of energy-dense foods and fuel, and increased use of mechanized transport. Relative social deprivation within urban areas is associated with increased risk of poor health (Figure 3.6).

Effective policy responses focus on good urban governance that positions sustainability, health and well-being, and social equality into urban planning and design (KNUS 2007). This is enabled by participation of communities themselves in the governance process. Urban design and policies that encourage active transport, rather than dependency on motorized vehicles, benefit both population health through increased physical activity and improved air quality and contribute to reduction in greenhouse gas emissions. Urban development that encourages social integration and builds trust between and within communities contributes to both improved health and reduced violence and

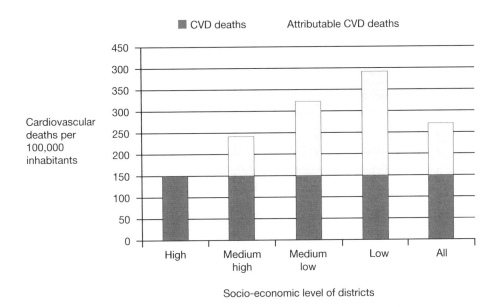

Figure 3.6 Cardiovascular deaths of people aged 45 to 64 and social inequalities: Porto Alegre, Brazil

Source: Bassanesi *et al.* 2008, reproduced with permission

Note: Darker shading indicates deaths attributable to poverty

criminality. Safe public spaces and green environments within urban areas contribute to mental and physical health and well-being.

Fair employment and decent work

> Work is the origin of many important determinants of health. Work can provide financial security, social status, personal development, social relations, and self-esteem and protection from physical and psychosocial hazards.
>
> (Marmot *et al.* 2008: 1663)

People need sufficient material resources gained from work or employment to provide the requirements for a healthy life. People with higher educational attainment or marketable skills are better placed than people with low education or with low skills to access good employment opportunities. Employment conditions that are insecure or precarious, and working conditions in which there is low control and little decision latitude, or where effort and rewards at work are imbalanced, can cause stress and poor health. Figure 3.7 shows the association between effort–reward imbalance at work and risk of poor health in six European countries. While there was variation between countries, high effort–reward imbalance was associated with increased risk of poor health outcomes (Figure 3.7).

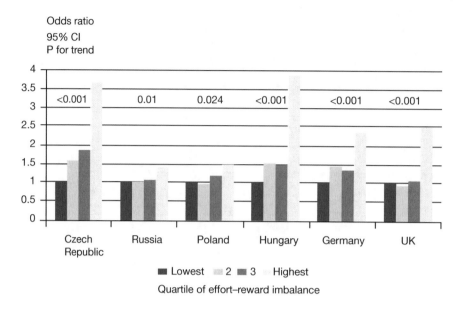

Figure 3.7 Risk of poor health by effort–reward imbalance at work in six countries

Source: Salavecz *et al.* 2010

Addressing employment opportunities is a basic requirement of national macroeconomic and development policy. A pattern of uneven economic development within countries may exacerbate regional inequities in health outcomes, such as urban–rural inequities.

In order to promote social equality, employment policies need to be inclusive and sustainable. A range of responses have been developed to support entry into employment in advanced economies, including active labour market policies that provide training and support to people seeking access to employment. Employment policies that focus on good work and provide a minimum income for healthy living have been emphasized (Marmot Review 2010).

In developing countries, a large proportion of the population works in the informal sector. South Asia and sub-Saharan Africa have the highest rates of informal sector working, at 77 per cent and 73 per cent of total employment, respectively (ILO 2008). By nature, the informal sector provides precarious employment, characterized by low incomes and a lack of financial and social security. An effective policy response focuses on protecting the rights of people working in the informal sector.

Social protection throughout life

Low living standards are a powerful determinant of health inequity. The fundamental principle of social protection is that all people need support at some point in their lives.

(Marmot *et al.* 2008: 1664)

The extent to which social welfare policies provide support for those in need affects levels of poverty in a country. Social protection systems that are universal and generous are associated with better population health (CSDH 2008). Figure 3.8 shows data from a study that examined the relationship between social welfare spending and age-standardized death rates from all causes in 18 European countries (Stuckler *et al.* 2010). Higher social spending per capita was associated with lower mortality rates, standard-ized by age.

Social protection policies may include a range of services and benefits in the form of cash transfers or other benefits such as food. Many developing countries have introduced systems based on conditional cash transfers (CCT), which distribute payments conditional on recipients making use of public services such as child health services and ensuring that their children attend school. An example is Brazil's CCT scheme, Bolsa Familia, which covers roughly 52 million people (about 25 per cent of the Brazilian population) and is targeted at poor families with children. Evidence shows that 25 per cent of the fall in the Gini coefficient measure of income inequality in Brazil since 2001 is attributable to Bolsa Familia (Santos *et al.* 2011). In addition, Bolsa Familia has increased food security, improved nutritional outcomes among children aged 12 to 59 months, and reduced school absence and child labour among older children (Santos *et al.* 2011). Brazil has responded to the need to support employ-ment among Bolsa Familia recipients by introducing the Proximo Passo programme, which aims to support people into work through training and job guarantee schemes (Santos *et al.* 2011).

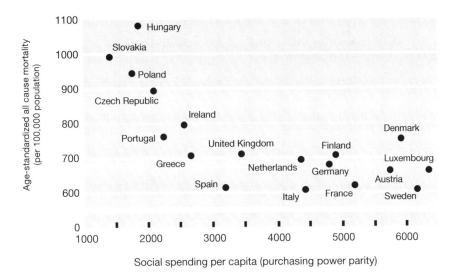

Figure 3.8 Relation between social welfare spending and all-cause mortality in 18 EU countries, 2000

Source: Stuckler *et al.* 2010, reproduced with permission from BMJ Publishing Group Ltd

Universal health care

The health care system is a determinant of health. Inequitable access to health care contributes to health inequities. This is most starkly manifest in inequities in maternal and infant mortality, which are largely avoidable through maternal and child health care services. While maternal and infant mortality rates have been declining worldwide, they remain high in many countries, especially among poorer groups. Where maternal and child health care services fail to reach the poor, progress in achieving improvements in population will inevitably be limited (Houweling *et al.* 2007). High maternal mortality rates in low-income settings are the end result of inequalities in economic and political power, including between men and women, which can be addressed at multiple levels (Sen and Östlin 2008).

Beyond health care, the health system has an important role in developing health promotion and ill health prevention strategies with partners outside the health sector. These might include school- or community-based health education and nutrition services.

Health equity in all policies, systems, and programmes

Every sector of government and society has the potential to affect health and health inequity. The CSDH argued that effects on health and health equity should be assessed to inform decision-making in all policies, systems and programmes. It is particularly important that policies are coherent, that is, that one policy (or set of policies) does not work against another. For example, a recent proposal in the United Kingdom to increase the speed limit on motorways from 70 miles per hour to 80 miles per hour, if enacted, might increase transportation efficiency but would increase both carbon dioxide emissions and the risk of road deaths.

Fair financing within and between countries

In countries at all stages of economic development, creating the conditions for health equity requires to a considerable extent the political will to invest in the social determinants of health, from early child development and education through living and working conditions to health care (CSDH 2008). Earlier sections in this chapter have outlined how poverty levels are influenced by the extent to which work provides sufficient income or resources for healthy living, and by the generosity of redistributive social protection systems.

Poverty levels can be reduced through progressive taxation and welfare systems; the extent to which this happens is a political choice. Figure 3.9 shows trends in the distribution of household income, including benefits, in the United Kingdom from 1978 to 2007/8 (Jones *et al.* 2009). The share enjoyed by the top 20 per cent increased rapidly from the late 1970s to the early 1980s from about 38 per cent to about 42 per cent of total income, then remained more or less constant. By contrast, the share enjoyed by the bottom 20 per cent declined from about 8 per cent of total income to 6 or 5 per cent and stayed there. The dotted line shows that taxation had no redistributive effect during this period. From 1997 the Labour government used the benefit system for redistribution (not shown in figure) (Marmot Review 2010).

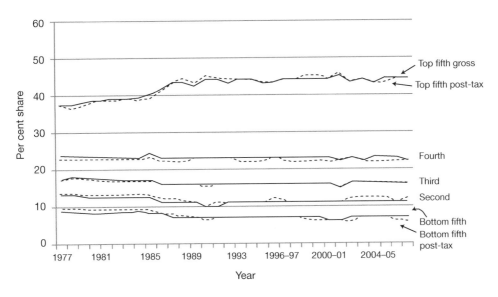

Figure 3.9 Percentage shares of equivalized total gross and post-tax income, by quintile groups for all households, 1978–2007/8

Source: Jones *et al.* 2009

In countries where the tax system is weak and revenue from direct taxation is low, more reliance is placed on other sources, including government borrowing and receipts from trade tariffs, to provide for government expenditure on public services. Low-income developing countries may be in weaker positions relative to countries with stronger economies to negotiate fair economic agreements. The CSDH argued that the impacts of economic agreements on health equity need to be assessed and taken into consideration in trade and investment negotiations (CSDH 2008).

Other sources of funding for public services in a number of developing countries come from multilateral and bilateral development assistance and debt relief. Notwithstanding agreement among donor countries to commit 0.7 per cent of GDP to official development assistance (ODA) and achievement of this by some countries, the overall level of ODA falls far short of this commitment as assessed by donor countries' combined gross national income (Figure 3.10).

Market responsibility

Markets can bring health benefits in the form of new technologies, goods, and services and improved standard of living. But the marketplace can also generate negative conditions for health, including economic inequalities, resource depletion, environmental pollution, unhealthy working conditions, and the circulation of dangerous and unhealthy goods.

(Marmot *et al.* 2008: 1666)

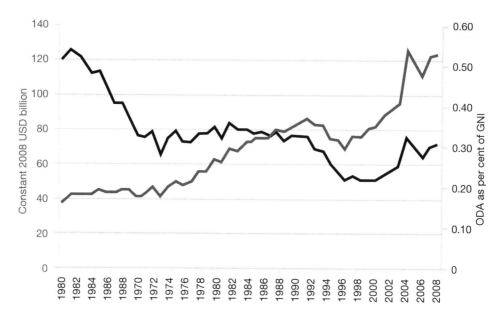

Figure 3.10 Flows of official development assistance, 1960–2010

Source: OECD 2010, reproduced with permission

Examining one of these disbenefits to health, economic inequalities, it is noteworthy that income inequality has been increasing in a number of advanced market economies. An analysis of long-term trends in labour market income before taxes in the United States showed how income inequality has risen over the past 30 years (Saez 2009) (Figure 3.11). This has been driven by a steady increase in the remuneration of top earners while incomes of lower-level workers have remained largely static. The proportion of total income paid to the top 10 per cent has increased from 34 per cent to 50 per cent over the last 30 years. Figure 3.11 shows that the top one per cent has taken its share of total income from roughly 9 per cent to 24 per cent over this period.

The main reasons for this trend have been the globalization of labour markets, reduction of the power of workers' unions, and broad social acceptability of income differentials (Saez 2009). Social movements in the United States and elsewhere have vociferously questioned the extremes of income inequality (*Economist* 2011).

Studies by Richard Wilkinson and Kate Pickett have examined the relationships between income inequality and a number of health and social outcomes in high-income countries and observed that higher income inequality is associated with lower life expectancy, higher child mortality, worse child well-being, higher rates of crime, and lower levels of trust between groups in society (Wilkinson and Pickett 2009).

Amartya Sen provided an insight into the link between income inequality and health: 'Relative deprivation in the space of incomes can yield absolute deprivation in the space of capabilities' (Sen 1992). Income inequalities may contribute to poor health outcomes through various mechanisms, for example, richer groups can afford to pay for private services in health and education, thus tending to residualize public services accessed by poorer groups.

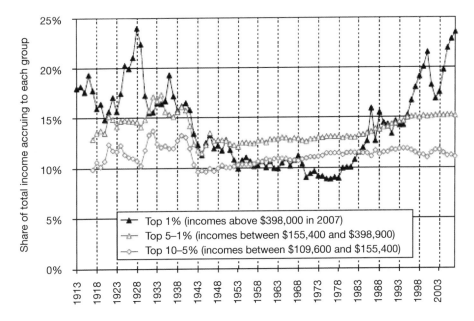

Figure 3.11 Trends in income share by top earners in the United States, 1913–2007

Source: Saez 2009, reproduced with permission

Gender equity

Inequalities in economic, political, and social power between men and women are important determinants of health for women and men.

> Gender inequality damages the health of millions of girls and women across the globe. It can also be harmful to men's health despite the many tangible benefits it gives men through resources, power, authority and control. These benefits to men do not come without a cost to their own emotional and psychological health, often translated into risky and unhealthy behaviours, and reduced longevity.
>
> (CSDH Women and Gender Equity Knowledge Network 2007: xii)

The roots of gender inequality lie in entrenched social and cultural norms that assign differential values and roles to men and women. Legislation to enforce the political, social, economic, and cultural rights of women has contributed to improving gender equality in many parts of the world. But many challenges remain, including gender inequalities in education, work, property ownership, and political participation.

Education of women and girls is seen as key to empowering women. Among women, evidence shows that more education delays marriage and leads to fewer children. Good quality education has other benefits for girls, building decision-making skills that enable them to have more control over their lives, to work outside the home and become economically independent, and plan for the future. Figure 3.12 shows how education contributes to gender relations between men and women with consequences for women's health and well-being. While there was great variation between countries,

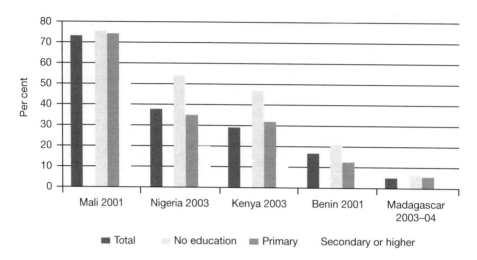

Figure 3.12 Percentage of married women who believe husband is justified to beat sex-refusing wife, by level of education: five countries

Source: Prepared by the authors using data from MEASURE DHS 2011

within countries women with more education were less likely to believe that a husband is justified in hitting or beating his wife if she refuses to have sex with him (MEASURE DHS 2011).

The health of men can also suffer as a result of effects that flow from gendered roles. In Russia, following the social upheaval that followed the collapse of the Soviet Union, men experienced higher mortality rates and alcoholism than women (Shkolnikov *et al.* 2001). This affected men with lower education in particular, leading to a widening of the gap in life expectancy among men (Murphy *et al.* 2006).

Political empowerment – inclusion and voice

For communities to achieve the conditions for health, it is of fundamental importance that mechanisms exist for full inclusion in decisions that affect them. Lack of voice in decision-making results from the exclusionary processes that drive inequalities, and lack of voice perpetuates inequalities. This is apparent in the histories of indigenous peoples in many countries (Indigenous Health Group 2007). While the health of indigenous peoples is well documented in some countries, including New Zealand, Canada, and Australia, relatively little data exist on the health of indigenous peoples in many parts of the world. 'Where data do exist, indigenous peoples have worse health and social indicators than others in the same society' (Indigenous Health Group 2007: 8).

One way to achieve better living conditions for disadvantaged communities is through processes that enable communities to control how local planning budgets are spent. This process, known as participatory budgeting, has been institutionalized in local governance in cities across Brazil over the last 25 years. The involvement of low socio-economic groups in the planning process through participatory budgeting has focused attention on their own priorities such as housing, education, street paving, and basic sanitation (IADB 2005).

Good global governance

The processes of globalization that have gathered pace since the 1970s have resulted in greater integration of markets and transnational flows of capital, goods, and services than ever before. Globalization affects the social determinants of health through its effects on employment and working conditions, urbanization, and availability of food, water, fuel, and essential medicines and on health systems (CSDH Globalization Knowledge Network 2007).

It is increasingly apparent that many processes that affect national populations are ungovernable by one country acting alone (Bell *et al.* 2010). Attempts by European countries to respond to the economic crisis in 2011 provide a notable case study in international decision-making. More broadly, the effects of climate change on human populations and broader biosystems require a globally consistent response.

Good global governance implies global decision-making forums that enable participation by all countries on an equitable basis. 'It is only through such a system of global governance, placing fairness in health at the heart of the development agenda and genuine equality of influence at the heart of its decision-making, that coherent attention to global health equity is possible' (CSDH 2008: 19).

Measure and understand the problem and assess the impact of action

Knowledge in itself is a powerful determinant of health and health equity – for example in the form of data about the distribution of health and the social determinants of health. Knowledge and values of social justice are the touchstones for effective action on social determinants of health. Lack of data often translates into lack of recognition that action should be taken.

In order to monitor progress in improving health and tackling health inequities, it is essential that data is disaggregated by sex, ethnicity/race, socio-economic status, and other social stratifiers. This applies to data systems at collected local and national levels, as well as to research projects (CSDH 2008).

Moving forward

Following the World Conference on Social Determinants of Health, held in Rio de Janeiro in October 2011, the political context became ripe for action. The Rio conference took forward the work of the WHO Commission on Social Determinants of Health by bringing together ministers and representatives from governments, UN agencies, the private sector, civil society, and academia to discuss how to align priorities and to commit to action on the social determinants of health.

The analysis and recommendations made by the CSDH have already helped to consolidate work by public health advocates in many countries and has stimulated a global movement for health equity (Marmot *et al.* 2011). A growing number of stakeholders in regions, countries, and local areas are examining the social determinants of health in their own context and what can be done to diminish social inequality in order to improve public health and reduce health inequities. Brazil established its own commission on social determinants of health in 2007. In the United Kingdom, the government commissioned the *Strategic Review of Health Inequalities* (Marmot Review

2010), which translated the CSDH recommendations into the English context. Many local areas in the United Kingdom, as well as third-sector organizations and institutions, have applied the analysis made by the Marmot Review to guide their strategies. Action on the social determinants of health is taking place around the world, including in Chile, Argentina, Brazil, Costa Rica, Australia, other countries in the Asia-Pacific region, and in Europe (Marmot *et al.* 2011).

The political declaration made by heads of government, ministers, and government representatives at the Rio conference expressed 'determination to achieve social and health equity through action on social determinants of health and well-being by a comprehensive intersectoral approach' (WHO 2011: 1). The global movement for health equity that has gathered momentum following the CSDH must ensure that governments move beyond rhetoric to reality.

References

Bassanesi, S.L., Azambuja, M.I., and Achutti, A. (2008) 'Premature mortality due to cardiovascular disease and social inequalities in Porto Alegre: from evidence to action', *Arquivos Brasileiros de Cardiologia*, 90 (6): 370–9.

Bell, R., Taylor, S., and Marmot, M. (2010) 'Global health governance: commission on social determinants of health and the imperative for change', *Journal of Law, Medicine and Ethics*, 38 (3): 470–85.

Commission on Social Determinants of Health (CSDH) (2008) *Final Report: Closing the Gap in a Generation: Health Equity through Action on the Social Determinants of Health*, Geneva: World Health Organization Commission on Social Determinants of Health.

Commission on Social Determinants of Health (CSDH) Early Child Development Knowledge Network (2007) *Early Child Development: A Powerful Equalizer*, Geneva: World Health Organization Commission on Social Determinants.

Commission on Social Determinants of Health (CSDH) Globalization Knowledge Network (2007) *Towards Health-equitable Globalisation: Rights, Regulation and Redistribution*, Geneva: World Health Organization Commission on Social Determinants of Health.

CSDH Women and Gender Equity Knowledge Network (2007) *Unequal, Unfair, Ineffective and Inefficient – Gender Equity in Health: Why it Exists and How we Can Change it*, Geneva: World Health Organization Commission on Social Determinants of Health.

Economist (2011) 'Capitalism and its critics: rage against the machine', *The Economist*, 22 October. Online, available at: http://www.economist.com/node/21533400 (accessed 14 July 2012).

Engle, P.L., Fernald, L.C., Alderman, H., Behrman, J., O'Gara, C., Yousafzai, A., de Mello, M.C. Hidrobo, M., Ulkuer, N., Ertem, I., and Iltus, S. *et al.* (2011) 'Strategies for reducing inequalities and improving developmental outcomes for young children in low-income and middle-income countries', *The Lancet*, 378 (9799): 1339–53.

Graham, H. (1987) 'Women's smoking and family health', *Social Science & Medicine*, 25 (1): 47–56.

Houweling, T.A.J., Ronsmans, C., Campbell, O.M.R., and Kunst, A.E. (2007) 'Huge poor-rich inequalities in maternity care: an international comparative study of maternity and child care in developing countries', *Bulletin of the World Health Organization*, 85 (10): 745–54.

Indigenous Health Group (2007) 'Social determinants and indigenous health: the international experience and its policy implications', paper presented at the Adelaide Symposium of the Commission on Social Determinants of Health, Adelaide, 29–30 April 2007.

Inter-American Development Bank (IADB) (2005) *Assessment of Participatory Budgeting in Brazil*, Washington, D.C.: Inter-American Development Bank. Online, available at: http://idbdocs.iadb. org/wsdocs/getdocument.aspx?docnum=995174 (accessed 13 July 2012).

International Labour Organization (ILO) (2008) *Global Employment Trends*, Geneva: International Labour Organization.

Jones, F., Annan, D., and Shah, S. (2009) *The Redistribution of Household Income 1977 to 2006/07*, London: Office for National Statistics.

Knowledge Network on Urban Settings (KNUS) (2007) *Our Cities, our Health, our Future: Acting on Social Determinants for Health Equity in Urban Settings*. Final Report of the Urban Settings Knowledge Network of the Commission on Social Determinants of Health, Geneva: World Health Organization.

Marmot Review (2010) *Fair Society, Healthy Lives: Strategic Review of Health Inequalities in England Post 2010*, London: Marmot Review.

Marmot, M.G., Shipley, M.J., and Rose, G. (1984) 'Inequalities in death – specific explanations of a general pattern?', *The Lancet*, 1 (8384): 1003–6.

Marmot, M.G., Smith, G.D., Stansfeld, S., Patel, C., North, F., Head, J., White, I., Brunner, E., and Feeney, A. (1991) 'Health inequalities among British civil servants: the Whitehall II study', *The Lancet*, 337 (8754): 1387–93.

Marmot, M., Friel, S., Bell, R., Houweling, T.A., and Taylor, S. (2008) 'Closing the gap in a generation: health equity through action on the social determinants of health', *The Lancet*, 372 (9650): 1661–9.

Marmot, M., Allen, J., Bell, R., and Goldblatt, P. (2011) 'Building the global movement for health equity: from Santiago to Rio and beyond', *The Lancet*, 379 (9811): 181–8.

MEASURE DHS (2011) *STATcompiler*. Online, available at: www.statcompiler.com (accessed 13 July 2012).

Murphy, M., Bobak, M., Nicholson, A., Rose, R., and Marmot, M. (2006) 'The widening gap in mortality by educational level in the Russian Federation, 1980–2001', *American Journal of Public Health*, 96 (7): 1293–9.

Nonoyama-Tarumi, Y., and Ota, Y. (2010) 'Early childhood development in developing countries: pre-primary education, parenting and health care', paper commissioned for the EFA Global Monitoring Report 2011, *The Hidden Crisis: Armed Conflict and Education*, Paris: United Nations Educational, Scientific and Cultural Organization.

Organisation for Economic Co-operation and Development (OECD) (2010) *The DAC: Fifty Years, Fifty Highlights*. Online, available at: http://www.oecd.org/dataoecd/22/26/47072129. pdf?contentId=47072130 (accessed 29 July 2012).

Population Reference Bureau (2007) *World Population Highlights*, Washington, D.C.: Population Reference Bureau.

Saez, E. (2009) *Striking it Richer: The Evolution of Top Incomes in the United States* (update with 2007 estimates), University of California Berkeley: Institute for Research on Labor and Employment.

Salavecz, G., Chandola, T., Pikhart, H., Dragano, N., Siegrist, J., Jöckel, K.H., Erbel, R., Pajak, A., Malyutina, S., Kubinova, R., Marmot, M., Bobak, M., and Kopp, M. (2010) 'Work stress and health in Western European and post-communist countries: an East–West comparison study', *Journal of Epidemiology and Community Health*, 64 (1), 57–62.

Santos, L.M.P., Paes-Sousa, R., Miazagi, E., Silva, T.F., and da Fonseca, A.M.M. (2011) *The Brazilian Experience with Conditional Cash Transfer: A Successful Way to Reduce Inequity and to Improve Health*, Geneva: World Health Organization. Online, available at: http://www.who.int/sdhconference/resources/draft_background_paper1_brazil.pdf (accessed 13 July 2012).

Sen, A. (1992) *Inequality Reexamined*, Oxford: Oxford University Press.

Sen, A. (1999) *Development as Freedom*, New York: Alfred A. Knopf.

Sen, G., and Östlin, P. (2008) 'Gender inequity in health: why it exists and how we can change it', *Global Public Health*, 3 (S1: 1–12.

Shkolnikov, V., McKee, M., and Leon, D.A. (2001) 'Changes in life expectancy in Russia in the mid-1990s', *The Lancet*, 357: 917–21.

Solar, O. and Irwin, A. (2010) 'A conceptual framework for action on the social determinants of health', *Social Determinants of Health Discussion Paper 2 (Policy and Practice)*, Geneva: World Health Organization.

Stuckler, D., Basu, S., and McKee, M. (2010) 'Budget crises, health, and social welfare programmes', *British Medical Journal*, 340: c.3311.

United Nations (UN) (2011) *World Population Prospects: The 2010 Revision*, New York: United Nations, Department of Economic and Social Affairs, Population Division.

United Nations Development Programme (UNDP) (2006) *Human Development Report 2006*, New York: United Nations Development Programme.

Wilkinson, R.G. and Pickett, K.E. (2009) *The Spirit Level: Why More Equal Societies Almost Always Do Better*, London: Allen Lane.

World Health Organization (WHO) (2011) *Rio Political Declaration on Social Determinants of Health*, Geneva: World Health Organization. Online, available at: http://www.who.int/sdhconference/declaration/Rio_political_declaration.pdf (accessed 14 July 2012).

4

EMBRACING COMPLEXITY

Toward platforms for integrated health and social service delivery

Andrew Ellner, Christine Pace, Scott Lee, Jonathan L. Weigel, and Paul Farmer

Kimberly, a 19-year-old, arrives in your office. She was referred to your inner-city primary care clinic from the local emergency room, where she was recently diagnosed with and treated for pelvic inflammatory disease, a common but serious disease of the female reproductive tract that is typically caused by untreated sexually transmitted infections such as gonorrhoea and chlamydia.

Given the nature of her recent problem, you ask more about her sexual history. Kimberly has a boyfriend with whom she is sexually active; they use condoms only occasionally, even though she strongly suspects he has other partners. When asked if she wants to become pregnant, she shrugs and says, 'If it happens, it happens'. Kimberly has other risk factors for health problems: she is overweight, she smokes half a pack of cigarettes each day and she shares a 12-pack of beer several nights a week with her boyfriend. 'It's a way to relax', she says.

The issue that Kimberly would most like to discuss with you today, however, is back pain that she has had for several years. She tells you that she developed this pain after being thrown down the stairs by her stepfather when she was 13 years old. When you examine her, you find she has mild tenderness of her lower back muscles, but you also notice two round scars on her arms. She tells you her stepfather inflicted them by rubbing out cigarette butts on her arms.

On further questioning, you learn that Kimberly never knew her biological father; while her mother was pregnant, he was incarcerated and later died in prison. When Kimberly was five, her mother married a man who 'had a temper' and often physically abused Kimberly and her siblings.

Kimberly's mother struggles with depression, diabetes, and obesity. Last year, with her mother mired in a particularly severe depressive episode and unable to work, Kimberly dropped out of high school just months before her graduation so that she could take on more hours at her job at the deli counter in a nearby supermarket. Now, with the economic downturn, the supermarket has been laying off staff; she fears she'll be next. All of these matters – usually condensed into a single line in a medical chart – seem relevant, if not causative, as you contemplate her symptoms, her history, and her physical exam. You remember, too, that other young patients – most of them also young people of colour – are in the waiting room.

As you end the encounter with Kimberly, you recommend ibuprofen and stretching exercises for the back pain. You note that she is drinking more than recommended amounts and that you are concerned about possible consequences, which include harm to a foetus if she becomes pregnant – the logical consequence of unprotected sex – as well as an alcohol use disorder. You also talk about birth control, but she says she has heard bad things about many of the forms of long-term contraception that you discuss. She will think about it, she says. You decide to discuss her smoking habit during her next appointment, which you arrange for next month.

As she leaves the office, you find yourself knitting your eyebrows in frustration. Despite your patient's polite promise to consider your advice, your own words feel meaningless in the face of the forces that shape her life and her decisions on a daily basis: poverty, unreliable employment, hopelessness, the stress of being a caretaker at such a young age, her memories of a violent childhood, gender inequality, and the profound disparities, many of them structured along racial and ethnic lines, in the city where you both live.

Why embrace complexity?

Physicians routinely encounter social forces embodied as illness among those they serve. Kimberly's case illustrates how 'medical' problems – sexually transmitted infection, back pain, the foreshadow of addiction – reflect social ills far beyond the control of doctors: gender disparities, psychosocial stress, histories of trauma and abuse, precarious family circumstances, poverty, racism. In the space between these so-called social determinants of health and the symptoms encountered by patients, physicians often find themselves caught between two paradigms. On one hand, they are trained to lay aside questions about a patient's background and to try to address his or her immediate needs. On the other, many physicians know that ignoring underlying causes of disease and disability leads to low-quality or inadequate patient care.

Compared to clinical medicine, public health has focused more on the social determinants of health. Nonetheless, most public health efforts are limited by focusing on a single disease or intervention – in the jargon, a 'vertical' approach – instead of tackling problems with an integrated systems approach. For example, a public health media campaign to discourage smoking might lead Kimberly to reconsider smoking, but would do little to mitigate the social stresses that, by her report, underlie her desire to smoke – nor would such a campaign address the other social forces that place Kimberly at high risk of both short- and longer-term health problems.

Physicians must of course give priority to the immediate manifestations of ill health rather than their social determinants. That is what we are trained to do, just as public health practitioners are trained to think beyond the immediacy of suffering. But too many health initiatives, we contend, focus narrowly on outmoded notions of disease and biomedicine. Despite evidence that health is principally determined by the interaction of genes and environment, and by behaviours and social conditions, many developed countries, particularly the United States, are struggling under the fiscal weight of health care systems designed with the delivery, by physicians, of biomedical technologies as the first (and sometimes only) principle (Chernew *et al.* 2010; Fuchs 1998). Moreover, perhaps partly because of their narrow focus on specific diseases or interventions, a significant proportion of resources dedicated to financing health programmes in low-income countries ends up supporting the work of international groups or local elites, rather than assisting people, like Kimberly, who are seeking to help themselves.[1] Sometimes well-intentioned health programmes squander an opportunity to help address the social and economic underpinnings of the very diseases that they seek to treat or control.

How might medicine and public health take on the diseases and conditions that threaten the well-being of individuals and communities while also addressing their social and economic roots? As a starting point, we explore the social determinants of health and examine how structural risks become embodied as illness and disease. We then consider examples of health interventions that address structural risk at different levels, and introduce a strategy of health system strengthening integrated with comprehensive social service delivery. Finally, we elaborate on three key pillars of the biosocial approach: accompaniment, partnerships, and continuous systems improvement and innovation.

Mechanisms mediating structural violence

Epidemiologists have mapped out the increased risk of ill health facing socially, economically, or politically disadvantaged individuals. In the United States, for example, African Americans have, in aggregate, significantly worse health indicators than white Americans (Williams and Mohammed 2009). Likewise, numerous studies demonstrate that, within developed nations, living in certain urban neighbourhoods puts individuals at increased risk for premature morbidity and mortality, relative to their fellow citizens (Diez Roux *et al.* 2001; Malmstrom *et al.* 2001; Pickett and Pearl 2001). In contrast, in developing nations, urban centres are the first to undergo the epidemiological transition from excessive premature morbidity and mortality due to predominantly infectious causes, to non-infectious chronic diseases like heart disease and lung cancer associated with longer life expectancy (Harpham and Molyneux 2001). Homeless populations in developed countries are also at risk: studies in North American and European cities find mortality rates among the homeless to be three to six times higher than those of the general population (Barrow *et al.* 1999; Hwang *et al.* 2009; Nordentoft and Wandall-Holm 2003). Finally, there is a vast gradient in all-cause morbidity and mortality between countries of varying wealth: the average life expectancy of developing nations is more than 30 years less than that of developed economies (Commission on Social Determinants of Health 2008).

In addition to factors such as race and place of residence, ample evidence suggests that social hierarchies impact health. In the Whitehall Studies, Michael Marmot and others demonstrated that health indicators declined on a steady gradient with social status in England and Wales in the twentieth century (see Chapter 3, Bell *et al.*, in this volume) (Marmot and Smither 1991; Marmot *et al.* 1978, 1984; Rose and Marmot 1981). With each successive decrement in civil service ranking, male British civil servants (all of whom had health insurance through the National Health Service) had increasing rates of all-cause premature morbidity and mortality, heart disease, lung cancer, accidents, suicides, and stroke, and decreasing rates of perceived health status. They also had increased rates of behavioural risk factors such as smoking, but behaviours alone were insufficient to explain the differences in health status.

These examples underscore what we call structural violence: the mechanisms by which large-scale social forces become embodied as adverse health outcomes among the poor and otherwise vulnerable (Farmer 1997, 2004a). Although evidence for the existence of structural risks is well documented, elucidating the precise mechanisms by which such risks become embodied by individuals and their communities as ill health is a more challenging task. Certainly, social, economic, and political disadvantage often constrain access to health care; but evidence suggests that access to care accounts for only part of the observed health disparities among communities on different rungs of development and social hierarchy (Commission on Social Determinants of Health 2008). Indeed, all facile claims of causality about aggregate health indicators must be approached with caution, especially those that scant the role of entrenched inequalities. Critical perspectives on structural risk must ask how large-scale social forces pattern the well-being of unequally positioned individuals in increasingly interconnected populations. Truly biosocial analysis must strive to take change and complexity into account, and must be global in scope, yet alive to local variation.

Despite the difficulty of defining the exact causal mechanisms underlying structural risk, it is useful to consider some of the forces that have been most well studied. An example is living environment. In developed nations, for example, poor communities often have less access to affordable, nutritious food than wealthier communities (Beaulac *et al.* 2009; Mari Gallagher Research and Consulting Group 2007). In developing nations, weak water and sanitation infrastructure predispose populations to epidemic diseases, such as cholera, from which most wealthy nations are sheltered.

Other contributors to structural risk may lie at a different, physiological level. Repeated external stress has been shown to lead to dysregulation of the neurohormonal axes. The Whitehall Studies found that cortisol awakening response and fibrinogen levels – a mediator and product, respectively, of the stress response – increased as socio-economic status decreased (Brunner *et al.* 1996; Kunz-Ebrecht *et al.* 2004). Animal studies offer further compelling evidence for the link between social status, stress, and ill health. In one of many studies on social hierarchy and the stress response, researchers found that socially dominant female monkeys who were moved to packs where they were socially subordinate had five times more atherosclerosis than their counterparts that did not change social status (Shively and Clarkson 1994).

Perhaps at least partially related to these mechanisms, a distinct body of literature shows a strong dose–response correlation between adverse childhood events, such as physical, sexual, or emotional abuse, and risk factors for several of the leading causes of death among adults, including obesity, physical inactivity, and substance abuse (Dube *et al.* 2003; Felitti *et al.* 1998). Such findings suggest a dynamic interrelationship between structural violence and physical and emotional violence; they also indicate that early child development may be a time of particular vulnerability to the health burdens of poverty, inequality, low social status, and other forms of structural risk. Among an insured and largely middle-class California population, individuals who experienced childhood trauma had higher rates of diabetes, chronic lung disease, and ischaemic heart disease – and also of cancer and premature mortality (Brown *et al.* 2009, 2010; Felitti *et al.* 1998). Although evidence is hard to come by, some have suggested that the health impacts of trauma exposure are even more devastating for survivors and witnesses of genocide, civil war, and other atrocities, which in recent years have disproportionately (but not exclusively) afflicted developing countries (Collier 2007; Johnson *et al.* 2008; Ranson *et al.* 2007). Those who care for war veterans in high-income countries are well aware of the high rates of premature morbidity and mortality in this population, though again it is difficult to explain such health indicators as a result of trauma or as a consequence of the fact that most veterans come from, and return to, social circumstances characterized by high burden of disease and constraints on care-seeking behaviour (Boehmer *et al.* 2004; Kang *et al.* 2002).

If low social status and exposure to trauma are associated with elevated levels of stress, it is not surprising that they are often also associated with high-risk behavioural 'choices'. Social mores and behavioural norms in an individual's environment shape his or her choices. But so do social conditions and other elements of structural risk (taken together, these contextual factors seem to constitute the modern term 'stress'). Risky behaviours – from alcohol, tobacco, or opioid abuse to over-eating, high-risk sex, and reckless driving – trigger spikes in dopamine and other neurotransmitters which can, in the short term, relieve stress and anxiety. 'It's a way to relax,' Kimberly said. Indeed, data show higher rates of alcohol and tobacco abuse among individuals who experienced adverse childhood events or war-related trauma (Johnson *et al.* 2008). Other 'behaviour'-related epidemics, such as obesity and tobacco use, also track with educational and socio-economic status. The latter is particularly unsurprising given the profound chronic stress of poverty (CDC 2009, 2010; Ford and Mokdad 2008). Alcohol and drug use disorders occur at higher rates among individuals at low education levels, although alcohol abuse is common across social strata and occupational class (Crum 2009). Moreover, the deleterious effects of substance use disorders are often greater for individuals who are already poor: they usually lack access to resources for recovery, and have little else to fall back on as their disease progresses.

Even after a cursory review, this literature problematizes not only facile claims of causality but also traditional distinctions between 'communicable' and 'non-communicable' disease. The former construct can of course be distinguished by the existence of microscopic, infectious agents that pass between individuals. But it is well known that large-scale social forces – such as poverty, racism, gender disparities, social hierarchies, urbanization, behavioural norms, and other components of structural risk we have discussed – pattern the transmission of infectious diseases (Dubos 1959; Farmer 1999). As reviewed above, a growing body of evidence underpins the notion that such social forces also shape the burden of non-communicable diseases, such as heart disease and cancer, among human populations. Ultimately, all pathologies spread through populations and manifest themselves as disease among individuals based on a combination of biologic and social mechanics. Only a fully biosocial approach can help us understand, and seek to address, the components of structural risk patterning disease and access to care around the globe.

From mechanisms to interventions

If structural violence refers to the harmful effects of large-scale social forces on individuals and populations, then 'structural interventions' might refer to efforts to mitigate the effects of such forces. Structural interventions, in other words, give individuals and communities the tools and opportunities to engage in healthy behaviours and to gain control over their lives. Tackling structural violence entails rebalancing the global distribution of riches and rights. But revolutions with this end have rarely (if ever) achieved it; most have triggered mass violence and erected new hierarchies in the place of old ones. Our focus eschews such grand schemes: we propose, rather, a model of integrated health and social service delivery.

In this model, structural approaches are aimed at addressing local (even individual) manifestations of the inequities that pattern premature morbidity and mortality around the globe; they target the mechanisms by which social, political, and economic forces become embodied as adverse health outcomes (Farmer 2004b). Structural interventions can act on different levels of the spectrum, from biological to social risk factors. Sometimes strictly medical interventions are the apposite modality of care: providing treatment for AIDS, diabetes, or depression might do more to help a patient achieve well-being than would securing him or her a job. On the other hand, distributing condoms and stern behaviour-change messages among poor women in urban settings will likely reduce risk of HIV infection less than would a stable job or generous loan that offers a chance at economic independence. But even this dichotomy between the medical and the social is misleading. A fully biosocial approach to redressing structural violence intervenes at multiple levels at once; it seeks to maximize the synergies between medical and social interventions.

Scholars have proposed classification systems for structural interventions (Blankenship *et al.* 2000; Cohen *et al.* 2000) that can be categorized on two dimensions: the *content* of an intervention and the *level* at which it operates. Blankenship's framework, for example, sorts structural interventions according to which of three content areas they target:

1 The *availability* of risk-taking as a behavioural option. Interventions in this category either penalize risk-taking behaviours or facilitate healthy behaviours (e.g. 'nudge' policies). Such interventions include taxing alcohol (targeting the individual), regulating the fat content of school lunches (targeting organizations), and building parks to increase access to exercise opportunities (targeting the environment).
2 The *acceptability* of a risk-taking or healthy behaviour. Interventions in this category aim to make risky behaviours less publicly acceptable and healthy ones more so. They generally target organizations (e.g. regulating tobacco advertisements) or environment (e.g. removing images of cigarettes from stamps).
3 The *accessibility* of certain behaviours. Interventions in this category seek to remedy inequalities of access by distributing products that enable healthy behaviours. Blankenship cites examples of free distribution of bicycle helmets or condoms, or banning sale of cigarettes in single-cigarette packages (which appeal mainly to low-income individuals).

These interventions function at various points along the chain of structural risk, linking social, political, and economic inequities to adverse health outcomes. They also target unhealthy behaviours at three levels: individuals, organizations, and environment. Coordinated efforts in each content area and at each level are necessary to begin to address the impact of deleterious large-scale social forces through policy and programmes.

We would, nonetheless, argue that this classification system leaves out an additional category of interventions that are even more 'structural'. Interventions that seek to give marginalized individuals and communities the tools and resources (and agency) to overcome institutionalized power imbalances – even when such imbalances are institutionalized in the health system itself – operate closer to the font of structural risk than those described above. Such interventions are often omitted from the health literature because they target the roots, not the symptoms, of structural violence; when carried out, they are also often integrated with conventional 'health' programmes (in the narrow sense of the term), which can make it difficult to disaggregate the marginal health effects of the former. However, a comprehensive and integrated structural approach – one that links interventions explicitly aimed at mitigating the effects of structural violence with biomedical approaches to health system strengthening – shows great promise for reducing premature morbidity and mortality and for triggering virtuous social cycles among impoverished communities. Practitioners of clinical medicine and public health can help guide such interventions because they witness the health effects of structural inequities every day; they also have unique access to populations whose health is undermined by structural violence.

Examples of structural interventions integrated with health service delivery

In the developing world, where poverty is often the single greatest barrier to health, there are many examples of systems that seek to integrate health service delivery with programmes to address social determinants of health. Indeed, some of the models of integrated health and social service delivery being scaled up in the United States today originated in poor countries, where the social determinants of health are more difficult to ignore.

In Haiti's Central Plateau, for example, Zanmi Lasante and Partners In Health, its American sister organization, have delivered community-based health care enriched by social services and hospital care, since the 1980s. Community health workers, or *accompagnateurs* in Haitian Creole, provide directly observed therapy for tuberculosis, AIDS, cancer, and other diseases, while also providing 'wraparound services' such as food assistance, access to safe drinking water, transportation fees, and job searching assistance. In some cases, Zanmi Lasante will help find or build patients new homes. This model of care has triggered virtuous social cycles across Haiti: neighbours began lending each other money or helping to care for one another's children; local procurement of agricultural produce for food supplementation has strengthened demand (Ivers *et al.* 2009; Louis *et al.* 2007; Walton *et al.* 2004). These spillover effects have been amplified by partnering with a microcredit organization, Fonkoze, which enables individuals to take out loans and begin small enterprises such as farmer and artisan collectives. In contrast to many other microlenders, Fonkoze also offers literacy sessions – most of which are taught by other borrowers – and workshops on reproductive health and business skills. Such social interventions complement improvements in basic health services and enhance the virtuous cycle noted above: families, no longer as burdened by high health care costs, are able to invest and save money, starting the long climb up the economic ladder. Such synergies between providing comprehensive health care services and also seeking to address social and structural roots of ill health have been transformative in a number of communities in Central Haiti where Zanmi Lasante and Fonkoze work.

The Prevention and Access to Care and Treatment (PACT) programme, a US-based arm of Partners In Health, has adapted this model to the urban United States – an example of 'reverse innovation'. PACT bolsters home-based medical care for poor patients with chronic diseases in Boston by offering wraparound services: food assistance, financial support for transportation fees or daycare costs, and psychosocial services, to name just a few. Community health workers have been shown effective in delivering such services while also providing directly observed therapy for AIDS, diabetes, hypertension, and other chronic illnesses (Behforouz *et al.* 2004); they are perhaps uniquely qualified to provide integrated health and social services in the communities in which PACT works. We have argued that this model of integrated community-based service delivery is the highest standard of care for chronic disease (Onie *et al.* 2012). Evaluations of the programme support such claims: 70 per cent of PACT's AIDS patients have had good treatment outcomes, including suppressed viral loads, normal CD4 counts, infrequent opportunistic infections, and few hospital visits. Cost reductions followed clinical improvement. An analysis of Medicaid claims data, for example, demonstrated a 16 per cent net savings for PACT patients, likely attributable to a substantial reduction in costly hospitalizations (Onie *et al.* 2012). This model has since been exported across the United States, including New York City, Miami, and the Navajo Nation.

The work of the Camden Coalition of Healthcare Providers, headed by Dr Jeffrey Brenner, employs a similar model to that of PACT. The Camden Coalition has sought to cut health care costs in Camden, New Jersey by providing high-quality, community-based care to the sickest (and often poorest) patients. These patients accounted for the lion's share of health care expenditures in the city's hospitals. Brenner's hypothesis, which is no surprise to health practitioners serving poor communities, was that providing comprehensive care for chronic illnesses and seeking to mitigate the impacts of structural violence – by addressing drug and alcohol abuse or housing containing moulds and other contaminants, for example – would both improve these patients' health outcomes and lessen the burden they place on the Camden health system (previously these sickest patients received most of their care from the emergency room, which is costly and poorly coordinated). The Camden Coalition's efforts have proved successful: the first cohort of patients made over 30 per cent fewer visits to the emergency room, and were hospitalized more than 50 per cent less often; their health care bills – which cost, on average, $1.2 million per patient per month before the Camden Coalition began providing services – decreased by over half (Brenner 2009). Few realize how costly it is to provide mediocre medical care to poor people in a rich country.

Medical–legal partnerships, pioneered at Boston Medical Center in 1993, are another example of structural interventions integrated with health services. Such partnerships bring legal services to health care facilities – especially those serving poor communities – in the United States. There are currently at least 81 medical–legal partnerships in the country, many of them funded by health care organizations and private donors. Through these programmes, medical providers can refer patients for legal assistance when patients face legal barriers to good health. Lawyers might help patients defend a right to housing free of contaminants that increase risk of respiratory illness, or to obtain a restraining order against a violent partner. They might also help patients address immigration issues that limit their access to legal employment (with fair compensation and health insurance). Many medical–legal partnerships also work at the broader policy level by lobbying state and federal governments on behalf of the communities they serve. In addition, a number of such partnerships offer supplementary training modules for medical providers about the social determinants of health. Evaluations of medical–legal partnerships have focused on the effects of such educational programmes, finding that supplementary training helps residents feel more empowered in screening their patients for legal problems that contribute to health disparities, and getting their patients the help they need (Cohen *et al.* 2010).

There are, too, many examples of community health centres and local primary health care systems that offer integrated health and social services. Codman Square Health Center and the Dorchester Multicenter House in Boston have founded a community organization that offers adult education classes (in computer skills, for example), teen recreational opportunities, and even discounted gym memberships through a partnership with a local fitness centre. For a patient like Kimberly, such low-cost and convenient opportunities could help her gain professional skills, find stable employment, and exercise.

This comprehensive approach to health care is gaining ground around the globe; in some countries, flexible health care financing encourages integrated structural interventions. In Australia, the state of Victoria has provided funding for local communities to organize primary care partnerships between different health care providers and community organizations. These partnerships have led to statewide standards for service coordination and increased access to health care. Because the partnerships are formed at the local level, they are able to respond nimbly to specific community needs. For example, during a drought in 2006, the primary care partnership in the shire of Campaspe worked with the local government to ensure that mental health and support services were available to farmers, a group traditionally reluctant to seek care (State of Victoria Department of Health 2010).

Health system strengthening done in conjunction with the provision of comprehensive social services aimed at removing the structural barriers to health and well-being can help communities break the cycle of poverty and disease. Recent models suggest that safety nets – basic health care or a minimal level of economic security – can help poor populations escape from 'poverty traps' in which they lack the baseline income to save, invest, and better their lot (Bonds *et al.* 2010; Plucinski *et al.* 2011). Often, poor households fall into poverty traps because, in the absence of safety nets, external shocks like acute illness, layoffs, price hikes, and droughts can deplete income sources and plunge them into debt. In fact, studies have found illness and health care costs among the chief causes of households falling into destitution in India, Uganda, and elsewhere (Krishna 2010). Buffers against such external shocks, such as public health measures and income supplements (e.g. cash transfers), have been shown to help reduce the occurrence and persistence of poverty traps; they appear most effective as complementary interventions (Plucinski *et al.* 2011). Recent research in Rwanda and elsewhere reinforces that comprehensive health investments, especially when integrated with social service delivery, can help break the cycle of poverty and disease (Bonds 2008; Rich *et al.* 2012). A robust health system bolstered with social services that provide these buffering effects can keep individuals and populations from falling into destitution and disease.

Building platforms for integrated biosocial service delivery

The programmes mentioned above have realized impressive outcomes by embracing the complexity by which large-scale social forces pattern the burden of illness and the availability of medical care. Many of these programmes have also simultaneously cut overall costs to the health system, highlighting a lesson that holds true in settings rich and poor: providing inadequate care for the poorest patients anywhere in the world is an expensive and unsustainable status quo.

Although delivery models differ, each of the programmes considered in the previous section seeks to address the structural roots of health care inequities while providing comprehensive services for acute and chronic medical needs. In so doing, these programmes break down boundaries between public health and biomedicine, between health care and other social services, and between 'vertical' and 'horizontal' interventions. The medical profession and global health community have reached a transformational moment: many countries and organizations have adopted the ambitious goal of providing comprehensive primary health care services. But to build durable health systems, health initiatives in countries rich and poor must further integrate biomedical and social service delivery. We propose an integrated biosocial delivery platform based on three principles: accompaniment, partnerships, and continuous systems improvement and innovation.

As noted, community-based health and social service delivery models offer the highest standard of care for chronic disease in rich and poor settings alike. This approach has been termed accompaniment (Behforouz *et al.* 2004). To accompany is to walk alongside another. However, for our purposes, we take it to mean caregiving in its comprehensive, true sense of the word – that is tailored to the specific needs of patients and their families. As many of the examples in the previous section illustrate, true accompaniment is often conducted by community health workers in the homes and communities of the intended beneficiaries. Community health workers are hired (and paid) to attend to provide medical care, especially for chronic illnesses, and psychosocial support; to help patients access healthier food, smoke and drink less, and start regular exercise; to address environmental barriers to good health, such as contaminants in their homes that can cause respiratory illnesses; and to help them find a decent and stable job, and access to credit. Accompaniment is what Dr Brenner and his colleagues have been doing in Camden, New Jersey; it is what Fonkoze's teams are doing in the rural reaches of Haiti. Accompaniment is how Partners In Health has delivered high-quality treatment for cancer and HIV and multidrug-resistant tuberculosis and many other chronic diseases in resource-poor settings from Haiti to Rwanda, Peru to Russia (Kotagal *et al.* 2009; Mitnick *et al.* 2003; Shin *et al.* 2006). Accompaniment is not a quick win; it is not easy, nor is it cheap. But it is the highest standard of care in settings poor and rich.

Closely related to accompaniment is the transformational potential of partnerships. Strong linkages with organizations focused on the social determinants of health – drug and alcohol rehabilitation programmes, nutrition and food access initiatives, mental health service providers, water and sanitation projects, microlenders – enable health care providers to deliver higher-quality care to populations whose health outcomes are most affected by structural risk. Effective partnerships allow providers to integrate structural and biomedical approaches, which can help break cycles of poverty and disease and build (or rebuild) health systems. A robust health and social service delivery system can help thousands of people live full lives in good health; it provides accompaniment to help individuals and communities anticipate, avoid, or overcome constraints to well-being and agency. Indeed, partnerships are themselves a form of accompaniment. Like community health workers accompanying patients with chronic diseases, partnerships must be nimble, open ended, long term; their approach must be determined not by the accompanying organization but by those being accompanied. A robust health system is a constant companion – an *accompagnateur* – to individuals and populations during their journeys through life.

Fully actualizing the principle of accompaniment and formation of partnerships might shake up the entrenched hierarchies of the medical profession, but it would also enhance its value. Doctors often have great (and perhaps undue) authority and responsibility within health systems and in society in general. In the United States and many other countries, myopic approaches to health care financing and regulation have reinforced the cult of the doctor by elevating specialized biomedical interventions at the expense of primary care services and community-based care (Onie *et al.* 2012). That prevention gets short shrift in the United States health system is rendered vivid by the status differential between, say, surgeons and nutritionists in the health profession. This doctor-centred paradigm has recently been challenged by health reformers who advise 'patient-centred' care and true partnerships between doctors, allied health professionals, and patients themselves (Rittenhouse and Shortell 2009). Discussions of 'task-shifting' – from doctors and nurses to community health workers, for example – in the global health literature rest on analogous arguments (Samb 2007). Such redistribution of authority and responsibility highlights a necessary cultural transformation in health care delivery in the twenty-first century.

The third pillar of the transformation in medicine and global health is embracing systems improvement and innovation as central to health care delivery – and, in particular, leveraging information technology to collect, analyze, and deploy health-related data to improve care. For too long, innovation in health care has been narrowly construed as biomedical advances, which are of course critical to developing new preventatives, diagnostics, and therapeutics. Novel information technology platforms are at times deemed research tools and, therefore, separated from the work of providing care. They should be integrated directly into health systems to create critical feedback loops in health care delivery (Krist *et al.* 2011; Mandl and Kohane 2008). Providers of all stripes can improve their performance, not to mention the performance of the health system as a whole, by monitoring and evaluating programmes and outcomes. Furnishing health systems with infrastructures of transparency and accountability can improve performance of health providers and make hospitals and clinics more responsive to specific patient needs; health information systems can also identify inefficient and wasteful uses of resources on a system level, and so cut costs while improving the coordination and quality of care (Chadhry *et al.* 2006; Chassin *et al.* 2010). As noted, the Camden Coalition started when system-wide data analysis revealed that the sickest patients in Camden were accruing unsustainably high costs to the system. In short, information technology linked to service delivery and research opens windows for disruptive innovation and continuous health system improvement (Blaya *et al.* 2010).

While collecting health information has traditionally been the responsibility – indeed, the burden – of health professionals, touch screen and mobile technologies offer the promise of decentralizing data collection and utilization to all health care workers and ultimately to patients themselves. Improved information technology systems would facilitate more nimble and patient-centred care: individuals who are (or are at risk of) decompensating from a medical or psychosocial perspective could be more rapidly identified and matched with individualized accompaniment (Coye *et al.* 2009); individuals who prefer and have less need for hands-on assistance could have access to the databases and tools needed to take control of their own health and well-being (Ahmed *et al.* 2011; Saberi and Johnson 2011; Schiel *et al.* 2011). Integrating rigorous data collection and analysis into service delivery will also yield important lessons for sector-wide health system reform. Such 'real-world' evaluative processes could complement traditional scientific research methods, such as the randomized controlled trial. Together these approaches could create critical feedback loops that assess the efficacy of individual interventions in highly controlled settings and also the integration of such interventions into systems of care that are constantly changing and improving in order to more effectively and equitably alleviate human suffering from disease.

Changing the narrative

An honest discussion of the limitations of any health system is always difficult, in large part because it is difficult to attach a value to a life – much less to non-mortal suffering. These limitations are felt sharply in a primary care clinic, such as the one in which Kimberly receives her care. Her most recent medical problem – pelvic inflammatory disease – is readily treated but much more can be done. In a matter of decades (if not years), without significant changes in behaviour, environment, and engagement in the health system, she will almost certainly be saddled with the diseases of urban poverty that contribute to a cycle of impoverishment and ill health; her children might also be born into this cycle of poverty and disease. Her primary care provider feels helpless, but addressing this patient's structural risk factors does not *need* to lie entirely outside the domain of her health care.

Five years have passed since you first met Kimberly and much has changed. Unfortunately, her life got worse before it got better. After becoming pregnant, she was physically assaulted by her boyfriend and had a miscarriage. She then fell into a major depression, complicated by alcohol and crack cocaine abuse.

Two years ago, after an eight-month hiatus between visits, the health record system notified you that Kimberly had recently visited several emergency rooms in the city complaining of abdominal pain. A social worker tried to phone her a number of times without reaching her. One of the clinic's newly hired community health workers, Stephanie, then went to visit Kimberly at home.

At first resistant, Kimberly cautiously agreed after the first visit that Stephanie could come back; Kimberly eventually also agreed to return to see you in clinic. Over the next months, Kimberly, Stephanie, and your team developed a trusting relationship. Kimberly disclosed her boyfriend's physical and emotional abuse, and your team worked with her and a lawyer to file a restraining order. A non-profit agency for women that has developed a partnership with your clinic gave Kimberly a loan, enabling her to rent her own apartment in another part of the city. Kimberly entered a day treatment programme for addiction, started an anti-depressant and began meeting regularly with the social worker for talk therapy.

Newly sober, Kimberly was able to get a job at the counter of a fast food restaurant and start paying back the loan. Although still struggling with her weight, she has begun exercising regularly. You know that her path will not be without twists, turns, and setbacks. But at least you now find yourself part of a team that will more effectively help her navigate these challenges, and you find yourself providing the type of care that had inspired you to become a physician in the first place.

Note

1   There is a long literature on the abuses of foreign aid. Economist William Easterly, for example, cites a study of four African countries that found 30–70 per cent of HIV drugs did not make it to patients (Easterly 2006: 259). Paul Collier mentions an even more dispiriting finding: only one per cent of health funding in Chad reached its intended destination in local clinics, according to a 2004 survey (Collier 2007: 67).

References

Ahmed, S., Bartlett, S.J., Ernst, P., Pare, G., Kanter, M., Perreault, R., Grad, R., Taylor, L., and Tamblyn, R. (2011) 'Effect of a web-based chronic disease management system on asthma control and health-related quality of life', *Trials*, 12 (1): 260.

Barrow, S.M., Herman, D.B., Cordova, P., and Struening, E.L. (1999) 'Mortality among homeless shelter residents in New York City', *American Journal of Public Health*, 89 (4): 529–34.

Beaulac, J., Kristjansson, E., and Cummins, S. (2009) 'A systematic review of food deserts, 1966–2007', *Preventing Chronic Disease*, 6 (3): A105.

Behforouz, H.L., Farmer, P.E., and Mukherjee, J.S. (2004) 'From directly observed therapy to accompagnateurs: enhancing AIDS treatment outcomes in Haiti and in Boston', *Clinical Infectious Diseases*, 38 (Suppl. 5): S429–36.

Blankenship, K.M., Bray, S.J., and Merson, M.H. (2000) 'Structural interventions in public health', *AIDS*, 14 (Suppl. 1): S11–21.

Blaya, J.A., Fraser, H.S., and Holt, B. (2010) 'E-health technologies show promise in developing countries', *Health Affairs (Millwood)*, 29 (2): 244–51.

Boehmer, T.K.C., Flanders, D., McGeehin, M.A., Boyle, C., and Barrett, D.H. (2004) 'Postservice mortality in Vietnam veterans', *Archives of Internal Medicine*, 164 (17): 1908–16.

Bonds, M.H. (2008) 'Breaking the disease-driven poverty trap; notes from the millennium villages project, Rwanda', *Consilience: The Journal of Sustainable Development*, 1: 98–111.

Bonds, M.H., Keenan, D.C., Rohani, P., and Sachs, J.D. (2010) 'Poverty trap formed by the ecology of infectious diseases', *Proceedings of the Royal Society: Biological Sciences*, 277: 1185–92.

Brenner, J. (2009) 'Reforming Camden's health care system – one patient at a time', *Prescriptions for Excellence in Health Care Newsletter*, (Suppl. 1) (5): 10. Online, available at: http://jdc.jefferson.edu/pehc/vol1/iss5/10 (accessed 22 July 2012).

Brown, D.W., Anda, R.F., Tiemeier, H., Felitti, V.J., Edwards, V.J., Croft, J.B., and Giles, W.H. (2009) 'Adverse childhood experiences and the risk of premature mortality', *American Journal of Preventive Medicine*, 37 (5): 389–96.

Brown, D.W., Anda, R.F., Felitti, V.J., Edwards, V.J., Malarcher, A.M., Croft, J.B., and Giles, W.H. (2010) 'Adverse childhood experiences are associated with the risk of lung cancer: a prospective study', *BMC Public Health*, 10: 20

Brunner, E., Davey Smith, G., Marmot, M., Canner, R., Beksinska, M., and O'Brien, J. (1996) 'Childhood social circumstances and psychosocial and behavioral factors as determinants of plasma fibrinogen', *The Lancet*, 347 (9007): 1008–13.

Centers for Disease Control and Prevention (CDC) (2009) 'Obesity prevalence among low-income, preschool-aged children – United States, 1998–2008', *Morbidity and Mortality Weekly Report*, 58 (28): 769.

Centers for Disease Control and Prevention (CDC) (2010) 'Vital signs: current cigarette smoking among adults aged ≥18 years – United States, 2009', *Morbidity and Mortality Weekly Report*, 59 (35): 1135.

Chadhry, B., Wang, J., Wu, S., Maglione, M., Mojica, W., Roth, E., Morton, S.C., and Shekelle, P.G. (2006) 'Systematic review: impact of health information technology on quality, efficiency, and costs of medical care', *Annals of Internal Medicine*, 144 (10): e12–22.

Chassin, M.R., Loeb, J.M., Schmaltz, S.P., and Wachter, R.M. (2010) 'Accountability measures – using measurement to promote quality improvement', *New England Journal of Medicine*, 363 (7): 683–8.

Chernew, M.E., Baicker, K., and Hsu, J. (2010) 'The specter of financial Armageddon – health care and the federal debt in the United States', *New England Journal of Medicine*, 362 (13): 1166–8.

Cohen, D.A., Scribner, R.A., and Farley, T.A. (2000) 'A structural model of health behavior: a pragmatic approach to explain and influence health behaviors at the population level', *Preventive Medicine*, 30 (2): 146–54.

Cohen, E., Fullerton, D.F., Retkin, R., Weintraub, D., Tames, P., Brandfield, J., and Sandel, M. (2010) 'Medical-legal partnership: collaborating with lawyers to identify and address health disparities', *Journal of General Internal Medicine*, May, 25 (Suppl. 2): S136–9.

Collier, P. (2007) *The Bottom Billion: Why the Poorest Countries are Failing and What Can be Done About It*, New York: Oxford University Press.

Commission on Social Determinants of Health (CSDH) (2008) *Closing the Gap in a Generation: Health Equity through Action on the Social Determinants of Health*, Geneva: World Health Organization.

Coye, M.J., Haselkron, A., and DeMello, S. (2009) 'Remote patient management: technology-enabled innovation and evolving business', *Health Affairs*, 28 (1): 126–35

Crum, R.M. (2009) 'The epidemiology of substance use disorders', in R.K. Ries, D.A. Fiellin, S.C. Miller, and R. Saitz, (eds) *Principles of Addiction Medicine*, 4th edition, New York: Lippincott Williams & Wilkins.

Diez Roux, A.V., Merkin, S.S., Arnett, D., Chambless, L., Massing, M., Nieo, F.J., Sorlie, P., Szklo, M., Tyroler, H.A., and Watson, R.L. (2001) 'Neighborhood of residence and incidence of coronary heart disease', *New England Journal of Medicine*, 345 (2): 99–106.

Dube, S.R., Felitti, V.J., Dong, M., Chapman, D.P., Giles, W.H., and Anda, R.F. (2003) 'Childhood abuse, neglect, and household dysfunction and the risk of illicit drug use: the adverse childhood experience study', *Pediatrics*, 111 (3): 564–72.

Dubos, R. (1959) 'Environment and disease', in R. Dubos (ed.) *Mirage of Health: Utopias, Progress, and Biological Change*, New Brunswick, NJ: Rutgers University Press.

Easterly, W. (2006) *The White Man's Burden: Why the West's Efforts to Help the Rest Have Done so Much Ill and so Little Good*, New York: Penguin.

Farmer, P. (1997) 'On suffering and structural violence: a view from below', in A. Kleinman, V. Das, and M. Lock (eds) *Social Suffering*, Berkeley, CA: University of California Press, 261–83.

Farmer, P.E. (1999) *Infections and Inequalities: The Modern Plagues*, Berkeley, CA: University of California Press.

Farmer, P.E. (2004a) 'An anthropology of structural violence', *Current Anthropology*, 45 (3): 305–26.

Farmer, P.E. (2004b) *Pathologies of Power: Health, Human Rights, and the New War on the Poor*, Berkeley, CA: University of California Press.

Felitti, V.J., Anda, R.F., Nordenberg, D., Williamson, D.F., Spitz, A.M., Edwards, V., Koss, M.P., and Marks, J.S. (1998) 'Relationship of childhood abuse and household dysfunction to many of the leading causes of death in adults: the adverse childhood experiences (ACE) study', *American Journal of Preventive Medicine*, 14 (4): 245–58.

Ford, E.S. and Mokdad, A.H. (2008) 'Epidemiology of obesity in the Western hemisphere', *Journal of Clinical Endocrinology and Metabolism*, 93 (11 Suppl. 1): S1–8.

Fuchs, V. (1998) *Who Shall Live? Health Economics and Social Policy*, Singapore: World Scientific.

Harpham, T. and Molyneux, C. (2001) 'Urban health in developing countries: a review', *Progress in Development Studies*, 1: 113–37.

Hwang, S.W., Wilkins, R., Tjepkema, M., O'Campo, P.J., and Dunn, J.R. (2009) 'Mortality among residents of shelters, rooming houses, and hotels in Canada: 11 year follow-up study', *British Medical Journal*, 339: b4036.

Ivers, L.C., Cullen, K.A., Freedberg, K.A., Block, S., Coates, J., and Webb, P. (2009) 'HIV/AIDS, undernutrition, and food insecurity', *Clinical Infectious Diseases*, 49 (7): 1096–102.

Johnson, K., Asher, J., Rosborough, S., Raja, A., Panjabi, R., Beadling, C., and Lawry, L. (2008) 'Association of combatant status and sexual violence with health and mental health outcomes in postconflict Liberia', *Journal of the American Medical Association*, 300 (6): 676–90.

Kang, H.K., Bullman, T.A., Macfarlane, G.J., and Gray, G.C. (2002) 'Mortality among US and UK veterans of the Persian Gulf War: a review', *Occupational and Environmental Medicine*, 59 (12): 794–9.

Kotagal, M., Lee, P., Habiyakare, C., Dusabe, R., Kanama, P., Epino, H., Rich, M., and Farmer, P. (2009) 'Improving quality in resource poor settings: observational study from rural Rwanda', *British Medical Journal*, 339: b3488.

Krist, A.H., Peele, E., Woolf, S.H., Rothemich, S.F., Loomis, J.F., Longo, D.R., and Kuzel, A.J. (2011) 'Designing a patient-centered personal health record to promote preventive care', *BioMed Central Medical Informatics and Decision Making*, 11: 73.

Krishna, A. (2010) *One Illness Away: Why People Become Poor and How They Escape Poverty*, Oxford: Oxford University Press.

Kunz-Ebrecht, S.R., Kirschbaum, C., Marmot, M., and Steptoe, A. (2004) 'Differences in cortisol awakening response on work days and weekends in women and men from the Whitehall II cohort', *Psychoneuroendocrinology*, 29 (4): 516–28.

Louis, C., Ivers, L.C., Smith Fawzi, M.C., Freedberg, K.A., and Castro, A. (2007) 'Late presentation for HIV care in central Haiti: factors limiting access to care', *AIDS Care*, 19 (4): 487–91.

Malmstrom, M., Johansson S.E., and Sundquist, J. (2001) 'A hierarchical analysis of long-term illness and mortality in socially deprived areas', *Social Science & Medicine*, 53 (3): 265–75.

Mandl, K.D. and Kohane, I.S. (2008) 'Tectonic shifts in the health information economy', *New England Journal of Medicine*, 358 (16): 1732–7.

Marmot, M.G., Rose, G., Shipley, M., and Hamilton, P.J.S. (1978) 'Employment grade and coronary heart disease in British civil servants', *Journal of Epidemiology and Community Health*, 32 (4): 244–9.

Marmot, M.G., Rose, G., and Shipley, M.J. (1984) 'Inequalities in death-specific explanations of a general pattern?', *The Lancet*, 323 (8384): 1003–6.

Marmot, M.G. and Smither, G.D. (1991) 'Health inequalities among British civil servants: the Whitehall II study', *The Lancet*, 337 (8754): 1387–93.

Mari Gallagher Research and Consulting Group (2007) *Examining the Impact of Food Deserts on Public Health in Detroit*. Online, available at: http://www.marigallagher.com/projects/2/ (accessed 13 September 2011).

Mitnick, C., Bayona, J., Palacios, E., Shin, S., Furin, J., Alcántara, F., Sánchez, E., Sarria, M., Becerra, M., Smith Fawzi, M.C., Kapiga, S., Neuberg, D., Maguire, J.H., Kim, J.Y., and Farmer, P. (2003) 'Community-based therapy for multidrug-resistant tuberculosis in Lima, Peru', *New England Journal of Medicine*, 348 (2): 119–28.

Nordentoft, M. and Wandall-Holm, N. (2003) '10 year follow-up study of mortality among users of hostels for homeless people in Copenhagen', *British Medical Journal*, 329 (7406): 81.

Onie, R., Farmer, P., and Behforouz, H. (2012) 'Realigning health with care: lessons in delivering more with less', *Stanford Social Innovation Review* (Summer 2012): 28–35.

Pickett, K.E. and Pearl, M. (2001) 'Multilevel analyses of neighbourhood socioeconomic context and health outcomes: a critical review', *Journal of Epidemiology and Community Health*, 55 (2): 111–22.

Plucinski, M., Ngonghala, C.N., and Bonds, M.H. (2011) 'Health safety nets can break cycles of poverty and disease: a stochastic ecological model', *Journal of the Royal Society Interface*, 8: 1796–803

Ranson, K., Poletti, T., Bornemisza, O., and Sondorp, E. (2007) *Promoting Health Equity in Conflict-affected Fragile States*, paper prepared for the Health Systems Knowledge Network of the World Health Organization's Commission on Social Determinants of Health.

Rich, M.L., Miller, A.C., Niyigena, P., Franke, M., Niyonzima, J.B., Socci, A., Drobac, P., Hakizamungu, M., Mayfield, A., Ruhayisha, R., Epino, H., Stulac, S., Cancedda, C., Karamaga, A., Niyonzima, S., Yarbrough, C., Fleming, J., Amoroso, C., Mukherjee, J., Murray, M., Farmer, P., and Binagwaho, A. (2012) 'Excellent clinical outcomes and high retention in care among adults in a community-based HIV treatment program in rural Rwanda', *Journal of AIDS*, 59 (3): e35–42.

Rittenhouse, D.R. and Shortell, S.M. (2009) 'The patient-centered medical home: will it stand the test of health reform?', *Journal of the American Medical Association*, 301 (19): 2038–40.

Rose, G. and Marmot, M.G. (1981) 'Social class and coronary heart disease', *British Heart Journal*, 45 (1): 13–19.

Saberi, P. and Johnson, M.O. (2011) 'Technology based self-care methods of improving antiretroviral adherence: a systematic review', *PLoS ONE*, 6 (11): e27533.

Samb, B. (2007) 'Rapid expansion of the health workforce in response to the HIV epidemic', *New England Journal of Medicine*, 357 (24): 2510–14.

Schiel, R., Kaps, A., and Bieber, G. (2011) 'Electronic health technology for the assessment of physical activity and eating habits in children and adolescents with overweight and obesity IDA', *Appetite*, 58 (2): 432–7.

Shin, S.S., Pasechnikov, A.D., Gelmanova, I.Y., Peremitin, G.G., Strelis, A.K., Andreev, Y.G., Golubchikova, V.T., Tonkel, T.P., Yanova, G.V., Nikiforov, M., Yedilbayev, M., Mukherjee, J.S., Furin, J.J., Barry, D.J., Farmer, P.E., Rich, M.L., and Keshavjee, S. (2006) 'Treatment outcomes in an integrated civilian and prison MDR-TB treatment program in Russia', *International Journal of Tuberculosis and Lung Disease*, 10 (4): 402–8.

Shively, C.A. and Clarkson, T.B. (1994) 'Social stress and coronary artery atherosclerosis in female monkeys', *Atherosclerosis, Thrombosis, and Vascular Biology*, 14: 721–6.

State of Victoria, Department of Health (2010) *Primary Care Partnerships: Achievements 2000 to 2010*, Melbourne: State of Victoria, Department of Health. Online, available at: http://www.health.vic.gov.au/pcps/ (accessed 26 September 2011).

Walton, D.A., Farmer, P.E., Lambert, W., Léandre, F., Koenig, S.P., and Mukherjee, J.S. (2004) 'Integrated HIV prevention and care strengthens primary health care: lessons from rural Haiti', *Journal of Public Health Policy*, 25 (2): 137–58.

Williams, D.R. and Mohammed, S.A. (2009) 'Discrimination and racial disparities in health: evidence and needed research', *Journal of Behavioral Medicine*, 32 (1): 20–47.

5

IDEOLOGICAL BARRIERS TO STRUCTURAL INTERVENTIONS

Toward a model of values-based interventions

Michael Sweat and Kevin O'Reilly

Introduction

Why is it that in current political discourse there is such strong resistance to implementation of new structural interventions, even in the face of overwhelming scientific evidence that they improve human health? The libertarian Cato Institute's *Handbook on Policy* dedicates an entire chapter, entitled 'The Nanny State' (Balko 2005) to indictments of such structural interventions as seat belt laws, requirements for motorcycle helmets, and bans on smoking in public. They raise concern that:

> once policymakers have bought the notion of a 'public health' in need of protection and nurturing by government, they can be comfortable giving the state pervasive control over nearly every facet of our lives – from mandating that we wear our seatbelts, to telling us what risks we should allow our children to take, to telling us what foods we should eat and how much and how often we should eat them.
>
> (Balko 2005: 270)

Regular updates on policy-based interventions are highlighted on their website under their 'Nanny State' section (The Cato Institute 2012) with a host of such articles as 'Busybodies of the World, Unite', 'Against the New Paternalism', and 'Puritans, Politicians, and Paternalism: Can We Take Back Control of Our Own Lives?'. The popular website, reason.com, hosts an online Nanny State forum (Reason Magazine 2012) that archives thousands of perceived overwrought government intrusions, including titles such as 'L.A.'s Insane War on the Porn Industry', 'Big Brother is Now Your Diet Coach', and 'Can the Government Force You to Eat Your Broccoli?'. A March 2012 national Harris Poll (Harris Interactive Poll 2012) found that 81 per cent of respondents in the United States agreed that individuals should 'be free to make their own decisions, even if they suffer as a result'. Clearly, there is resistance to structural interventions among many, and if we as public health practitioners want to utilize structural interventions, we should understand and come to terms with this resistance.

The concept of improving human health through structural interventions is not new. In fact, the origins of the field of public health are grounded in structural interventions.

Yet it appears the attractiveness of regulation and policy-based interventions has waned under modern democratic capitalism. We believe that this is largely due to four key factors: (1) an affinity for a market-centric ideology that promotes resistance to policies which encumber individual and corporate choices through state intervention; (2) resistance to programmes that address inequalities and the redistribution of resources; (3) failure to recognize that individual risk taking frequently results in the costs of those behaviours being socialized; and (4) limits in current theories of structural interventions with regard to mechanisms of social change and the role of individual agency and values. Let us begin with a brief history of structural interventions, and evidence for their profound impact on health.

Physical environment and social ecology affect health

The structure of the environment strongly affects some of the most salient factors in the production of health, including physical activity, diet, stress, social support, and recreation. Some health problems such as chronic disease, addiction, violence, injury, and sexually transmitted infections are particularly sensitive to structural forces (Blankenship et al. 2000). When we succumb to illness, structural forces also affect the willingness and capacity to seek treatment, most notably within the health system, but also within the institutions of the family and workplace. For example, it has been found that one of the best predictors of treatment seeking for malaria is accessibility to a hospital (Muller et al. 2003). In Tanzania it was found that sustaining antiretroviral treatment for AIDS was associated with social support from the family and community (Roura et al. 2009). It is thus not surprising that some of the most potent strategies to improve health are found in interventions that address the structure of the environment, commonly referred to as 'structural interventions'.

As noted by many (Blankenship et al. 2000; Farley and Cohen 2005), structural interventions are not new, especially those that focus on the physical environment. In 1854 John Snow, known as the father of epidemiology, initiated a classic structural intervention by removing the handle of the contaminated Broad Street water pump in London, effectively halting a cholera epidemic in the area (Johnson 2006). In the early days of public health as a discipline, hygiene-based interventions were the most common strategies utilized. These took the form of water and sewage treatment, rodent control, garbage collection and disposal, and mosquito eradication, among others (Rosen 1993). With ever-increasing industrialization and urbanization, public health initiatives shifted to also embrace a broad array of safety-oriented interventions, such as engineering safer roads (Montgomery 1988), housing (Petroski 2012), occupational environments (Aldrich 1997), and consumer products (Arnold 2009).

Later, advances in public health through structural interventions were made with the expansion to laws, policies, and regulations addressing the ecology of risk (Cheng 2005). The list is long, but includes laws and regulations on such things as alcohol sales, cigarette sales, urban zoning, traffic law enforcement, regulation and nutritional labelling of food products, regulation of pharmaceutical drugs, access and affordability of nutritious food, access to public transportation, developing public parks and recreational facilities, noise ordinances, poverty eradication, and access to low-cost community health services. The trend toward legislating risk reduction was driven to some degree by the growing capacity to identify the associations between structural factors and health outcomes that came with large-scale systematic collection of health status data. For example, the National Health Interview Survey was initiated by the United States Census Bureau in 1957, and these data provided the first national comprehensive overview of the distribution and predictors of health and illness (Khrisanopulo 1963). Analysis of these national health data by demographic, behavioural, and geographic variables enabled identification of factors associated with healthy outcomes, and provided an empirical rationale for such laws and policies.

There is clear evidence that living in environments with regulations and programmes that ensure access to high-quality and low-cost food (Mikkelsen and Chehimi 2007), housing (Thomson *et al.* 2010), a living wage (Bhatia and Katz 2001), transport (Dora and Phillips 2000), recreation (Brownson *et al.* 2001), and health care (Moonesinghe *et al.* 2011) results in significant improvements in health. One excellent example of a comprehensive, multi-country structural intervention is the World Health Organization European Healthy Cities Network. This initiative, active in over 90 cities across Europe, specifically addresses inequalities in health and poverty and implements interventions relevant to the social, economic, and environmental determinants of health (Barton *et al.* 2003). This is achieved though coordinated efforts to foster political commitment, leadership, specific institutional changes, and the development of inter-sectoral partnerships.

Multiple health intervention theories now incorporate structural components, although to varying degrees. The primacy of structural factors in theoretical models varies largely based on how distal or proximal the theory is to individual risk. For instance, intervention theories related to psychological cognitive processes – highly proximal to individuals – typically pay only minimal, if any, attention to structural factors. Examples include the Health Belief Model (Janz and Becker 1984), and the Theory of Reasoned Action (Fishbein 1980). These theories are grounded in a rational actor paradigm, assuming that if people have accurate information they will make positive and rational decisions about their health. On the other extreme are ecological theories. There are many examples (McLaren and Hawe 2005), perhaps most notably the Ecological Systems Theory (Bronfenbrenner 1979). These theories are highly distal to individuals, with focus primarily on higher-order effects, and rarely address cognitive processes of the individual. There are also meso-level theories whose unit of analysis and action are groups and social networks. Examples of these include social capital-based strategies (Bourdieu 1986; Putnam 2000), popular opinion leader interventions (Kelly *et al.* 1991), and programmes that foster social support (Vaux 1988). These theories are hybrids in that individual health benefits are seen as realized or mediated through social networks proximal to individuals, with the individual reducing risk and improving health as a consequence of participation in social groups.

Ideology

Placing structural interventions, and resistance to them, in perspective requires some understanding of the historical forces that have shaped contemporary ideology on the role of state control and the values of egalitarianism and individual freedom. Ideology is a critical factor in the successful implementation of structural interventions, both with regard to their development and in generating the requisite public support and resources to implement and sustain them. Ideology is a comprehensive belief system that informs our view of the world and filters our understanding of actions and intentions. It provides a logical and coherent value system for filtering our cognitive experience, guides our evaluations of events, and offers a framework for action (Mullins 1972). In the first half of the twentieth century, world wars were fought over ideology, which realigned the economic and political world order. The great ideological shifts that were experienced in the last century, and the associated world wars that were fought, primarily reflect tensions over opposing beliefs about two key factors: (1) the legitimate role of state power; and (2) the degree of social and economic equality that should be fostered in society (Chirot and Merton 1986).

By the beginning of the twentieth century, the almost universal establishment of the modern nation state – a phenomenon consolidated in the nineteenth century – together with the accumulation of vast state wealth from dramatic increases in industrial production, led to an impressive increase in the capacity of centralized governments to enact reforms (Chirot and Merton 1986). As Chirot and Merton (1986) describe, stronger cultural ties fostered by nationalism, improved communication technologies, democratization, and increased participation in civil society and economic life put great demands on states to address long-standing social and economic inequalities. These trends precipitated competing ideologies over the role and scope of state power, and tolerance for social and economic inequality.

With regard to state power, on one extreme are beliefs that central government power corrupts markets, fosters economic inefficiencies, usurps local control, unfairly redistributes wealth, and constrains individual liberty. On the other end of this spectrum is the belief that state power can and should be used as an instrument of positive social change to address institutionalized inequalities, balance and mediate competing market interests, plan and regulate essential economic functions, establish minimum living standards, and guarantee equal rights and opportunities.

An equally polarized continuum exists in ideologies regarding inequality. At one extreme is the belief that people are born or created with different and complementary roles and capacities, that poverty is a result of laziness and deficient values, and that inequality serves as a motivating factor in society, enriching those who deserve it the most and punishing those who do not try hard enough. On the opposite extreme are beliefs in radical equality, with any private property representing an unfair distribution of resources, all hereditary and familial advantages anathema to fairness, and inequality viewed as suppressing economic vigour and social mobility. Obviously, for both of these constructs (the role of government power and equality) there are gradations of beliefs across the entire spectrum. At the same time it should be noted that many people adhere to extreme ideological beliefs, leaving little room for recognition of the middle ground that exists between the extreme positions. In addition, it is those who hold extreme views on these issues of state power and promotion of equality who also vie strongly for public influence.

When we bring these two ideological continuums on state power and equality together, what emerges is a framework for examining modern political discourse on structural interventions through an ideological lens. This is depicted in Figure 5.1. On the far extremes we find the largely failed ideologies of anarchism, feudalism, fascism, and communism – each with a combination of extreme ideological orientations on state power and social equality. Anarchism, with its utopian belief that the total elimination of the state will engender full equality in society; feudalism, which embraced beliefs in absolute inequality based on heredity, and weak state power; fascism, which espoused total state control and a command economy together with inequality based on the believed superiority of select national, racial, and ethnic groups; and finally, communism, which promised complete equality through complete state control. In the great battles over these ideologies in the mid-twentieth century it was the centrist ideologies that prevailed, and it is here that we can position the current debates regarding the feasibility of implementing structural interventions.

While centrist beliefs have emerged as the contemporary mainstream ideologies, ideological variants remain as an artefact of these long-standing conflicts over the appropriate degree of state power, and value of fostering social and economic equality. The extreme differences in orientation seen in mainstream ideologies of the last century have been dramatically muted in intensity, yet still persist.

In Europe we find quite high acceptance of state power, and also the belief that the state should take an activist stance to promote equality. American ideology is generally less accepting of concentrated state power and tolerates inequality to a much higher degree. In both the United States and Europe there are internal differences as well, with conservatives less accepting of state power and having less activist policies regarding equality than liberals and social democrats, respectively.

There is also a growing movement toward libertarianism in the United States, which is openly hostile to state power and is not supportive of active state efforts to diminish inequality. In fact, in the United States, it is libertarians who are most vocal and hostile toward structural interventions, as evidenced by the quote from the Cato Institute's

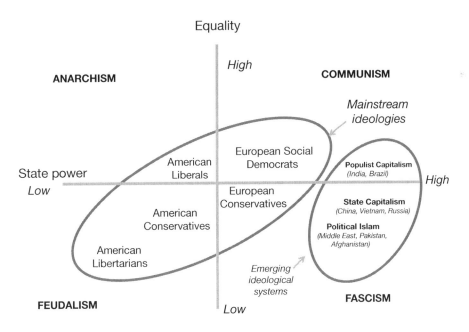

Figure 5.1 Framework for examining modern political discourse through an ideological lens

Source: Adapted from Chirot and Merton 1986, reproduced with permission

official policy guide cited earlier. Interestingly, extreme ideological beliefs related to state power often lead to support for policies which would appear counterintuitive, such as support for gay marriage by American libertarians, evidenced in the 2010 Libertarian Party platform that states that 'Sexual orientation, preference, gender, or gender identity should have no impact on the government's treatment of individuals, such as in current marriage' (The Libertarian Party 2010). In this seemingly paradoxical case, it is the radical belief that there is virtually no legitimate sphere of government regulation for private behaviour that lends support to gay marriage. This policy position has little to do with the desire to actively enhance equality, except in the belief that all should be equally left alone by government.

In addition to the mainstream ideologies highlighted, there are also newly emerging alternative ideologies and political-economic systems, most notably state capitalism in China, Vietnam, and Russia; political Islam in the Middle East; and strong and rising capitalist economic systems coupled with populist political movements in Brazil and India (Kupchan 2012). Interestingly, these emerging ideological systems tend to be high in state control, but low in realized equality. As Kupchan (2012) suggests, these systems do not adhere to the democratic, secular, and free market ideologies seen among the economic powers of North America, Western Europe, Japan, and Oceania. How these rapidly emerging systems will ultimately align on the state power/equality continuums remains to be seen. The state capitalist models of China and Russia certainly rank high with regard to state power, but are low in terms of income and participatory equality. Significant levels of state power are seen in India and Brazil. They also have high degrees of participatory equality coupled with high income inequality, and a rapidly growing middle class. Political Islam represents a highly disparate collection of ideologies, with many countries highly embedded in the capitalist world system, with strong state power, low levels of equality, and a newly emergent trend toward democratic participation (Anderson 2011). In countries with economic and political systems based on state capitalism and political Islam there is a high degree of state power that facilitates the capacity to enact structural interventions, yet the low levels of participatory equality limits pressure for activist policy. The populist capitalist democracies engender high degrees of bottom-up pressure for reform, generating significant pressures for activist and redistributive policy, yet they concurrently have an extremely high degree of social and economic inequality.

Implications for structural interventions

So how does this distribution of ideological systems, with their varying affinity for state-sponsored intervention and willingness to redress social inequality, relate to the capacity to implement structural interventions? Foremost, it is important to recognize that structural interventions typically are state-sponsored or state-sanctioned, and they frequently attempt to redress inequalities. The poor do not eat enough nutritious food and we believe it is linked to cost and access – so we regulate fast food outlets, use zoning and incentives to eliminate food deserts, and provide financial aid to poor families to buy healthy food. Gun violence results in significant death and disability, especially in poor urban areas – so we regulate access to guns, build public housing that is less prone to violence, and incarcerate those who commit crimes. Smoking cigarettes is one of the leading causes of morbidity and mortality, especially among the less educated and those who started smoking at an early age – to address this we raise taxes on cigarettes, limit tobacco sales to adults, and ban smoking in public spaces. Each of these structural interventions has elements of state sponsorship and/or attempts to remedy inequality, the two key touchstones of major ideological divides and battles of the past century.

One key lesson from the heated ideological wars of the past is that centrist ideologies prevailed. The extremes of feudalism, anarchism, communism, and fascism have largely failed as ideologies and have little popular appeal globally. Moreover, there is a persistent trend in history, albeit with fits and starts, toward greater equality, and ideologies that support enhanced equality. Yet the intensity of debates over state power continues, largely unabated. This leads us to believe that advocating for structural change to improve health is best sought by first stressing the need to eliminate health disparities, and second seeking centrist policy positions as they relate to state power. It is difficult to argue against equality, and policies that engender extreme degrees of state power are likely to face significant resistance. It is slow incremental policy changes, strongly linked to reductions in health disparities, that will likely become implemented, institutionalized, accepted, and sustained.

One important defining feature of the major ideological conflicts of the past century is the evolution of divergent definitions on the meanings of 'freedom' and 'responsibility'. On the left, 'freedom' is frequently articulated as freedom of expression and dissent, with 'responsibility' realized through collective action to assure minimum human needs, often through state intervention. In contrast, on the right, 'freedom' is now typically defined as freedom *from* state intervention, with absolute 'responsibility' assigned to individuals. As a case in point, the slogan for a popular United States Tea Party organization named FreedomWorks is 'Lower Taxes. Less Government. More Freedom' (FreedomWorks 2012). There is, however, a paradox to the logic that freedom is synonymous with individual responsibility. Simply put, it is morally bankrupt and impractical to hold people individually responsible for themselves when they are denied the freedom to do so. Amartya Sen writes about this dilemma eloquently when he notes:

> Responsibility *requires* freedom. ... The argument for social support in expanding people's freedom can, therefore, be seen as an argument *for* responsibility, not against it. ... The alternative to an exclusive reliance on individual responsibility is not, as is sometimes assumed, the so-called nanny state. There is a difference between 'nannying' an individual's choices and creating more opportunity for choice.
>
> (Sen 2008: 276)

This emphasis on choice that Sen highlights is insightful. He points out that only when people have agency in their decisions are they free, and only then can they be held responsible for themselves. You cannot expect people with no range of choice to choose good health behaviours. This is the great appeal of structural interventions – they have the potential to create the opportunity for positive health decisions. In addition, structural interventions that dictate policies without incorporating the voice of those affected limit both freedom and responsibility. We believe that this line of reasoning needs to be made more forcefully, and that the role of agency of those affected needs to be incorporated into the theoretical models of structural interventions. Another important aspect of 'choice' is the generation of a false sense of choice, prevalent in modern markets. As

Farley and Cohen describe, there is an amazing variety of products available in modern supermarkets, but the majority are processed foods, with ever-shrinking space allocated to fresh fruits and vegetables (Farley and Cohen 2005). This creates the false sense of choice to consumers, who actually have a vast choice between bad options.

Another aspect of responsibility that merits exploration with regard to structural interventions is that when moral hazard is present there is a greater tolerance for state-sanctioned regulation. Moral hazard, as defined by economist Paul Krugman, is 'any situation in which one person makes the decision about how much risk to take, while someone else bears the cost if things go badly' (Krugman 2009: 63). In these situations, where the outcomes of private risk are socialized, there is typically a much greater tolerance for government regulation. This was seen with the 2008 global banking crisis. There was a societal willingness to allow the government to bail out banks, which took horrendous risks, as their collapse would have led to systemic risk to the entire financial system, resulting in private risk and socialized cost. The significant resistance to large-scale publicly funded bailouts of the banks was overcome, even in the most conservative sectors of society, when it became clear that failure to act would have resulted in enormous damage to the overall financial system. These financial institutions were too big to fail.

A lesson to learn from these events is that when regulations of private health risks are linked to the public costs of not regulating, there is likely to be greater public support for regulation. The larger the socialized cost of private risk, the greater the willingness to regulate and support structural interventions. An excellent example of this is the significant resistance to regulation of public smoking behaviour that occurred for many years. This did not change until smoking in public was linked to the health effects of passive smoke, as well as to the costs of medical care for smokers incurred by society at large. Likewise, quite coercive regulations such as mandated vaccination and isolation of those with serious infectious diseases are generally quite acceptable to the public, largely because they mitigate the potential for moral hazard with private risk/socialized impact.

Values-based interventions

Prevailing theories on structural interventions also frequently lack several critical elements: (1) they often neglect the voice and agency of those affected; (2) the proposed interventions lack linkage to a plan for generating social change; and (3) they typically do not have clear articulation of the values that undergird them. We believe that the best intervention outcomes will occur, and will be most likely to be implemented and sustained, when there is strong voice from those affected in the design of interventions; when there is thought given to the process of generating social change; and when core values underpinning the intervention are defined and codified. A key element of this strategy is promotion of consensus among affected individuals and communities in articulating core values that are then acted upon through bottom-up pressure to codify structural change. Eschewing extreme ideology, values-based interventions seek consensus and middle ground. Despite this fact, values-based interventions share key features with many of the ideologies discussed previously. Like libertarianism, this strategy favours choice over coercion. Like free market capitalism, it acknowledges the wisdom of groups armed with information over key individuals in taking decisions about best courses of action. Unlike other ideological approaches, values-based interventions highlight communitarianism and the collective good in an effort to find a balance between individual rights, individual freedoms, and collective benefits.

One excellent example of a values-based intervention is the Sonagachi Project (see Chapter 10, Swendeman and Jana, in this volume). Values-based interventions have grown out of the experiences of community development and mobilization among sex workers in Sonagachi, a red light district of Kolkata, India (Jana *et al.* 2004), and later among high-risk groups across six states of India under the Avahan project (Chandrasekaran *et al.* 2008; Rao 2010), an HIV prevention effort funded by the Bill and Melinda Gates Foundation. In the Sonagachi red light district, early efforts toward HIV prevention focused on convincing sex workers to use condoms with all clients. It quickly became apparent that in a system that controlled their lives and choices, the average sex worker lacked the skills and certainly the power to make such demands. Operating from a firm values basis, the leaders of the Sonagachi Project were able to collectivize the women practising sex work in the red light district despite the fact that little aside from their circumstances linked them together. By exploring and respecting the experiences and opinions of all involved, the project was able to come up with a very different set of priorities from those that it had been using for HIV prevention. Intervention efforts continued to include basic HIV prevention efforts but expanded to include other issues considered by the community to be important, such as literacy classes, child vaccination programmes, and social protection issues, including banking and insurance. Presenting clear and factual information about HIV and its risks allowed the focus on HIV prevention to remain. By listening respectfully to the other important problems that sex workers faced on a daily basis, the project was able to craft possible solutions for community acceptance. Some solutions had ancillary benefits for HIV prevention as well. For example, sex workers faced the near impossibility of opening bank accounts, and as a result experienced grave difficulties in managing their funds. Theft was frequent, as was fraud and usury as independent agents posing as bankers often embezzled the money or offered loans at exorbitant interest rates. Faced with daily rents for their lodging and place of work, some sex workers would agree to riskier 'no condom' sex late in the evening after a slow day with no customers. A collective organization was formed by the sex workers and their children, some of whom had earned university degrees and gained experience in business. Using the collective model, sex workers who had encountered a low earning day were now able to make low- to no-interest loans to cover their daily expenses. By involving, respecting, and listening to the concerns of sex workers, key problems that may have gone unnoticed or have seemed unrelated to the goal of HIV prevention were identified, solutions acceptable to the women concerned were found, and individual risks were reduced through the development of a structural solution.

The attractiveness of values-based interventions stems in large part from the merging of structural interventions with the empowerment of individuals to make informed choices. By involving those who experience the health or social problems in the decision-making process, the 'top-down' approach, often decried by libertarian ideology, is muted. By incorporating the 'bottom-up' perspective, new related problems, which may otherwise have been missed, can be identified, with the promise that creative, acceptable solutions can also be found. By harnessing the wisdom and power of groups, structural interventions can be implemented that avoid many of the pitfalls identified by critics.

The process of developing and implementing values-based interventions should not be proscriptive. Instead, it should operate from recognition of key values, foremost among them egalitarianism. Through collective action, the actors and beneficiaries of any action should be identified so that all perspectives and opinions can be heard. This process facilitates coalescing different groups of people, often from very different backgrounds and perspectives, around what becomes identified as a common or shared problem or concern.

The power of values-based interventions comes from the ability to identify factors beyond the control of any one individual that may increase risk of an adverse health outcome, or conversely, factors that may diminish that risk. These interventions are also valuable in that they may be less narrowly focused on the most proximal issues in a problem, but can identify vitally important distal issues as well. This community development mechanism to generating structural change has the added benefit of fostering social capital among those most affected, which in itself has documented health benefits. In addition, it gives voice to those most affected, and reduces resistance to policies that come to bear on the population.

Structural interventions are powerful tools that have been at the core of some of the most effective public health accomplishments over time. They are becoming more and more challenging to develop, however, as ideological positions become more rigid and strident. Of particular concern in these ideological debates is the balance between central authority or control and the agency of individuals. Values-based interventions offer the possibility of addressing key public health concerns, a widely shared goal, by striking a balance between these two concerns.

Summary and conclusion

Societal acceptance of structural interventions to improve health mirrors important ideological divisions that have strongly defined development of the prevailing political and economic systems in the modern era. Despite strong evidence of their efficacy, concerns over the acceptable scope of state power and state activism to mitigate inequality generate significant resistance to implementing structural interventions. In fact, there has been such strong polarization of opinion over these issues in many developed economies that we now have competing definitions of the meaning of 'freedom' and 'responsibility'. The political left defines freedom primarily in terms of freedom from deprivation, and responsibility as a communal duty. The political right defines freedom as liberty from government interference, and responsibility as an individual mandate. Lost in the ideological debates is the role of individual agency and values, and the irony that without social protection for greater freedoms, individuals typically lack the agency to make responsible decisions. It is clear, however, that when individual risk behaviours result in socialized costs (moral hazard) there is a much greater willingness to tolerate state intervention. And it should be noted that in the heated ideological battles of the past century, it is centrist ideologies that have prevailed, with gradual acceptance of equality as a moral standard. Therefore, an important lesson learned from history is that structural interventions are most likely to be widely supported when they are based on the promotion of equality, engender values of enhanced agency, and mitigate the socialization of the costs of individual behaviours.

Perhaps one of the most interesting developments with regard to structural interventions is the variation in their acceptance globally. The most significant resistance to structural interventions now comes from the global North in advanced capitalist economies, the very locations where structural interventions originally developed in tandem with the emergence of highly organized bureaucratic economic systems. Interestingly, now perhaps the greatest willingness to implement structural interventions is found in newly emerging economies. It is here also that some of the most innovative structural interventions are being developed. In Brazil (Paes-Sousa *et al.* 2011) and Mexico (Bustamante 2011; Sosa-Rubi *et al.* 2011), for example, there has been a willingness to implement conditional cash transfers to address inequality and health disparities. Structural interventions to address health issues are widely accepted in Brazil and India, especially when they address health disparities and are perceived to improve the overall quality of life. In Asia and Latin America, there have been major efforts in recent years to reduce HIV through structural interventions that recognize sex work as a legitimate enterprise, for example the Sonagachi Project described earlier in this chapter (Jana *et al.* 2004). It remains to be seen how sustained these efforts will be within these newly emerging models of economic development in the global South, and whether the established economies of the global North will continue their historical support for innovation in developing and implementing structural interventions to improve their citizens' health.

References

Aldrich, M. (1997) *Safety First: Technology, Labor, and Business in the Building of American Work Safety, 1870–1939*, Baltimore, MD: Johns Hopkins University Press.

Anderson, L. (2011) 'Demystifying the Arab Spring: parsing the differences between Tunisia, Egypt, and Libya', *Foreign Affairs*, May/June.

Arnold, N.S. (2009) *Imposing Values: An Essay on Liberalism and Regulation*, New York: Oxford University Press.

Balko, R. (2005) 'The nanny state', in D. Boaz (ed.) *Cato Handbook on Policy*, 6th edition, Washington, D.C.: Cato Institute.

Barton, H., Mitcham, C., and Tsourou, C. (eds) (2003) *Healthy Urban Planning in Practice: Report of the WHO City Action Group on Healthy Urban Planning*, Copenhagen: World Health Organization Regional Office for Europe. Online, available at: http://www.euro.who.int/__data/assets/pdf_file/0003/98400/E82657.pdf (accessed 15 August 2012).

Bhatia, R. and Katz, M. (2001) 'Estimation of health benefits from a local living wage ordinance', *American Journal of Public Health*, 91 (9): 1398–402.

Blankenship, K.M., Bray, S.J., and Merson, M.H. (2000) 'Structural interventions in public health', *AIDS*, 14 (Suppl. 1): S11–21.

Bourdieu, P. (1986) 'The forms of capital', in J.G. Richardson (ed.) *Handbook of Theory and Research for the Sociology of Education*, New York: Greenwood Press.

Bronfenbrenner, U. (1979) *The Ecology of Human Development: Experiments by Nature and Design*, Cambridge, MA: Harvard University Press.

Brownson, R.C., Baker, E.A., Housemann, R.A., Brennan, L.K., and Bacak, S.J. (2001) 'Environmental and policy determinants of physical activity in the United States', *American Journal of Public Health*, 91: 1995–2003.

Bustamante, A.V. (2011) 'Comparing federal and state healthcare provider performance in villages targeted by the conditional cash transfer programme of Mexico', *Tropical Medicine & International Health*, 16 (10): 1251–9.

Chandrasekaran, P., Dallabetta, G., Loo, V., Mills, S., Saidel, T., Adhikary, R., Alary, M., Lowndes, C.M., Boily, M.C., and Moore, J. (2008) 'Evaluation design for large-scale HIV prevention programmes: the case of Avahan, the India AIDS initiative', *AIDS*, 22 (Suppl. 5), S1–15.

Cheng, E.K. (2005) 'Structural laws and the puzzle of regulating behavior', *Northwestern University Law Review*, 100 (2): 655–718.

Chirot, D. and Merton, R.K. (1986) *Social Change in the Modern Era*, San Diego, CA: Harcourt Brace Jovanovich.

Dora, C. and Phillips. M. (2000) 'Transport, environment and health', *WHO Regional Publications, European Series, No. 89*, Rome: World Health Organization.

Farley, T. and Cohen, D. (2005) *Prescription for a Healthy Nation: A New Approach to Improving our Lives by Fixing our Everyday World*, Boston, MA: Beacon Press.

Fishbein, M. (1980) 'A theory of reasoned action: some applications and implications', *Nebraska Symposium on Motivation*, 27: 65–116.

Freedomworks (2012) *FreedomWorks: Lower Taxes. Less Government. More Freedom.* Online, available at: http://www.freedomworks.org/ (accessed 14 August 2012).

Harris Interactive Poll (2012) *Many Americans Ambivalent over Laws Aimed at Healthy Living: Poll* [Press Release], Norwalk, CT: Harris Interactive. Online, available at: http://www.harrisinteractive.com/NewsRoom/PressReleases/tabid/446/mid/1506/articleId/986/ctl/ReadCustom%20Default/Default.aspx (accessed 12 August 2012).

Jana, S., Basu, I., Rotheram-Borus, M.J., and Newman, P.A. (2004) 'The Sonagachi Project: a sustainable community intervention program', *AIDS Education and Prevention*, 16 (5): 405–14.

Janz, N.K. and Becker, M.H. (1984) 'The health belief model: a decade later', *Health Education Quarterly*, 11: 1–47.

Johnson, S. (2006) *The Ghost Map: The Story of London's Most Terrifying Epidemic – and How it Changed Science, Cities, and the Modern World*, New York: Riverhead Books.

Kelly, J.A., St. Lawrence, J.S., Diaz, Y.E., Stevenson, L.Y., Hauth, A.C., Brasfield, T.L., Kalichman, S.C., Smith, J.E., and Andrew, M.E. (1991) 'HIV risk behavior reduction following intervention with key opinion leaders of population: an experimental analysis', *American Journal of Public Health*, 81 (2): 168–71.

Khrisanopulo, M.P. (1963) 'Origin, program, and operation of the US National Health Survey', *Vital Health Statistics*, 1: 1–41.

Krugman, P.R. (2009) *The Return of Depression Economics and the Crisis of 2008*, New York: W.W. Norton.

Kupchan, C. (2012) 'America's place in the new world', *New York Times*, 7 April 2012.

McLaren, L. and Hawe, P. (2005) 'Ecological perspectives in health research', *Journal of Epidemiology and Community Health*, 59 (1): 6–14.

Mikkelsen, L. and Chehimi, S. (2007) *The Links between the Neighborhood Food Environment and Childhood Nutrition*, Princeton, NJ: Robert Woods Johnson Foundation.

Montgomery, J.A. (1988) *Eno: The Man and the Foundation: A Chronicle of Transportation*, Westport, CT: Eno Foundation for Transportation.

Moonesinghe, R., Zhu, J., and Truman, B.I. (2011) 'Health insurance coverage – United States, 2004 and 2008', *Morbidity and Mortality Weekly Report Surveillance Summary*, 60 (Suppl.): 35–7.

Muller, O., Traore, C., Becher, H., and Kouyate, B. (2003) 'Malaria morbidity, treatment-seeking behaviour, and mortality in a cohort of young children in rural Burkina Faso', *Tropical Medicine & International Health*, 8 (4): 290–6.

Mullins, W.A. (1972) 'On the concept of ideology in political science', *American Political Science Review*, 66 (2): 498–510.

Paes-Sousa, R., Santos, L.M., and Miazaki, E.S. (2011) 'Effects of a conditional cash transfer programme on child nutrition in Brazil', *Bulletin of the World Health Organization*, 89: 496–503.

Petroski, H. (2012) *To Forgive Design: Understanding Failure*, Cambridge, MA: Belknap Press of Harvard University Press.

Putnam, R.D. (2000) *Bowling Alone: The Collapse and Revival of American Community*, New York: Simon & Schuster.

Rao, P.J. (2010) 'Avahan: the transition to a publicly funded programme as a next stage', *Sexually Transmitted Infections*, 86 (Suppl. 1): i7–8.

Reason Magazine (2012) *The Nanny State*, Los Angeles: The Reason Foundation. Online, available at: http://reason.com/topics/nanny-state (accessed 31 August 2012).

Rosen, G. (1993) *A History of Public Health*, Baltimore, MD: Johns Hopkins University Press.

Roura, M., Busza, J., Wringe, A., Mbata, D., Urassa, M., and Zaba, B. (2009) 'Barriers to sustaining antiretroviral treatment in Kisesa, Tanzania: a follow-up study to understand attrition from the antiretroviral program', *AIDS Patient Care and STDs*, 23: 203–10.

Sen, A. (2008) 'Individual freedom as a social commitment', in S.M. Kwok and M.A. Wallis (eds) *Daily Struggle: The Deepening Racialization and Feminization of Poverty in Canada*, Toronto: Canadian Scholars' Press.

Sosa-Rubi, S.G., Walker, D., Servan, E., and Bautista-Arredondo, S. (2011) 'Learning effect of a conditional cash transfer programme on poor rural women's selection of delivery care in Mexico', *Health Policy and Planning*, 26: 496–507.

The Cato Institute (2012) *The Nanny State*, Washington, D.C.: The Cato Insititute. Online, available at: http://www.cato.org/nanny-state (accessed 14 August 2012).

The Libertarian Party (2010) *Libertarian Party Platform [Article 1.3: Personal Relationships]*. Online, available at: http://www.lp.org/platform (accessed 14 August 2012).

Thomson, H., Thomson, S., Sellstrom, E., and Petticrew M. (2010) 'Housing improvements for health and associated socio-economic outcomes (Protocol)', *Cochrane Database of Systematic Reviews*, 9: CD008657.

Vaux, A. (1988) *Social Support: Theory, Research, and Intervention*, New York: Praeger.

6

GETTING THE BALANCE RIGHT

Agency and structure in HIV prevention

Peter Aggleton, Jean Shoveller, Kate Shannon, Thomas Kerr, and Rod Knight

Introduction

The 1986 Ottawa Charter for Health Promotion stressed the significance of the relationship between social structures and the actions of individuals and communities, if efforts to promote health are to succeed. The Charter signalled the importance of ensuring equal opportunities and resources to enable all people to achieve their fullest health potential. Put quite simply, people cannot 'achieve their fullest health potential unless they are able to take control of those things which determine their health' (WHO 2011).

Later, within the context of HIV, Oussama Tawil *et al.* (1995) built on ideas to draw attention to the possibilities of environmental interventions that make healthy choices easier choices. Alongside greater concern for the political context within which health-promoting interventions occur, the foundations were laid for a major shift in the manner in which HIV prevention and health promotion were conceived. Hitherto, the dominant ethos had been for programmes and interventions to address apparent 'deficits' of one kind or another – in knowledge and understanding, in skills of sexual communication and negotiation, and in 'correct' values and attitudes to protect against infection. Surveys of HIV- and AIDS-related knowledge, attitudes, beliefs, and reported practices were undertaken, sometimes (but not always) accompanied by interventions to make good what was apparently lacking in the individuals surveyed.

Throughout the 1990s, growing concern with context and the 'located-ness' of social and biomedical interventions against HIV encouraged a more sophisticated understanding of what was needed to achieve HIV prevention success. Increasingly questioned were individualistic models of cognitive, attitude, and behaviour change and the assumption that there might be magic bullet interventions to protect people against HIV regardless of time and place. In their place, new frameworks emerged that focused as much attention on the setting or context within which people found themselves as on their knowledge, attitudes, and skills (Dowsett and Aggleton 1999; Ingham and van Zessen 1997).

In recognition of the fact that some communities, groups and individuals are made vulnerable to HIV by large-scale 'structural' factors such as poverty, gender inequality, racism and xenophobia, sexual discrimination, population movement, and so on, HIV prevention experts talked increasingly of the need to simultaneously tackle *social vulnerability* and *individual risk* (UNAIDS 1998). Attention has moved progressively toward the broader political, economic, and social factors influencing social vulnerability to HIV.

Bride price, lack of inheritance rights, violence, sexual abuse, and gender inequality were among the key factors identified as causing women throughout sub-Saharan Africa to be especially vulnerable to HIV (Lawson 1999). In the United States, racial inequalities are among the many influences causing Black and Hispanic peoples to be disproportionately represented among HIV cases (Millett *et al.* 2006, 2011; Mizuno *et al.* 2012). Religious and cultural homophobia throughout Asia, Africa, and Latin America is responsible for making men who have sex with men unable to access the services they need (Beyrer 2008; van Griensven *et al.* 2009). In many locations worldwide, criminalization of drug use contributes to HIV risk (Kerr *et al.* 2005).

By the early 2000s, the frame of reference had begun to shift to social exclusion and human rights. Lack of access to housing, employment, as well as health and other services was viewed as contributing to the heightened vulnerability to HIV among injecting drug users, refugees, internally displaced people, and other mobile populations. The criminalization of sex work and drug use was seen as contributing to sex workers' and drug users' continuing vulnerability to HIV. Lack of concern for human rights, including the right to education, was seen as influencing the increased risks that many young people faced.

The World AIDS Campaigns of 2001 and 2002 ensured a clearer focus on the interface between the structural and the behavioural determinants of HIV-related vulnerability and risk. Through their emphasis on the nature and origins of HIV-related stigma, they drew attention to the deep-seated causes of discrimination and social exclusion. In a highly influential paper, Parker and Aggleton (2003) argued that contrary to popular belief, stigmatizing responses to HIV have their origins less in the minds and behaviours of 'bad' individuals (although individuals may be involved in their expression) than in the deeper inequalities of society.

Negative social responses to HIV are influenced by the inequalities of gender, age, class, race, and sexuality that structure much of social life today. As Jonathan Mann (1987) so aptly put it nearly 30 years ago, HIV has the capacity to systematically exploit the fault lines of an already unequal world. But if HIV-related stigma and discrimination drew attention to the negative aspects of the epidemic, the responses of diverse communities highlighted the potential for HIV to do 'good', triggering solidarity, compassion, and care.

In a review of the responses of diverse community groups such as The AIDS Support Organization (TASO) in Uganda, Grupo Pela Vidda in Brazil, the Sonagachi Project in India, and the Gay Men's Health Crisis in New York, Aggleton (2002) was able to identify a number of factors each of these responses had in common. These included (1) dense and overlapping networks of membership and communication; (2) the presence of individual and community trust; (3) a pervasive sense of inequity and injustice that calls for a response; and (4) cultural templates of success in the form of community initiatives that others can emulate. Positive responses such as these – on a global scale – have literally made HIV and AIDS unlike any disease before it. The global and local response to HIV has been and remains exceptional in many respects.

There also has been growing interest in structural approaches to HIV prevention (see, for example, Auerbach *et al.* 2011; Rao Gupta *et al.* 2008; Sumartojo 2000).

These approaches seek to change political, economic, social, cultural, organizational, and environmental factors affecting HIV-related risk. While different frameworks for understanding exist (see Rao Gupta *et al.* 2008 for a recent review), HIV prevalence has been shown to be associated with migration and location of residence (Gould 1993; Lurie *et al.* 2003), past exposure to domestic violence, and being orphaned, among other variables (Hallman 2005; Ravi *et al.* 2007). Structural factors act as barriers to individually oriented forms of HIV prevention. Thus, the fear and/or experience of HIV-related stigma and discrimination may discourage people from disclosing their HIV serostatus (Maman and Medley 2007), seeking HIV counselling and testing (Kalichman and Simbayi 2003), and negotiating condom use (Jewkes *et al.* 2006).

Structural programming addresses factors influencing individual behaviour rather than the behaviour itself. Examples of different instances of structural intervention include legal actions to combat discriminatory practices, such as the repeal in 2009 of Section 377 of the Indian Penal Code, which hitherto criminalized homosexual activity but was then adjudged to violate the rights to life, liberty, and equality as guaranteed by the Constitution of India (Misra 2009). Other structural interventions, such as the IMAGE study in South Africa, have provided women with microcredit to start their own income-generating activities, reducing intimate partner violence and lessening women's dependency on men (Pronyk *et al.* 2008) (see Chapter 14, Pronyk *et al.* in this volume).

The Sonagachi Project in Kolkata was a community-oriented programme to address the needs of sex workers (see Chapter 10, Swendeman and Jana, in this volume). By mobilizing and empowering sex worker groups by responding to the community's expressed needs, the project was able to build the kinds of trust and reciprocity that are central to HIV prevention success. Likewise, efforts to promote risk reduction among injecting drug users through clean syringe and needle exchange programmes have a structural component. Not only do they require policy and legal changes in countries where the possession or use of certain drugs is illegal, but they also seek to intervene in the environment surrounding drug injection by providing users with access to clean needles, syringes, and equipment, thereby reducing infection risk.

It would, however, be wrong to think that structural programmes and interventions imply that individuals play no role in reducing their HIV risk and vulnerability. It is the interplay between the individual and the wider community or society – between agency and structure – that demonstrates the potential of people to change their worlds. Using three case studies that describe efforts to address HIV risk reduction, each within the Canadian context (which is sometimes erroneously assumed to be or portrayed as relatively free of inequities in HIV risk), we will illustrate the intimate relationship between structure and the actions of individuals and communities, highlighting how it is vital to take these factors into account when devising and evaluating interventions.

Sex work

Sex work offers the opportunity to reveal the mechanisms and processes implicated in actions and responses that attempt to balance the need to address risk at multiple levels, including the individual or interpersonal levels (e.g. social norms), institutional or organizational levels (e.g. community mobilization), and at the structural level (e.g.

legal reforms and innovative housing/workplace models related to sex work). The aim of this first case study is to illustrate the potential for structural interventions to be linked to other types of programme strategies (e.g. grassroots, community-based actions) to address multiple forms of inequality, including the risk of violence, which is frequently linked to HIV and sex work. The examples show how interventions that address structure need not be conceptualized or actualized as attempts by experts to limit the agentic practices of vulnerable subgroups in an effort to 'improve' behaviour in the name of reducing HIV risk. They highlight how those who are relatively privileged (e.g. researchers) and those who are less privileged (e.g. sex workers) can *both* have roles in creating spaces where the modus operandi of most previous interventions (i.e. 'targeting' intervention recipients with primarily individualized prevention strategies) is re-balanced.

Linking structural intervention and agentic practice

Although the buying and selling of sex itself have never been illegal in Canada, legislation passed by the Federal Government in 1985 prohibits communication or solicitation for the purposes of sexual transaction in public spaces (Goodyear *et al.* 2005; Lowman 2000, 2004). The law also prohibits living off the avails of prostitution, or operating a brothel, which severely limits sex workers' abilities to work indoors in safer and quasi-supervised settings (Pivot Legal Society 2004). Together, these laws ensure that sex work takes place within a largely prohibitive environment.

Growing research both in Canada and globally suggests that approaches that focus on arrest and prosecution detrimentally affect sex workers, pushing them beyond the reach of public health. Policy dialogue and actions have focused on removal of criminal sanctions surrounding prostitution as a promising means for addressing harms and promoting agency in negotiating risks, such as HIV, among sex workers (Goodyear and Cusick 2007). In 2009, two legal challenges were launched in Canada calling for removal of key criminal code provisions related to prostitution as a violation of the Canadian Charter of Rights and Freedom, particularly the security of the person.

In late 2010, Ontario's provincial court struck down important provisions in Canada's prostitution laws, specifically those against keeping a common bawdy house, communicating for the purposes of prostitution, and living on the avails of the trade. The landmark Ontario ruling drastically changed the landscape related to structural interventions (e.g. criminalized prostitution laws) and simultaneously marked empowered roles for sex workers in creating policy dialogue and space for structural-level change (e.g. legal reforms).

Although opinions differ among reform advocates, a basic tenet that seems to apply across stakeholders is that successful legal reforms must acknowledge sex workers' agentic practices (e.g. their right to work in safe environments) while concomitantly addressing structural-level factors (e.g. vulnerability to prosecution for soliciting) that constrain agency. Linking the ways in which structural interventions and agency can be simultaneously expressed and valued is integral to efforts to reduce HIV vulnerability amongst sex workers and their clients – something that is particularly important in the area of street-based sex work, considering its associated symbolic, structural and cultural/social violence (Amnesty International 2004; Cler-Cunningham and Christensen 2001).

Balancing outsider and insider contributions

Much has been written about the importance of participatory action research and the value of partnerships with marginalized populations, emphasizing the need to reduce power imbalances between 'outside experts' and 'insider experts' (Bernier *et al.* 2006). Community-based HIV prevention research partnerships initiated in 2005 between the British Columbia Centre for Excellence in HIV/AIDS and sex work organizations have attempted to offer an alternative to conventional public health approaches to HIV risk reduction by recognizing knowledge as co-constructed through the 'lived experiences' of sex workers, the 'insiders', and researchers, the 'outsiders'. Current and former sex workers have also been employed to engage in leadership and implementation of all aspects of these projects, from conceptualization and the development of research questions, to joint research and operational programming, and knowledge translation in the form of community dialogues, policy briefs, and research dissemination.

The emphasis is on action being research-driven and informed by community and theory alike, with value placed on documenting the lived experiences of sex workers and the complex and dynamic pathways between upstream and downstream effects of structural processes, agentic practices, and negotiations of HIV risk. In this way, these efforts illustrate how structural actions, such as interventions, are not solely something that experts 'do' to other so-called vulnerable subgroups, but rather that grassroots, community-based actions are integral to addressing any and all forms of HIV risk, including structural, cultural/social, and symbolic forms of violence. These approaches also illustrate how those who are relatively privileged, such as the researchers, have an important role to play in creating spaces where agency can be expressed and valued.

Injecting drug use

Numerous factors exogenous to the individual interact with agentic practices to increase vulnerability to HIV among injecting drug users. Concomitantly, agency and structure affect interventions to ameliorate injection-related HIV risk. In particular, among people who inject drugs, structural factors may act as barriers to individually oriented forms of HIV prevention, producing unintended and untoward consequences. To explore these issues in some depth, we will use examples from Vancouver, Canada to demonstrate how well-intentioned interventions such as needle and syringe exchange often fail to address structural realities, thereby failing to reach their full potential and sometimes resulting in unintended negative outcomes such as elevated HIV risk and increased HIV incidence. The cases chosen highlight the complexities of the interplay between agency and structure, noting that each alone is a necessary, but insufficient, condition for successful HIV reduction programming.

Structural barriers to individual–oriented prevention

Providing sterile syringes to people who inject drugs is now widely regarded as an essential component of an evidence-informed public health response. It is frequently characterized as a strategy that targets specific behaviours (e.g. the borrowing and lending of used syringes) that are affected by both agency and structural factors. However, even as these intervention efforts attempt to address the nexus of structure and agentic practices, a failure to address a fulsome set of structural features (e.g. policing practice, trends in drug use, norms within injecting communities, illegalities related to drug possession) can limit the effectiveness of structural interventions and produce unintended *elevations* in HIV risk.

In Vancouver, for example, early efforts to decrease syringe sharing focused on one-for-one needle *exchange*, rather than clean syringe distribution (without exchange requirements), in large part due to concerns among local residents and businesses that the programme would prompt an increase in discarded syringes in the neighbourhood. In the face of local concern, only one fixed syringe outlet was opened. Coincident with a local rise in cocaine injection (a drug which is typically injected many times per day due to its short half-life), the limited scope of syringe provision as a singularly robust HIV risk intervention was revealed (Strathdee *et al.* 1997; Wood *et al.* 2002).

Even after programmatic changes were made to redress rules such as one-for-one exchange, police crackdowns and other police practices, for example searches resulting in syringe confiscation, fuelled a reluctance to access sterile syringe sources as well as syringe borrowing (Werb *et al.* 2008; Wood *et al.* 2003). Even as more cutting-edge interventions, such as a supervised injecting sites, have emerged in Vancouver, the combination of the cultural logics of local injectors (e.g. injection in public spaces), rules governing the site (lack of assisted injecting) (Small *et al.* 2007), and ongoing criminalization of drug use, make the sustained reduction of blood-borne HIV infection risk among drug users a vexing proposition.

Sustaining HIV risk reduction

The case of injecting drug use also highlights the complex interaction between agency and structure, whereby no single intervention to alter legal and regulatory mechanisms, improve operational features of public health interventions, or even reorient local drug-using cultures is sufficient for producing the conditions required for successful and sustained HIV risk reduction.

Part of the complexity here lies in the fact that the interactions between agency and structure in this realm have great potential to constrain conventional public health efforts and produce unanticipated outcomes (e.g. increased police presence within public injecting venues, such as alleys, leading to rushed and increasingly unsafe injection practices to avoid arrest). Adding to this intricacy is the fact that many structural factors thought to contribute to HIV risk within the Vancouver context are rooted in sectors other than public health and, in particular, within the criminal justice system.

Taking action to reduce HIV risk thereby demands yet another set of actors to be engaged and mobilized to act, for example by advocating for legal reforms regarding drug possession or altering norms that promote confrontational dynamics between injectors and the police. Well beyond the immediate influence of public health, the sustained reduction of HIV risk is inextricably linked to these and other interventions, which demand both structural and individual actions. Each of those links to other sectors reveals a fresh set of structural-level constraints, including political risks, bureaucratic recalcitrance, and stigma and discrimination toward injecting drug users.

Young people and sexuality

Young people who identify as lesbian, gay, bisexual, transgender, or queer (LGBTQ) in Canada have improved health compared to previous generations (Houzeau and Ryan 2011; Ryan and Futterman 2001). However, their HIV risk remains shaped by social context and structural conditions, as well as by their individual behaviour (Groneberg and Funke 2011). The complexity of navigating HIV risk as sexual lives become established is exacerbated for some young people who are either learning to hide their sexuality or cope with a stigmatized identity (Saewyc 2011). Compared to their heterosexual peers, some LGBTQ youth remain at increased risk of HIV as well as various forms of social alienation, discrimination, and violence (McCreary Centre Society 2007).

Recent experiences provide an opportunity to examine actions that aim to address discrimination through social cohesion and social change by addressing cultural and social norms (Shoveller *et al.* 2006), while simultaneously improving knowledge and individual decision-making skills. CampOUT! is a social, health, and educational intervention designed to improve health and reduce HIV risk for young people who are LGBTQ – as well as their heterosexual allies – who live in British Columbia, Canada. It aims to tackle simultaneously social vulnerability *and* individual risk by promoting solidarity, compassion, and caring social norms. The initiative focuses on enhancing aspects of social and cultural capital required for successful and healthful lives beyond the camp experience. It adopts a strengths-based, rather than a 'deficit-fixing' approach to enhancing young people's sexual rights.

Social cohesion and social change

As an emphasis on the structural determinants of HIV risk has grown, so too have efforts to address its inherently cultural and ideological aspects (e.g. homophobia). Although more attention has been paid to the ways in which these social aspects structure adult populations' HIV risk (e.g. through the work of Gay Men's Health Crisis in New York), some new actions hold promise for addressing social cohesion and social change to reduce HIV risk among young people. In CampOUT!, for example, approximately 60 camper members (LGBTQ youth ages 14–21) as well as youth and adult camp leaders (both LGBTQ and allies) have the opportunity to explore and understand the health, social, spiritual, and educational issues and concerns facing sexual minority individuals. Leadership skills are honed to realize personal potential and to create social change to address homophobia and heterosexism. As an action designed to address social cohesion and inspire social change, the camp asks every participant – including campers, camp leaders, advisory committee members, and sponsors – to make a commitment to apply and share their new knowledge and skills (including HIV risk reduction) and to help and improve their 'home' communities. Each year, the camp receives extensive and positive media coverage, ultimately normalizing and contributing to the de-stigmatization of non-heterosexual identities.

Social and cultural capital

Together, the camp's sponsors and partners (e.g. financial institutions, community organizations, media outlets, the University of British Columbia) simultaneously generate and deploy significant amounts of social and cultural capital to promote social change and reduce homophobia and heterosexism. In using material and symbolic resources, the camp and its supporters also aim to alter other institutions, including the educational system, by promoting Gay-Straight Alliances and attempting to influence curriculum content (although much progress remains to be achieved there).

Camp planners have been challenged to 'get the balance right' with regards to agency and structure. Stressing agency in some aspects (e.g. by asserting that everyone has a unique path along which to contribute to positive social change that better protects young people's rights to healthy sexual lives), the camp also emphasizes engagement with social structures. For example, campers are invited to engage in critical and innovative ways by connecting with the wider community (e.g. peers, friends and families) and institutions (e.g. schools and the health care system) to build solidarity and compassion as means to address HIV, and to promote a rights-based approach to young people and sexuality.

CampOUT! offers a promising strategy to address social norms and institutional/structural-level changes related to homophobia and heterosexism, but it has yet to be rigorously evaluated in terms of its capacity to reduce HIV risk. Evaluation of these kinds of actions is challenging regarding study design and funding, and novel public health intervention research methods. For example, advances in quasi-experimentation may be required to deal appropriately with the complexities associated with documenting the impact of these kinds of HIV risk prevention actions. What this type of action does indicate, however, is the importance of attempting to concomitantly address the *interactions* between structure and agency (Rhodes and Simic 2005), particularly within everyday practices.

Some concluding comments

This chapter stresses the importance of striking the balance between agency and structure in HIV prevention and, like others (Rao Gupta *et al.* 2008; Strathdee *et al.* 2010), we argue that the greatest traction for reducing HIV risk exists at the *nexus* of structure and agency. However, theoretical, methodological, political, and philosophical challenges remain in appreciating how HIV risk is shaped concomitantly by structural and agentic practices (Rhodes 2009). The frameworks outlined in Auerbach *et al.* (2011) offer promise in this respect, by distinguishing more clearly between causal processes and units of change in the theorization of how particular outcomes may be achieved, and by outlining the kinds of information needed at different implementation stages.

Rooted in grassroots experiences globally and from within Canada, there is good evidence for promoting actions that draw on a multiplicity of strategies – combining the strengths of structural and agentic approaches for any given setting and/or population of interest. Getting the balance right between structure and agency in HIV prevention is likely to demand much of researchers and interventionists in terms of theory development and interdisciplinary application (Blankenship *et al.* 2006) to fully implement the vision of *combined* approaches. It is not our view, however, that such an exercise need be academic or 'scholastic', especially when rooted in the experiences of diverse communities and affected groups globally, and when conducted in partnership with community organizations working closely with and for such groups.

As the HIV epidemic morphs and as contexts change, so too must actions to address HIV-related vulnerability and risk. The progression from basic syringe and needle exchange approaches to more comprehensive, complex, and encompassing interventions illustrates how the structure–agency nexus can be addressed to continually improve efforts to more effectively address injecting drug use and HIV risk. Likewise, recent projects on sex work and HIV in Canada highlight the necessity of working closely with community groups to ensure that agentic practice can become the motor for more enduring structural change. Forging alliances – both structurally and in terms of meaningful partnerships with individual actors – is also central to success, as our work with LGBTQ young people and their allies demonstrates.

Finally, the case examples described above, as well as additional examples in other settings, demonstrate that a strictly linear approach may be insufficient – and in some instances harmful – to addressing structure and agency as they affect HIV-related vulnerability and risk (Auerbach *et al.* 2011). Successful interventions depend upon an emergent knowledge base that sufficiently accounts for the real-world and ever-changing complexities associated with getting the balance right between structure and agency.

Acknowledgements

We would like to acknowledge Taylor Basso for his assistance in preparing the manuscript.

References

Aggleton, P. (2002) 'Towards a new paradigm for prevention success: the importance of social capital', Background paper prepared for an Expert Consultation on Social Exclusion, Social Capital and HIV/AIDS, Coppet, Switzerland, 24 October 2002.

Auerbach, J., Parkhurst, J., and Caceres, C. (2011) 'Addressing social drivers of HIV/AIDS for the long-term response: conceptual and methodological considerations', *Global Public Health*, 6 (Supplement 3): S293–309.

Amnesty International (2004) *Stolen Sisters: A Human Rights Response to Violence and Discrimination against Indigenous Women in Canada*, Ottowa: Amnesty International Canada.

Bernier, J., Rock, M., Roy, M., Bujold, R., and Potvin, L. (2006) 'Structuring an inter-sector research partnership: a negotiated zone', *Social and Preventive Medicine*, 51: 335–44.

Beyrer, C. (2008) 'Hidden yet happening: the epidemics of sexually transmitted infections and HIV among men who have sex with men in developing countries', *Sexually Transmitted Infections*, 84 (6): 410–12.

Blankenship, K.M., Friedman, S.R., Dworkin, S., and Mantell, J.E. (2006) 'Structural interventions: concepts, challenges, and opportunities for research', *Journal of Urban Health*, 83: 59–72.

Cler-Cunningham, L. and Christensen, C. (2001) *Violence Against Women in Vancouver's Street-level Sex Trade and the Police Response*, Vancouver: Providing Alternatives Counselling and Education Society.

Dowsett, G. and Aggleton, P. (1999) 'Young people and risk-taking in sexual relations', in Joint United Nations Programme on HIV/AIDS (ed.) *Sex and Youth: Contextual Factors Affecting Risk for HIV/AIDS*, Geneva: Joint United Nations Programme on HIV/AIDS. Online, available at: http://data.unaids.org/Publications/IRC-pub01/jc096-sex_youth_en.pdf (accessed 23 April 2012).

Goodyear, M. and Cusick, L. (2007) 'Protection of sex workers', *British Medical Journal*, 334: 52–3.

Goodyear, M., Lowman, J., Fischer, B., and Green, M. (2005) 'Prostitutes are people too', *The Lancet*, 366: 1264–5.

Gould, P. (1993) *The Slow Plague: A Geography of the AIDS Epidemic*, Oxford: Blackwell.

Groneberg, M. and Funke, C. (eds) (2011) *Combatting Homophobia: Experiences and Analyses Pertinent to Education*, Berlin: Lit Verlag.

Hallman, K. (2005) 'The effects of orphaning and poverty on sexual debut in KwaZulu Natal, South Africa', IUSSP Seminar on Poverty and AIDS, University of Cape Town, South Africa, 12–14 December 2005.

Houzeau, M. and Ryan, B. (2011) 'Translating legal equality to school reality in Canada', in M. Groneberg and C. Funke (eds), *Combatting Homophobia: Experiences and Analyses Pertinent to Education*, Berlin: Lit Verlag.

Ingham, R. and van Zessen, G. (1997) 'Towards an alternative model of sexual behaviour', in M. Cohen, G. Guizzardi, D. Hausser, and L. Van Campenhoudt (eds) *Sexual Interactions and HIV Risk: New Conceptual Perspectives in European Research*, London: Taylor and Francis.

Jewkes, R., Dunkle, K., Nduna, M., Levin, J., Jama, N., Khuzwayo, N., Koss, M., Puren, A., and Duvvury, N. (2006) 'Factors associated with HIV serostatus in young rural South African women: connections between intimate partner violence and HIV', *International Journal of Epidemiology*, 35: 1461–8.

Joint United Nations Programme on HIV/AIDS (UNAIDS) (1998) *Expanding the Global Response to HIV/AIDS through Focused Action. Reducing Risk and Vulnerability: Definitions, Rationale and Pathways*, Geneva: Joint United Nations Programme on HIV/AIDS.

Kalichman, S. and Simbayi, L. (2003) 'HIV testing attitudes, AIDS stigma, and voluntary HIV counselling and testing in a black township in Cape Town, South Africa', *Sexually Transmitted Infections*, 79 (6): 442–7.

Kerr, T., Small, W., and Wood, E. (2005) 'The public health and social impacts of drug market enforcement: a review of the evidence', *International Journal of Drug Policy*, 16: 210–20.

Lawson, A.L.-G. (1999) 'Women and AIDS in Africa: sociocultural dimensions of the HIV/AIDS epidemic', *International Social Science Journal*, 51: 391–400

Lowman, J. (2000) 'Violence and the outlaw status of (street) prostitution in Canada', *Violence Against Women*, 6: 987–1011.

Lowman, J. (2004) 'Reconvening the federal committee on prostitution law reform', *Canadian Medical Association Journal*, 171: 47.

Lurie, M., Williams, B., Zuma, K., Mkaya-Mwamburi, D., Garnett, G., Sturm, A.W., Sweat, M.D., Gittelsohn, J., and Abdool Karim, S.S. (2003) 'The impact of migration on HIV transmission in South Africa', *Sexually Transmitted Diseases*, 30: 149–56.

Maman, S. and Medley, A. (2007) *HIV Status Disclosure to Sexual Partners: Barriers and Outcomes for Women*, Geneva: World Health Organization, Department of Gender and Women's Health.

Mann, J. (1987) Statement at an informal briefing on AIDS to the 42nd Session of the United Nations General Assembly, 20 October, New York.

McCreary Centre Society (2007) *Not Yet Equal: The Health of Lesbian, Gay, & Bisexual Youth in BC*, Vancouver: McCreary Centre Society.

Millett, G.A., Peterson, J.L., Wolitski, R.J., and Stall, R. (2006) 'Greater risk for HIV infection of black men who have sex with men: a critical literature review', *American Journal of Public Health*, 96 (6): 1007–19.

Millett, G.A., Ding, H., Marks, G., Jeffries, W.L., Bingham, T., Lauby, J., Murrill, C., Flores, S., and Stueve, A. (2011) 'Mistaken assumptions and missed opportunities: correlates of undiagnosed HIV infection among black and Latino men who have sex with men', *Journal of Acquired Immune Deficiency Syndrome*, 58 (1): 64–71.

Misra, G. (2009) 'Decriminalising homosexuality in India', *Reproductive Health Matters*, 17 (34): 20–8.

Mizuno, Y., Borkowf, C., Millett, G.A., Bingham, T., Ayala, G., and Stueve, A. (2012) 'Homophobia and racism experienced by Latino men who have sex with men in the United States: correlates of exposure and associations with HIV risk behaviors', *AIDS & Behavior*, 16 (3): 724–35.

Parker, R. and Aggleton, P. (2003) 'HIV and AIDS-related stigma and discrimination: a conceptual framework and implications for action', *Social Science & Medicine*, 57: 13–24.

Pivot Legal Society (2004) *Voices for Dignity: A Call to End the Harms Caused by Canada's Sex Trade Laws*, Vancouver: Pivot Legal Society.

Pronyk, P., Kim, J., Abramsky, T., Phetla, G., Hargreaves, J., and Morison, L., (2008) 'A combined microfinance and training intervention can reduce HIV risk behaviour in young female participants', *AIDS*, 22 (13): 1659–65.

Rao Gupta, G., Parkhurst, J.O., Ogden, J.A., Aggleton, P., and Mahal, A. (2008) 'Structural approaches to HIV prevention', *The Lancet*, 372: 764–75.

Ravi, A., Blankenship, K., and Altice, F.L. (2007) 'The association between history of violence and HIV risk: a cross-sectional study of female prisoners in Connecticut', *Journal of Women's Health Issues*, 17 (4): 210–16.

Rhodes, T. (2009) 'Risk environments and drug harms: a social science for harm reduction approach', *International Journal of Drug Policy*, 20: 193–201.

Rhodes, T. and Simic, M. (2005) 'Transition and the HIV risk environment', *British Medical Journal*, 331: 220–3.

Ryan, C. and Futterman, D. (2001) 'Social and developmental challenges for lesbian, gay and bisexual youth', *SIECUS Report*, 29: 5–18.

Saewyc, E.M. (2011) 'Research on adolescent sexual orientation: development, health disparities, stigma, and resilience', *Journal of Research on Adolescence*, 21: 256–72.

Shoveller, J.A., Johnson, J.L., Savoy, D.M., and Wia Pietersma, W.A. (2006) 'Preventing sexually transmitted infections among adolescents: an assessment of ecological approaches and study methods', *Sex Education*, 6: 163–83.

Small, W., Rhodes, T., Wood, E., and Kerr, T. (2007) 'Public injection settings in Vancouver: physical environment, social context and risk', *International Journal of Drug Policy*, 18: 27–36.

Strathdee, S.A., Patrick, D.M., Currie, S.L., Cornelisse, P.G., Rekart, M.L., Montaner, J.S., Schechter, M.T., and O'Shaughnessy, M.V. (1997) 'Needle exchange is not enough: lessons from the Vancouver injecting drug use study', *AIDS*, 11 (8): F59–65.

Strathdee, S.A., Hallett, T.B., Bobrova, N., Rhodes, T., Booth, R., Abdool, R., and Hankins, C.A. (2010) 'HIV and risk environment for injecting drug users: the past, present, and future', *The Lancet*, 376: 268–84.

Sumartojo, E., 2000. 'Structural factors in HIV prevention: concepts, examples, and implications for research', *AIDS*, 14 (Suppl. 1): S3–10.

Tawil, O., Vester, K., and O'Reilly, K.R. (1995) 'Enabling approaches for HIV/AIDS prevention: can we modify the environment and reduce the risk?', *AIDS*, 9: 1299–306.

Van Griensven, F., de Lind van Wijngaarden, J.W., Baral, S., and Grulich A. (2009) 'The global epidemic of HIV infection among men who have sex with men', *Current Opinion in HIV and AIDS*, 4 (4): 300–7.

Werb, D., Wood, E., Small, W., Strathdee, S., Li, K., Montaner, J., and Kerr, T. (2008) 'Effects of police confiscation of illicit drugs and syringes among injection drug users in Vancouver', *International Journal of Drug Policy*, 19: 332–8.

Wood, E., Tyndall, M.W., Spittal P.M., Li, K., Hogg, R.S., O'Shaughnessy, M.V., and Schechter, M.T. (2002) 'Needle exchange and difficulty with needle access during an ongoing HIV epidemic', *International Journal of Drug Policy*, 13: 95–102.

Wood, E., Kerr, T., Small, W., Jones, J., Schechter, M.T., and Tyndall, M.W. (2003) 'The impact of police presence on access to needle exchange programs', *Journal of AIDS*, 34: 116–18.

World Health Organization (WHO) (2011) *The Ottawa Charter for Health Promotion*. Online, available at: http://www.who.int/healthpromotion/conferences/previous/ottawa/en/index.html (accessed 15 August 2011).

Part 2

DESIGNING AND IMPLEMENTING STRUCTURAL INTERVENTIONS

7

INTEGRATING WATER AND SANITATION INTERVENTIONS FOR HEALTH

A case study from eThekwini Municipality

Elisa Roma, Neil Macleod, and Christopher Buckley

Introduction

South Africa is a country of many contrasts. Although classified as a middle-income economy with a GDP of R710 billion (mid–2011 estimates) (StatsSA 2011), South Africa has an income Gini coefficient of 57.8, with 26.9 per cent of its 50.5 million population living with a purchasing power parity of US $1.25 per day or less (UNDP 2010). The image of South Africa as a progressive nation clashes with figures reporting 23 per cent (11,615,000) of its population lack access to basic sanitation and 9 per cent (4,455,000) have no access to appropriate water (UNDP 2010).

Analysis of eThekwini Municipality's strategy to provide basic water and sanitation cannot occur without its contextualization within South African political and socio-economic history. Today's picture of South Africa partly reflects the legacy left by apartheid (1948–94), where poverty and inequality were mirrored in the scant provision of basic services that prioritized the needs of selected minorities (Earle *et al.* 2005). Service policies implemented until 1994 left a skewed distribution of water and sanitation (WATSAN) services, with 12 million people lacking adequate supplies of drinking water and 21 million people lacking basic sanitation (DWAF 1994). At the dawn of the new democracy, the government led by the African National Congress acknowledged the importance of restoring balance by equally providing basic services to all citizens, among which the improvement of water and sanitation was a pivotal response to poverty and social underdevelopment. This aspiration for change in South Africa is reflected in its Bill of Rights (1996) and the legal framework, as well as the principle of 'some for all' rather than 'all for some' adopted in the country's WATSAN service delivery policy (DWAF 1994: 8).

The national response to address backlogs in WATSAN service delivery has shown promising results, with a reported increase in access to water infrastructures from 59 per cent in 1994 to 97 per cent in 2009, and access to sanitation from 49 per cent in 1994 to 79 per cent in 2009 (DWAF 2010). Although remarkable, these numbers not only report delivery statistics which do not take into account system quality, but also are insufficient to achieve the nation's ambitious goal of providing universal access by 2014. National progress in service delivery, in fact, struggles to keep up with challenges dictated by fast-paced urban migration, increased water demand in water stressed conditions, and a background of high incidences of human immunodeficiency virus (HIV) and tuberculosis (TB).

This chapter reviews the main challenges faced by South Africa in improving health and WATSAN conditions of the poor, and the structural approaches undertaken to address these challenges, by presenting the case study of one of its most progressive municipalities: eThekwini. A discussion of eThekwini's strategic approach in addressing the provision of basic water and sanitation is preceded by analysis of those structural changes in the national legislation that shaped the municipality's interventions.

Structural changes to the nation's water and sanitation framework

During apartheid, the economic divide between the rich and the poor coincided with the demarcation between those with access to adequate piped water and sewerage systems and those without. The democratic reconstruction of the country in 1994 focused on formalizing citizens' right to water and sanitation and establishing access to these services according to the principle of equity. The *Water Supply and Sanitation Policy* white paper on community water and sanitation (DWAF 1994) set the premise for such an equitable policy by endorsing the principle of 'some service for all' to describe the access to basic WATSAN services as a human right for all citizens, irrespective of their race, and pledged to fulfil this promise by 2001 (DWAF 1994). Furthermore, although sanitation had just materialized on the national political agenda, basic sanitation was defined as a household ventilated improved pit (VIP) latrine, constructed according to agreed standards. The right to access basic water and sanitation outlined in the white paper was reiterated with legal enforcement into the Constitution of the new Republic of South Africa (RSA 1996).

The achievement of universal basic water and sanitation provision was strategically orchestrated through the reorganization of municipalities' structures to devolve them greater responsibilities and make them financially viable for service provision. One of the legacies inherited from the previous government was a provincial and municipal demarcation defined according to racial lines to manage segregation and limit the burden of service provision (Cottle and Deedat 2002). Thus, the process of boundary redefinition served the purpose of expanding equitable service provision to reach all racial groups. The Water Service Act 108 of 1997 (RSA 1997) was the legislative base that substantiated the constitutional rights to access to basic WATSAN services for all. Furthermore, the Act assigned to those municipalities designated as Water Service Authorities (WSAs) the responsibility for providing access to at least basic water and sanitation within the national policy context.

Although considerable progress has been made, by the end of 2001 the government's pledge of free basic WATSAN services to all was clearly proving to be a daunting task, with 18 million people still estimated to lack access to sanitation (DWAF 2001). Moreover, WATSAN service demand was exceeding municipalities' ability to supply, leading to increasing backlogs. Acknowledging the struggle of the indigent population in affording water and sanitation, President Mbeki announced a free basic WATSAN policy provision, consisting of 6 kilolitres of drinking water per household per month (DWAF 2001). The Free Basic Water programme was funded by the national government through equitable share schemes (i.e. financial arrangements paid to municipalities for provision of basic services) and infrastructure grants for municipalities as well as from internal subsidies from water tariffs.

The innovative decision-making progress initiated with Mbeki's pledge was further highlighted by the severe cholera epidemic threatening the lives of thousands of poor South Africans. This public health threat for the first time brought an urgent national focus on sanitation issues. In the second *White Paper for Water and Sanitation* (DWAF 2001), the government redefined the concept of sanitation to incorporate not only its hardware (technical aspects) but also its software components (health and hygiene awareness and behaviour). The principles of free basic water and sanitation outlined in the paper were formalized in the *Strategic Framework for Water Services* (DWAF 2003), which set a strategic vision by pledging the achievement of new national targets – basic water for all by 2008 and basic sanitation for all by 2010 (DWAF 2001) – and outlining the necessity of incorporating health and hygiene promotion in the sanitation subsidy. The *Strategic Framework for Water Services* defined basic water and sanitation provision as the first step in the service ladder and requested WSAs to provide higher service levels (i.e. household waterborne sanitation and ground tank supply) where technically and financially feasible (DWAF 2010).

Challenges to water and sanitation provision in eThekwini

eThekwini Municipality (EM) is located within KwaZulu-Natal province and occupies an area of 2,297 square kilometres, with a population of 3.5 million (StatsSA 2007). Established in December 2001, EM incorporated the seven local authorities in the previous Durban metropolitan area as well as part of the old Ugu, Ndlovu, and Ilembe regional council areas. As a result of this reorganization, in 2002 eThekwini became the municipal WSA, with the eThekwini Water and Sanitation Unit (EWS) acting as the area's water service provider, responsible for taking measures to address the universal right to free basic water and sanitation within its jurisdiction (EWS 2004).

Since 2002, EWS has embraced a progressive response in adapting national legislation to address environmental challenges and water and sanitation demand, quantified in the backlogs of 205,947 households lacking sanitation, and 54,292 households without water in June 2011 (Figure 7.1). These challenges, having originated in political, environmental, and socio-economic dynamics, are discussed in the following sub-sections.

Boundary expansion and urbanization

In the past decade, EM has undergone a profound geo-political reorganization which has significantly impacted on the management of WATSAN demand within its jurisdiction. As a result of a two-staged expansion process begun in 1996, eThekwini municipal boundaries were enlarged by 68 per cent of their original size, with a population increase of 9 per cent (Figure 7.2). Within this process eThekwini incorporated 75,000 new households, 80 per cent of which were not served by adequate water and sanitation (Gounden *et al.* 2006). This progressive reorganization, enacted to redistribute resources to poorer peripheries, generated immense equity challenges for the provision water and sanitation to unserved people and management of existing infrastructures to a dispersed population (Eales 2010).

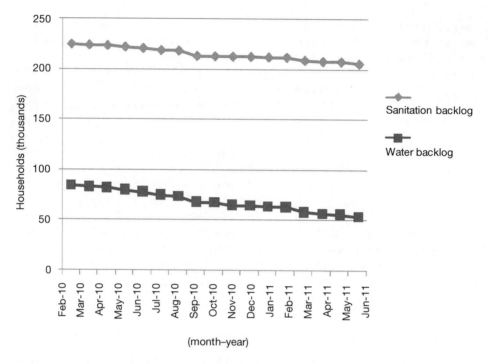

Figure 7.1 Household WATSAN backlog (based on 2007 population)

Source: EWS 2011a

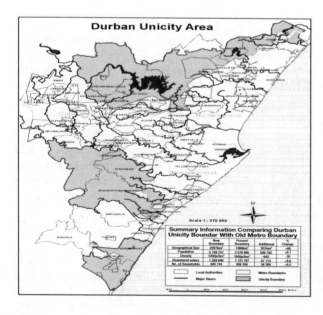

Figure 7.2
eThekwini boundary expansion

Source: EM 2008, reproduced with permission

The incorporation of new areas was accompanied by environmental challenges, health risks and infrastructural problems such as lack of sanitation coverage, and lack of health and hygiene education. In the years immediately preceding the expansion, the province of KwaZulu-Natal was plagued by a cholera epidemic, with official provincial statistics reporting 105,389 cases and 219 documented deaths (case fatality rate = 0.21 per cent) for the period from August 2000 to July 2001 (Mudzanani *et al.* 2003). The city of Durban itself recorded 2,456 cases with a case fatality rate of 1.18 per cent (DOH 2001). Several risk factors were associated with this epidemic: inefficient health services in rural areas; use of contaminated water from highly polluted rivers for drinking purposes; inappropriate water storage techniques; poor sanitation coverage; and lack of appropriate hygiene behaviour, such as hand-washing (Mugeru and Hoque 2001).

The burden of expanding appropriate services to disadvantaged areas has been further exacerbated by the fast-paced urbanization process recorded since the end of apartheid. It is estimated that a quarter of eThekwini population lives in 550 densely populated (1,437 people/km^2) informal settlements, formed as result of the influx of people of African ethnicity from rural areas into Durban in search of job opportunities. Informal settlements are slums, developed within urban and peri-urban areas, characterized by semi-permanent dwellings made of corrugated iron, wood, or wattle and daub and often located in privately owned land (Marx and Charlton 2003). Lack of basic services – such as water, sanitation, electricity, and roads – often characterizes these areas. Where sanitation facilities are missing, open defecation is still widely practised.

Targeting the unserved population in informal settlements generates great pressure on EWS, especially in terms of efficient infrastructure delivery to a fast growing population (0.7 per cent per annum). Most of the people living in informal settlements have family and houses in rural areas and temporarily occupy rented shacks within easy reach of employment. In other cases, however, informal settlements became 'urban containers' for unemployed people who migrated into the city hoping for a better future. As a result of high mobility and population density and poor environmental conditions, addressing water and sanitation backlogs in informal settlements is a complicated and dynamic issue (Eales 2010).

Environmental pollution and water stress

South Africa is classified as water stressed, with an uneven availability of water resources across the country (UNEP 2002). In line with global trends, recent forecasts for eThekwini have predicted that manufacturing, chemical, and other industrial production will trigger increased water demand (EM 2007), which will eventually outpace resource availability. Concurrent with the industrial demand for water is the national mandate to provide free water and sanitation to poor citizens, who aspire to the same service standards as the rich population. For disadvantaged communities, indoor flush toilets and piped water supply are not only a service provided by the government, but also a symbol of dignity and of social redemption from the service discrimination suffered before 1994 (Eales 2008).

Beyond the demand and political pressure for water, EM faces environmental pollution and degradation of its water resources. Recent bio-monitoring programmes of its 18 main rivers revealed poor ecosystem status, with some classified as endangered, due to anthropogenic activities including illegal sand mining, industrial pollution, solid waste dumping, and wastewater contamination (EM 2011). Through the establishment of the 'Green Rivers' programme in 2010, EWS aims to improve poor river water quality by means of an integrated approach which minimizes river pollution to acceptable levels (i.e. *E. coli* 400–2000 cfu/1000mL) (EWS 2011b). One of the main causes of river pollution is reported to be the presence of informal settlements located adjacent to rivers. Particular issues are the proximity of pit latrines and wastewater pollution to communal standpipes (vertical pipes extending from water supply systems) and public taps in informal settlements. Thus, strategic sanitation interventions in disadvantaged areas significantly contribute to transforming the overall water quality of municipal watercourses.

HIV and tuberculosis

Provision of appropriate water and sanitation in South Africa is also crucial for providing care to the approximately 6 million people living with HIV (PLWH) (UNDP 2010). HIV in the country is clustered within people of African ethnicity, with infection rates of 13.9 per cent (Kane-Berman and Macfarlane 2009). Although HIV prevalence rates have decreased over the past years, the national life expectancy at birth (52.0 years) has significantly declined to levels that are lower than the least developed countries' average (57.7 years) (UNDP 2010).

KwaZulu-Natal has the highest proportion of the HIV and AIDS pandemics in the country (Day *et al.* 2010), and eThekwini has the greatest HIV prevalence among women attending antenatal clinics in the country (approximately 40 per cent) (Day *et al.* 2010). HIV prevalence must be analyzed in the context of TB infection, with PLWH being highly susceptible to TB and to extensively drug-resistant (XDR) TB. eThekwini is burdened with concurrent epidemics of HIV and TB, with the highest number of cases (40,000) recorded in 2008 (Day *et al.* 2010).

The negative impacts of poor water and sanitation are magnified for PLWH and TB patients. Diarrhoea is reported as the most common waterborne disease affecting PLWH, thus highlighting the necessity of providing PLWH a sufficient amount of clean water and adequate sanitation to address the health risks resulting from their weakened immune system. A recent study (Clacherty and Potter 2007) on the experience of caregivers of PLWH in South Africa reports that a minimum of 200 litres of water per person per day is necessary to satisfy the basic needs of PLWH, such as drinking, washing clothes, and bathing. Furthermore, having adequate sanitation facilities located close to a patient's house is important to avoid having to walk long distances.

Structural approaches to water and sanitation in eThekwini

In response to the health, environmental, and urban challenges described in the previous section, EWS has developed a progressive integrated approach that includes research and implementation of new WATSAN technologies, as well as providers' engagement with technology users, with increased considerations for their health and the sustainability of the systems delivered (Figure 7.3).

The basis of EWS's approach is the recognition that the combined provision of water and sanitation and safe disposal of human waste are necessary to promote citizens' public health, as well as to minimize environmental pollution. Since 2002, EWS has pledged

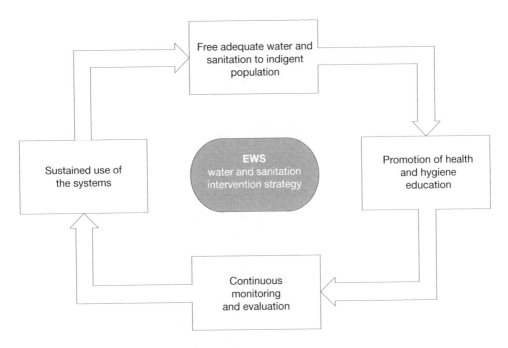

Figure 7.3 eThekwini water and sanitation strategy

Source: authors' elaboration

to provide combined free basic WATSAN services to all indigent people (i.e. living in a unit valued less than R190,000/US $26,700). EWS policy allows for supply of the first 9 kilolitres of water free of charge, while free access to potable water in informal settlements is provided via standpipes or community ablution blocks (CABs). CABs are temporary shared sanitation facilities adapted from converted steel shipping containers and fitted with two or more toilets, urinals, washbasins, showers, and an external laundry area. CABS are provided in urban and peri-urban informal areas of eThekwini Municipality, where basic provision of water and sanitation is lacking. The minimum standard of sanitation provided in rural areas is urine diversion toilets (UDTs), water-less sanitation facilities installed at household level. UDTs separate urine from faecal matter at source by diverting urine to a pedestal and collecting faeces in a pit. Finally, any ventilated improved pit (VIP) latrine in the municipality is emptied every five years free of charge.

The following sub-sections illustrate the main integrated WATSAN approaches adopted by eThekwini Municipality to implement and maintain the aforementioned systems.

The waterborne edge demarcation and appropriate water and sanitation

Reflections over the causes of the recent cholera epidemic acknowledged the importance of providing both water and sanitation solutions as a combined measure to break the disease cycle. To implement an appropriate public health strategy, EWS coined the concept of the 'waterborne edge', a line drawn on a map that separates areas where sanitation systems can be reticulated to the existing sewer lines from other areas (mainly

Figure 7.4
eThekwini waterborne edge

Source: Gounden 2009,
reproduced with permission

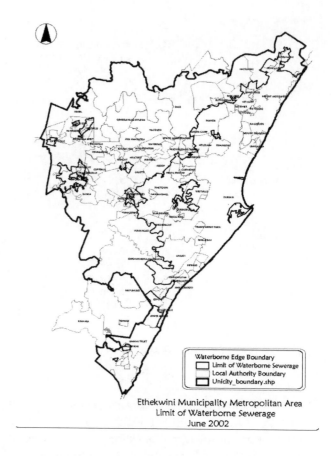

Waterborne Edge Boundary
☐ Limit of Waterborne Sewerage
☐ Local Authority Boundary
☐ Unicity_boundary.shp

Ethekwini Municipality Metropolitan Area
Limit of Waterborne Sewerage
June 2002

peri-urban and rural) where the provision of waterborne sanitation is not financially or technically feasible (Gounden *et al.* 2006).

Communal water and sanitation facilities in informal settlements

To address the dynamic WATSAN backlogs in informal settlements within the waterborne edge, EWS has delivered a combined WATSAN package in the form of community ablution blocks (CABs), connected to the sewer system, with wastewater being reticulated to the nearest wastewater treatment plant. The purpose of the urban WATSAN strategy is to improve health and environmental conditions, prioritizing those people living in informal dwellings who will not receive government housing within the next 20 years (EM 2006). Design parameters for CABs vary, as local contractors tender to design, construct, and deliver the facilities. Two blocks (one for male and one for female) serve up to 75 households within a 200 metre radius.

Since 2008, 222 CABs have been implemented and an additional 1,100 are planned for delivery by 2013 (EWS 2011b). The CAB implementation process is supported by continuous independent and municipal evaluations of infrastructural appropriateness, economic sustainability, and user satisfaction of the systems. In response to a recent assessment (Roma *et al.* 2010) reporting lack of cleanliness, vandalism, and toilet blockages at CABs, EWS adopted innovative management and technical improvements. Among these, toilet paper is distributed for free to each facility to prevent blockages often caused by the use of newspapers for anal cleaning purposes; and copper-based taps are being replaced with plastic ones to avoid theft. Finally, as opposed to previously adopted schemes where CAB caretakers worked on a voluntary basis, permanently employed caretakers supervise and clean the facilities daily.

Water and sanitation solutions outside the waterborne edge

In those areas located outside the waterborne edge, sparsely populated communities require a service delivery approach of a different nature. To address this challenge, EWS provided a comprehensive household-based package, which included a ground water tank and a urine diversion toilet (UDT). The tank, whose inlet is controlled by a float valve, is filled daily and maintained by the householders (EWS 2011b). Each household is provided with 200 litres of drinking water per day supplied by an automated electronic bailiff to a 200 litre plastic ground tank, positioned near the house. To accommodate the recent increase in free water supply provision from 6 to 9 kilolitres per month (300 litres per day), existing ground tanks are being substituted with metred yard taps.

Household water supply is accompanied by the provision of a UDT, a waterless sanitation system designed to separate urine and faeces in a healthy and environmentally sustainable manner. Since 2003, EWS has installed an estimated 75,000 UDTs. The UDT as designed and developed by EWS is a double-vault ventilated system, where urine is collected separately and diverted via the soak away into the soil, and faeces are collected in a sealed chamber constructed above or slightly below the ground. A pedestal is positioned above one vault, while the other is kept sealed until use. Once the first vault is full, it is sealed, the content allowed to dry and the pedestal is moved over to the empty vault (EWS 2003). When the second vault is full, the first one is emptied by the household or by a local private contractor and its content buried. Independent evaluations have routinely been conducted to examine effectiveness of education activities, user acceptance, and health impacts of UDTs (Gounden *et al.* 2006). A longitudinal study on 1,160 households highlighted areas where technical problems emerged (HSRC 2004). As a result of this study, improvements were introduced to toilet design: a plastic sliding slab substituted the cement slab, the vent pipe was lengthened, and the roof overhang was increased. A further study evaluating the health impacts of UDTs provided evidence of associations between disease outcomes in relation to the provision of UDTs, water provision, and hygiene education. A prospective cohort study on a total of 1,337 households was conducted in three matched intervention and control areas. Results showed significantly decreased health risks in the intervention compared to the control areas. Specifically, diarrhoea incidence rates in the intervention areas (11.7 per 1,000 persons per day) were significantly lower than in control areas (16.0 per 1,000 persons per day) (Lutchminarayan *et al.* 2007).

Human waste disposal

The EWS pledge to improve environmental health involves the management of sanitation facilities installed by the previous local authorities. Although South African national policy defines VIPs as an acceptable basic level of sanitation, in eThekwini Municipality, the provision of VIP systems has been substituted by UDTs. Academic research based on local VIP latrines has found that their ability to hygienically separate human waste, control nuisance, and prevent pathogen transmission can be affected by poor design and maintenance (Foxon *et al.* 2008). Furthermore, the requisite pit-emptying not only represents a costly option (approximately US $252), but spatial and topographic considerations make emptying with tanker trucks a daunting task. Conversely, the more economical alternative of manually emptying pits creates health hazards, as it requires eThekwini staff to manually excavate the latrine's pit in order to dig out the sludge. Examinations of facemasks used by workers emptying full VIP latrines showed a high load of helminth eggs (Foxon *et al.* 2008).

When EWS became the WSA it faced the issue of 50,000 VIP latrines needing to be emptied. Since 2007, 32,000 VIP latrines have been emptied by contractors and subcontractors employed by the municipality. To address potential health issues among workers, medical examinations were conducted routinely. Furthermore, appropriate equipment (gloves, overalls, hard hats, boots, and gas masks) was distributed. In rural and sparsely populated areas, disposal of human waste is achieved by onsite burial, while in densely populated areas the sludge is transported using drum-barrows and the contents buried in trenches (EM 2011).

Sustainable water and sanitation

In recognition of the importance of sustainable systems in improving the living conditions and health of users, EWS adopted two holistic approaches targeting education and job creation linked to water and sanitation. Education and awareness programmes and the creation of local water and sanitation entrepreneurs are instrumental in the municipal mandate to address poverty and provide sustainable solutions to communities.

WATSAN education and awareness schemes

eThekwini recognizes the importance of education in improving users' satisfaction and awareness of health and hygiene, preventing anthropogenic pollution, and correcting behaviour linked to misuse and wastage of water and sanitation. Since 1997 EWS has created a comprehensive network of educational activities, which comprises multiple approaches to target various WATSAN users, such as communities in rural areas and informal settlements, teachers, and schoolchildren. The programme's core principle rests on the creation of a mutual trust relationship between the WSA and its beneficiaries through multiple approaches. Household visits in the pre- and post-implementation stages of service delivery are the most frequently adopted approach. Visits are conducted by EWS health promoters, education officers, community facilitators, and appropriately trained community members. An example is the extensive education adopted in the implementation of UDTs. During multiple visits, community facilitators provide households with a pre-implementation brief on the provision of water and sanitation; education on disease cycle and hygiene behaviour; use of and best practices with UDTs; ground tank operation; and maintenance of systems installed. To strengthen messages delivered in person, street theatre performances, workshops, and focus groups are routinely conducted in communities and schools. Drama is employed to deliver powerful health messages employing simple language and comedy to groups of people in public places (such as taxi ranks, shopping centres, and health clinics) in areas nearby informal settlements, rural communities, and schools.

eThekwini's long-term vision of service sustainability also reflects the priority placed on educating future generations on the importance of water, sanitation, and health, by including these subjects into school curricula. Since 2004, EWS has developed the 'environment and sustainable schools' scheme, an accredited training development programme targeting school teachers and students. The course aims to strengthen teachers' environmental knowledge and skills, enhance their ability to transmit this knowledge to pupils, and encourage schools to adopt initiatives that improve the environment. Since the programme's inception, 90 teachers have completed the accredited course and more than 2,000 copies of school activity packs focusing on the importance of hand-washing and pit latrine maintenance have been distributed (EWS 2011b).

Local water and sanitation job creation

The EWS mandate to provide sustainable water and sanitation services also involves training and job creation schemes. Since 2004, EWS has cooperated with the national Expanded Public Work Programme (EPWP) (DPW 2009), whose goal is to reduce unemployment by creating full-time equivalent jobs through the public and community services. The 'EPWP contractor and learnership' scheme aims to build the capacity of local contractors, formed through an open selection process, while simultaneously giving them suitable work experience in local municipal projects. In the rural areas, local people are trained in the construction of UDTs and ground water tanks and subsequently employed. Furthermore, within each rural area, local businesses were sourced and trained in the supply of concrete blocks and bricks for toilets. Since the beginning of the programme until 2009, 500 local contractors have been employed and trained to build onsite toilets; 300 facilitators and health promoters from local communities have been trained; and 30,000 people have been contracted as local labour in project areas (EWS 2009).

In the urban areas of eThekwini, an equivalent sustainable business programme has been created and linked to the construction of CABs. Eight small local contractor companies have been working with four major contractors in the construction of communal water and sanitation facilities and are mentored by professional consultants in aspects of business operation. Furthermore, local community facilitators and caretakers are employed to provide education and take care of the facilities, respectively. Since the launch of the CAB project in informal settlements, the sustainable sanitation business programme has generated 4,000 jobs, providing skills in water and sanitation and, more generally, uplifting poor and marginalized communities. Job creation in the WATSAN sector enables EWS to perpetuate the benefits of educational activities as well as create necessary skills to operate and maintain the systems installed in communities.

Lessons learned and replicability

Since becoming the WSA, eThekwini has faced daunting challenges that have undermined progress in providing basic water and sanitation to the people under its jurisdiction. A decade later, despite the presence of dynamic backlogs and health challenges, EWS has achieved outstanding results in improving the living conditions of its citizens by adapting progressive strategies that have influenced national policies. To date, 674,000 more people have access to water, and the sanitation backlog has been reduced by 50 per cent from 1996 figures (EM 2011). This success must be viewed in the context of progressive WATSAN legislation coupled with a long-term vision of sustainable service provision.

In its effort to provide adequate services, EWS does not embrace a one-policy-for-all approach; rather, it investigates, designs, and conceptualizes various policies. The identification of the 'waterborne edge', subsequently adopted at the national level, is an illustration of a case-based policy intervention. The implementation of waterless sanitation systems outside the waterborne edge was the result of appropriate decision-making determined by health priorities and financial and environmental considerations pertaining exclusively to those rural areas outside the waterborne edge. As previously discussed, the limited support for the intervention registered by a portion of users led EWS to develop appropriate community-based participatory strategies to gather users' feedback and design interventions to increase acceptance, use, and maintenance of the systems. At the basis of the EWS strategy is a process of learning from previous experiences, which are technically monitored and evaluated through the users' voice. The adoption of ad hoc programmes to channel users' feedback is an essential component of the EWS sustainability mandate.

The case-based intervention policy fits within a long-term vision of sustainable service provision. The municipal approach of investing in a comprehensive educational programme targeting communities, schools, and teachers is fundamental in shaping environmental consciousness and the appropriate hygiene behaviour of present and future generations. Furthermore, this policy is in line with the municipality's pledge to provide water and sanitation facilities that are sustainably used and maintained by their users. At the same time, the creation of small entrepreneurships and WATSAN jobs reinforces the educational messages within communities and give rise to a skilled labour force in the water and sanitation sector, which will be available to provide maintenance and operational support. Noticeably, the municipality's demand-responsive approach based on research and development, efficient service delivery, and progress monitoring represents a positive example to those South African municipalities with lower performance, struggling to keep up with their financial debts and public health threats (Eales 2010).

In many ways, eThekwini Municipality epitomizes a national and global model for integrated service delivery. By learning and engaging with research groups and international organizations, EWS produced progressive WATSAN policies which have often been adopted by other municipalities and adapted to national policies.

Acronyms

DWAF   Department of Water Affairs and Forestry
EM   eThekwini Municipality
EPWP   Expanded Public Work Programme
EWS   eThekwini Water and Sanitation
PLWH   People Living with HIV infection
UDT   Urine Diversion Toilet

UNDP   United Nations Development Programme
VIP   Ventilated Improved Pit (latrine)
WATSAN   Water and Sanitation
WSA   Water Service Authority

References

Clacherty, A. and Potter, A. (2007) 'Integrating health and hygiene education in the water and sanitation sector in the context of HIV/AIDS', TT 316/07, Pretoria: Water Research Commission.

Cottle, E. and Deedat, H. (2002) 'The cholera outbreak: a 2000–2002 case study of the source of the outbreak in the Madlebe Tribal Authority areas, Uthungulu region, KwaZulu-Natal', RDSN and ILRIG. Online, available at: www.hst.org.za/uploads/files/cholera.pdf (accessed 21 June 2011).

Day, C., Monticelli, F., Barron, P., Haynes, R., Smith, J., and Sello, E. (eds) (2010) *The District Health Barometer 2008/2009*, Durban: Health Systems Trust. Online, available at: http://www.hst.org.za/publications/district-health-barometer–200809 (accessed 11 June 2011).

Department of Health (DOH) (2001) *Cholera Update in KwaZulu-Natal, November 2001*, Epidemiology Unit, Department of Health, KwaZulu-Natal. Online, available at: http://www.kznhealth.gov.za/cholera5.pdf (accessed 30 June 2011).

Department of Public Works (DPW) (2009) *Expanded Public Works Programme: Five Year Report 2004–2005/2008–2009*, Pretoria: Department of Public Works. Online, available at: http://www.epwp.gov.za/index.asp?c=Home (accessed 13 August 2011).

Department of Water Affairs and Forestry (DWAF) (1994) *Water Supply and Sanitation Policy, White Paper*, Cape Town: Department of Water Affairs and Forestry.

Department of Water Affairs and Forestry (DWAF) (2001) *The White Paper on Basic Household Sanitation*, Cape Town: Department of Water Affairs and Forestry. Online, available at: ftp://ftp.hst.org.za/pubs/govdocs/acts/1998/act36.pdf (accessed 24 May 2011).

Department of Water Affairs and Forestry (DWAF) (2003) *Strategic Framework for Water Services. Water is Life and Sanitation is Dignity*, Cape Town: Department of Water Affairs and Forestry. Online, available at: http://www.durban.gov.za/durban/services/water_and_sanitation/policies_and_guidelines/wsdp/statframeworksept2006 (accessed 24 May 2011).

Department of Water Affairs and Forestry (DWAF) (2010) *Annual Report 2009/2010*, Cape Town: Department of Water Affairs and Forestry.

Eales, K. (2008) 'Rethinking sanitation improvement for poor households in urban South Africa', paper presented at the IRC Symposium: Sanitation of the Urban Poor Partnership and Governance, Delft, November 2008.

Eales, K. (2010) 'Water Services in South Africa: 1994–2009', in B. Schreiner and R. Hassan (eds) *Transforming Water Management in South Africa: Designing and Implementing a New Policy Framework, Global Issues in Water Policy*, vol. 2, Dordrecht: Springer.

Earle, A., Goldin, J., and Kgomotos, P. (2005) *Domestic Water Provision in the Democratic South Africa – Changes and Challenges*, Uppsala: The Nordic Africa Institute.

eThekwini Municipality (EM) (2006) *Integrated Development Plan: 2010 and Beyond*, Durban: eThekwini Municipality. Online, available at: http://www.durban.gov.za/durban/government/policy/idp/idp/idp2011/idp1 (accessed 28 April 2011).

eThekwini Municipality (EM) (2007) *Durban's Sustainability Best Practice Portfolio. Water Special Edition 2007/2008*, Durban: eThekwini Municipality. Online, available at: http://www.durban.gov.za/durban/services/development-planning-and management/epcpd/documents/Sustainability%20Best%20Practice%20Special%20Edition%20Water.pdf (accessed 11 August 2011).

eThekwini Municipality (EM) (2008) *Approach to the Planning of Sanitation Services*, Durban: eThekwini Municipality, unpublished document.

eThekwini Municipality (EM) (2011) *Integrated Development Plan: Five Years 2011–2016*, Durban: eThekwini Municipality. Online, available at: www.durban.gov.za/durban/government/policy/idp/idp/idp2011/idp1 (accessed 18 August 2012).

eThekwini Water and Sanitation Unit (EWS) (2003) *Business Plan for the Delivery of Basic Water and Sanitation in eThekwini Municipal Area*, Durban: eThekwini Municipality.

eThekwini Water and Sanitation Unit (EWS) (2004) *Water Services Development Plan*, vol. 2, Durban: eThekwini Municipality.

eThekwini Water and Sanitation Unit (EWS) (2009) *Job Creation and Skills Development: Rural Water and Sanitation Programme*, Durban: eThekwini Municipality, unpublished document.

eThekwini Water and Sanitation Unit (EWS) (2011a) *Water Services Development Plan*, Durban: eThekwini Municipality, unpublished document.

eThekwini Water and Sanitation Unit (EWS) (2011b) *Revised Water and Sanitation Backlog Based on 2007 Photography*, Durban: eThekwini Municipality, unpublished document.

Foxon, K., Brouckaert, C., Rodda, N., Nwaneri, C., Balboni, E., Couderc, A., and Buckley, C. (2008) *Scientific Support for the Design and Operation of Ventilated Improved Pit Latrines (VIPs) and the Efficacy of Pit Latrine Additives*, Report TT 357/08, Pretoria: Water Research Commission.

Gounden, T., Pfaff, B., McLeod, N., and Buckley, C. (2006) 'Provision of free sustainable basic sanitation: the Durban experience', paper presented at the 32nd Water, Engineering, and Development Centre International Conference, Colombo, 2006.

Gounden, T. (2009) *Sustainable Sanitation in eThekwini Municipality*, unpublished document.

Human Science Research Council (HSRC) (2004) *Assessment of the Effectiveness of the Education Programme for Households Receiving Sanitation and Water*, Durban: Human Science Research Council.

Kane-Berman, J. and Macfarlane, M. (eds) (2009) *South Africa Survey 2008/2009*, Johannesburg: South African Institute of Race Relation.

Lutchminarayan, R., Knight, S., and Stenstrom T. (2007) 'Comparative study evaluating the health outcomes of sanitation, water and hygiene education in eThekwini municipality, Durban, South Africa', paper presented at the International Conference on Sustainable Sanitation Dongsheng, China, August 2007.

Marx, C. and Charlton, S. (2003) 'Urban slums report: the case of Durban, South Africa', in UN-HABITAT, *Global Report on Human Settlements 2003, the Challenge of Slums*, London: United Nations Human Settlement Programme.

Mudzanani, L., Ratsaka-Mathokoa, M., Mahlasela, L., Netshidzivhani, P., and Mugero, C. (2003) 'Cholera', in P. Ijumba, C. Day, and A. Ntuli (eds) *South Africa Health Review 2003/2004*, Durban: Health System Trust. Online, available at: http://www.hst.org.za/publications/south-african-health-review–200304 (accessed 8 July 2011).

Mugeru, C. and Hoque, A. (2001) *Review of Cholera Epidemic in South Africa, with Focus on KwaZulu-Natal Province*, Epidemiology Unit, Department of Health. Online, available at: www.kznhealth.gov.za/cholerareview.pdf (accessed 1 June 2011).

Roma, E., Buckley, C., Jefferson, B., and Jeffrey, P. (2010) 'Assessing users' experiences of shared sanitation facilities. A case study of community ablution blocks in Durban, South Africa', *Water SA*, 36 (5): 589–94.

Republic of South Africa (RSA) (1996) *Constitution of the Republic of South Africa, No. 108 of 1996*. Online, available at: http://www.info.gov.za/documents/constitution/1996/a108–96.pdf (accessed 2 May 2011).

Republic of South Africa (RSA) (1997) *Water Services Act. Act No.108, 1997*. Online, available at: http://www.info.gov.za/view/DownloadFileAction?id=70766 (accessed 4 March 2011).

Statistics South Africa (StatsSA) (2007) *Community Survey 2007: Statistical Release Basic Results Municipalities, P0301.1*, Pretoria: Statistics South Africa. Online, available at: www.statssa.gov.za (accessed 11 June 2011).

Statistics South Africa (StatsSA) (2011) *Gross Domestic Product: First Quarter 2011. Statistical Release P0441*, Pretoria: Statistics South Africa. Online, available at: http://www.statssa.gov.za/

publications/statspastfuture.asp?PPN=P0441&SCH=5250 (accessed 11 June 2011).

United Nations Development Programme (UNDP) (2010) *Human Development Report 2010. The Real Wealth of Nations: Pathway to Human Development*, New York: United Nations Development Programme.

United Nations Environment Program (UNEP) (2002) *Vital Water Graphics – an Overview of the State of the World's Fresh and Marine Waters*, Nairobi: United Nations Environment Program.

8

CITY PLANNING AS A STRUCTURAL DETERMINANT OF HEALTH

Toward healthy urban governance in the century of the city

Jason Corburn

City planning is a discipline and professional practice that includes political processes, institutions, and discourses that generate policies, rules, and physical plans that shape where we live, learn, work, and play in cities and towns. Yet city planning is much more than rules and regulations concerning land use and the built environment: planners regularly make discretionary decisions that shape the implementation of formal rules; can provide greater public access to (or stymie) forums for democratic decision-making; and interpret national and even global ideologies about urbanization and development. In these ways, city planning helps structure the distribution of social, physical, and economic 'goods and bads' that influence human health and explain persistent urban health inequities. In other words, city planning acts as a structural determinant of health through its formal and informal institutions, its micro and macro politics, and how these intersect with our day-to-day activities, from access to employment and food to the qualities of our neighbourhoods and housing to the allocation and distribution of social and health care services.

The twenty-first century is the century of the city; the United Nations (UN) Population Reference Bureau predicts that by 2050, 70 per cent of the world's population will be living in metropolitan areas (UN DESA 2012). Thus, city planning must be understood as part and parcel of global health. In the nineteenth century, city planning emerged as a modern profession and discipline with close ties to public health initiatives, including tenement housing reforms, the construction of urban water supply and sewerage systems, and the design of parks and playgrounds. While having similar visions of the equitable and healthy city, the work of professionals in each field diverged throughout the twentieth century, which has contributed to the persistence of health inequities for many poor and minority urban populations. Efforts in the early years of the twenty-first century, aimed at reconnecting city planning and public health, have been limited and largely focused on a narrow framing of the intersection of the fields, such as whether and how the built environment might change behaviours to increase physical activity and related health outcomes. The built environment and health framing tends to ignore the politics of planning and, as I will highlight in this chapter, important lessons from each field's modern history.

Throughout this chapter, I identify at least three lessons from each field's modern history that present challenges for reconnection around the structural determinants of urban health inequities, including an overemphasis on: (1) physical changes for improving social conditions; (2) scientific rationality; and (3) professionalization and fragmentation of the disciplines. Building on the historic review and these themes, the chapter suggests a set of reconnection strategies and practices for moving toward 'healthy and equitable city planning'. This will require continued critical engagement with the histories of the fields along with new issues and problem framings, investigative and analytic techniques, and inclusive and deliberative public processes that together can generate new norms, discourses, and practice for greater health equity. In short, healthy city planning will require new commitments to inject health and social justice into *urban governance*. Healthy urban governance will mean that the decision-making processes and institutions that shape places are altered to focus on equity, and that new decisions ensure a more equitable distribution of the positive, physical, and social characteristics of places that promote urban health.

Early connections between city planning and health: 1840s–1890s

In the 1820s, French epidemiologist Louis René Villermé highlighted that the wealthier the Parisian neighbourhood – or *arrondissement* – the lower the mortality rate and likelihood of illness. By 1842, Edwin Chadwick would build on Villermé's work and publish the *Report on the Sanitary Conditions of the Labouring Population in Great Britain*, documenting that the 'gentry and professional' classes lived longer than 'labourers and artisans' (Chadwick 1842: 87). Miasma – filth or dirty air – was the leading theory of disease causation, and sanitary commissions were created in European and American cities to clean up urban environments with the hope of arresting infectious disease epidemics (Duffy 1990). Sanitary engineers tended to address urban health issues by employing new technologies to remove waste by, for instance, piping it away from cities into rivers and oceans (Melosi 2000). When removing the miasma did not seem to reduce disease, the sick were removed from society. *Contagion*, the belief in the direct passage of poison from one person to another, led to large quarantines of immigrants and justified state-sponsored interventions in the economy.

Research and practice linking planning and public health during this era included the sanitary survey, park and playground planning, and the work of settlement houses. Intensive spatial and social surveys of urban environments were the epidemiologic methods of this era, such as the sanitary maps of Bethnal Green and Liverpool prepared by Chadwick and the 1878 Memphis sanitary survey that described every street, structure, and individual lot within the city to determine the environmental conditions that might 'breed' diseases (Peterson 1979: 90). Progressive Era park and playground movements advocated for urban play spaces next to schools so that gymnasiums, reading rooms, and baths could all be used for children's recreation, literacy, and hygiene.

The women of Hull House in Chicago, influenced by the burgeoning Chicago School of Sociology that initiated the study of neighbourhood effects on well-being, worked with residents to document unsanitary neighbourhood and workplace conditions and advocated on behalf of immigrants for new social policies (Hull House Residents 1895). The researchers at Hull House, particularly Florence Kelley, borrowed methods from public health researchers in England at the time, namely Charles Booth, to conduct some of the first community health surveys that included neighbourhood mapping of both non-infectious and infectious diseases in the United States.

By the end of the nineteenth century, many urban health interventions focused on physical removal of both 'environmental miasmas' – garbage, waste water, air pollution, etc. – and 'undesirable and sick' people. For sanitarians, the local solution to pollution was removal and dilution, but the downstream environmental health impacts were often ignored (Tarr 1996). Housing reformers were split between those advocating physical improvements, such as bathrooms, ventilation, and fire escapes, and those calling for the construction of safe and affordable housing. Many housing and sanitary reforms were grounded in the belief that technological and design innovations could not only improve living conditions but also make 'immoral' slum dwellers more orderly and healthy (Fairfield 1994).

Germ theory and planning 'the city scientific': 1900s–1940s

By the turn of the new century, it was well known in public health that both miasma and contagion failed to explain certain aspects of urban health, such as why, with ubiquitous filth, epidemics only occurred sometimes and in some places. By this time, the driving ideology in public health shifted to *germ theory*, which stated that microbes were the specific agents that caused infectious disease (Susser and Stein 2009). Medical treatment and disease management began to replace strategies of physically removing harms, and public health shifted toward laboratory research and interventions aimed at eliminating bacteria, such as vaccinations and chlorination of municipal drinking water supplies. Separate municipal bureaucracies emerged during this era to manage these urban improvement schemes, such as water service delivery infrastructure, sewage systems, public housing, parks and recreation, school-based health, and others, resulting in greater fragmentation and segmentation of work in public health and city planning (Peterson 1979).

Public health, social justice and the emergence of American city planning

Social inequalities kept the fields of planning and public health somewhat linked. In 1906, W.E.B. Du Bois published *The Health and Physique of the Negro American* and used data from census reports, vital statistics, and insurance company records to generate some of the first documentation of the poor health status of African Americans living in both southern and northern cities in comparison to white Americans. Du Bois questioned whether improvements in science, technology, housing, and other services were benefiting all Americans and concluded that racial health disparities were a result of social conditions – not eugenic ideas of inherent racial inferiority that were commonly accepted at the time (Du Bois 1906).

As American planners prepared for their first national conference in the early years of the twentieth century, Benjamin Marsh and his group, the New York Committee on the Congestion of Population (CCP), argued that city planning ought to more explicitly embrace a social justice agenda. In a 1908 article entitled *City Planning in Justice to the Working Population*, Marsh argued that American planning ought to make 'the right of the citizen to leisure, to health, to care in sickness, to work under normal conditions, and to live under conditions which will not impair his health or efficiency' a 'foresight' rather than an afterthought (Marsh 1908: 1514). Yet, Fredrick Law Olmsted, Jr., the first president of the American City Planning Institute and its conference, responded by defining the field as primarily concerned with the means of 'circulation', the distribution of public space and the development of private land (Olmsted 1910: 69). As Peterson (2003: 249) has noted, 'while Marsh battled for justice, Olmsted focused more on planning itself, especially ways to build it up as a technically effective field'. The comprehensive, rational, and aesthetically focused 'City Beautiful' ideas of Olmsted Jr. took hold, while the human health and social justice concerns of Marsh and the CCP largely fell off the agenda. By the Fifth National City Planning Conference in 1913, entitled 'The City Scientific', American planning had defined itself largely as a technocratic profession aimed at designing efficient cities (Fairfield 1994).

The biomedical model, housing policies and the fractured city: 1950s–1990s

By mid-century, the driving theory in public health would shift again to the *biomedical model* of disease (Susser and Stein 2009). This model combined laboratory science with a focus on individuals and attributed morbidity and mortality to molecular-level pathogens brought about by lifestyles, behaviours, hereditary biology, or genetics. The biomedical model would provide public health with explanations for emerging chronic diseases such as heart disease, and shifted research and interventions to personal health 'risk factors', e.g. smoking, diet, and exercise. At the same time, 'New Deal' programmes would help usher in the era of the 'bureaucratic city', where a new set of impersonal public institutions, staffed by newly credentialed professionals, would help to increase disciplinary boundaries and further separate planning from public health (Duhl and Sanchez 1999).

A series of Federal Housing Administration policies would help to physically and socially fracture poor urban communities of colour in the 1940s and 1950s by refusing to insure mortgages for older homes and razing poor communities of colour under the guise of 'urban renewal'. Planners and public health practitioners often justified the labelling of an area as blighted and thus subject to demolition by using healthy housing and neighbourhood guidelines recommended in the 1948 American Public Health Association (APHA) publication entitled *Planning the Neighborhood*, which offered design guidelines for 'healthy' new neighbourhoods but no guidance to *improve* existing housing (APHA 1948). The result was widespread displacement of the urban poor and policies that acted to shut out people of colour from the health-promoting benefits of suburban living, such as home ownership, capital accumulation, access to better-funded schools, and participation in the growing suburban economy.

Urban activism and rejection of rational planning

Social movements in the 1950s and 1960s pushed back against the displacement and inequities perpetuated by federal housing and other urban policies. Social movements helped pass important legislation that would improve the health of all populations, but especially the urban poor and people of colour, such as Medicaid and civil rights laws. During this time, planning and urban policymakers, supported by federal War on Poverty programmes, turned back to improving neighbourhoods, and the Office of Economic Opportunity supported a national network of community health centres (CHC), the first two of which were located in Columbia Point, Boston and Mound Bayou, Mississippi. The CHC model focused on providing both immediate care and preventative services for the poor, instead of treating people and sending them back into the living and working conditions that made them sick in the first place. According to Jack Geiger, a physician and leader of the health centre movement, CHCs aimed to take a holistic view of health by 'writing prescriptions for the building blocks of health' such as food, rent, jobs, and sanitation (Geiger 2005).

By the mid–1980s, academics, government agencies, and the World Health Organization (WHO) came together to create the Healthy Cities programme to re-invigorate the linkages between city planning and public health (Duhl and Sanchez 1999). Focused primarily in Europe, the Healthy Cities programme enrolled cities to draft 'healthy city plans' and share examples of the opportunities and barriers for planning more healthy cities (Barton *et al.* 2009). By the 1990s, public health researchers began to re-conceptualize explanations for the distribution of disease across populations to explain health disparities, energizing the field of social epidemiology (Krieger 2011). Place inequities – such as residential segregation, urban divestment, and environmental injustices – began to be seen by epidemiologists by the early twenty-first century as linked social determinants of health that may help explain distributions of death and disease across different population groups and places and issues needing urgent policy attention.

Toward healthy and equitable urban governance

As this brief review has suggested, reconnecting city planning and public health to address structural inequities must be attentive to the political – not just the scientific, technical, and physical design – challenges of *healthy urban governance*. Healthy urban governance demands more than just governmental reform, but includes such political processes as identifying and framing new policy issues; generating appropriate standards of evidence; constituting some social actors as 'experts'; adjudicating scientific uncertainty and different knowledge claims; securing public accountability for decisions; and implementing and monitoring policies. Governance practices are, in short, the rules, norms, and processes for exercising power over collective actions and, when inattentive to social inequalities, often sort populations into unequal outcomes by upholding existing distributions of resources like political power, wealth, and knowledge (Corburn 2009).

The key challenge for reconnecting planning and public health in the twenty-first century is to learn from each field's history and jointly develop strategies that address the root causes of poor health, not just devise interventions aimed at specific diseases or individual behaviours. Grappling with the political challenges of reconnecting the fields demands that, for instance, planners experiment with new institutional designs which can handle cross-disciplinary conflicts over political power, social justice, and health values; such as when a state- or private-sector-sponsored development project clashes with the health objectives of a local community. Planners will also need to critically question the adequacy of existing norms and institutions that help determine how practitioners use or abuse power, respond to or even resist market forces, work to empower some groups and disempower others, promote multi-party decision-making, or simply rationalize decisions already made.

Health impact assessment: preventing, not displacing urban health risks

The first lesson from the histories of planning and public health for healthy urban governance is that removal and displacement of 'problems' does not necessarily improve urban health and may leave the most vulnerable groups and places worse off. Health impact assessment (HIA) is one example of a precautionary practice that can help reconnect planning and public health and prevent problem displacement. Now widely used for healthy urban planning in Europe, HIA is both an analytic tool and political process that might bring together the built and social environmental factors that influence urban health. The San Francisco Department of Public Health (SFDPH) has used HIA to assess a proposed living wage ordinance, new housing proposals, and rezoning plans. During one HIA process, called the Eastern Neighborhoods Community Health Impact Assessment (ENCHIA), the SFDPH organized a participatory planning process that included over 40 governmental and non-governmental organizations for evaluating the positive and negative human health impacts from a proposed rezoning plan. During the ENCHIA process, stakeholders collaboratively defined the elements of a healthy place, discussed how land use does or does not influence these elements, and investigated how a set of rezoning proposals and potential alternatives might influence the health of the largely low-income, immigrant communities of the Mission and South of Market neighbourhoods in San Francisco (Corburn 2009).

One outcome of the ENCHIA process was the Healthy Development Measurement Tool (HDMT), an analytic method outlining the broad social indicators, land use development goals, and quantitative and qualitative data for healthy urban development (www.thehdmt.org). The HDMT is now being used by the city's planning agency, private developers, and community-based organizations to evaluate the extent to which new development projects and land use plans will promote health equity (Corburn 2009). While no panacea, HIA is beginning to bring together government agencies, advocacy organizations, and researchers that rarely work together, suggesting that it may be a process for breaking-down 'disciplinary boundaries' and other institutional barriers confronting efforts to reconnect planning and public health.

Integrated, spatial planning for returning inmates

Healthy and equitable city planning must also address the urban 'epidemic' of incarceration and prisoner re-entry. American jail populations are disproportionately young, urban, African American and Latino men – the same groups that have the poorest health. Incarceration has created a planning and public health challenge by spatially concentrating both the removal of young men from families and the workforce and the social stress that accompanies inmates' return to their neighbourhood. The constant cycle of incarceration and re-entry in American cities in particular has brought the health issues of prisons into the neighbourhood, including infectious disease, addiction, mental health problems, and routine physical violence. Yet, returning inmates face homelessness, family evictions from public housing, denial of food stamps, terminated Medicaid benefits, and regular workplace discrimination (Freudenberg *et al.* 2005; Rich *et al.* 2011).

In New York City, a neighbourhood-focused reintegration project, called the Community Reintegration Network, is working to address the strains on public safety, community health, family stability, and municipal budgets that come from neighbourhood concentrations of former inmates. As a partner in this coalition, the Vera Institute of Justice launched Project Greenlight, which prepares inmates for release and reintegration by matching them with programmes and organizations in their home community, including supportive and special needs housing, drug-treatment programmes, job training, and health clinics (Brown and Campbell 2005). While these initiatives aim to build one-stop locations for housing, job training, and social and health services, city planners have a unique opportunity to reconnect with the social justice roots of the profession by participating in community-based re-entry programmes, and might offer their knowledge of spatial and social programming to help reduce recidivism. In the twenty-first century, incarceration and re-entry must become planning and public health issues so that, for instance, municipal funds are redirected to provide the place-based housing, education, employment, and social services necessary to prevent recidivism and reduce the spatial impacts of incarceration.

New institutions for healthy and equitable city planning

A second set of related lessons from the histories of urban planning and public health is that an over-reliance on technological solutions and physical designs, without accompanying institutional change, fails to protect the most vulnerable population groups. Healthy city governance will depend, in part, on robust community-based institutions. The histories of planning and public health suggest that, for instance, economic development in the absence of community-based institutions may fail to improve living conditions because local institutions can help ensure that the benefits of development are distributed to meet the needs of local people. For example, a coalition of community-based organizations called the Figueroa Corridor Coalition successfully negotiated a community benefit agreement (CBA) with the Los Angeles Arena Land Company, a private developer, over the Staples Center Phase II project in downtown Los Angeles. The CBA is a legally binding agreement guaranteeing that the developer include affordable housing and public amenities such as new parks and that the new commercial establishments hire local residents at a living wage (Gross *et al.* 2002). Reminiscent of struggles for early twentieth century workplace and neighbourhood improvements, organized labour unions are acting as integral partners in shaping these agreements, recognizing that their members increasingly come from low-income communities and are working in service sector jobs.

Tempering professional models with lay expertise

A final lesson from the histories of urban planning and public health is that when interventions ignore what local people know, how they move through the world, and their subjective experiences with illness and their environment, the interventions ultimately fail. Local knowledge, including the experiences and narratives shared by populations living with persistent hazardous exposures, chronic diseases, and social marginaliza-tion, is a valuable form of 'expertise' that can improve scientific analyses, the relevance of health-promoting interventions, and the democratic character of public decisions (Corburn 2005). Drawing from the lessons of Progressive Era neighbourhood surveys and the neighbourhood health centre movement, twenty-first century planning and public health might re-embrace local knowledge by promoting and supporting networks of community health workers (CHWs).

Often called *promotoras de salud*, CHWs are frontline lay health outreach workers that organize neighbourhood residents around health issues and provide health education, basic disease screening, and translation and interpretation services. CHWs often act as the bridge-builders between poor, minority, and immigrant communities and profes-sional health services and institutions. Since CHWs live in the places within which they work, they have a keen awareness of local culture and practices, and often have lived experiences of how macro-social structures impact the daily lives of local residents. Ultimately, CHWs tap local knowledge to improve health by building community, stimulating informal networks, formal associations, and other connections between socially dissimilar persons or groups that can be crucial for securing both immediate health-promoting resources and organizing long-term policy advocacy coalitions.

An asthma prevention and management programme in Brooklyn, New York, relies on CHWs to organize residents and understand the barriers asthmatics and their fami-lies face in managing this disease. The Community Health Educator (CHE) team at an organization called El Puente[1] is working in the Latino neighbourhoods of south Williamsburg, Bushwick, and Bedford-Stuyvesant, performing home visits and holding community-wide focus groups to assist families in managing asthma. During a series of focus group meetings, the CHE team heard from local women that many asthmatic families were turning to home and herbal remedies in place of physician-prescribed medications to control asthma (Ledogar *et al.* 2000). When asked why, local people, many of whom were Spanish speakers and Dominican immigrants, said that the time-tested herbal treatments acted as a familiar practice in a world where asthma caused unparalleled social and economic disruption to families and communities by forcing children to miss school, adults to miss work, and families to fall further into poverty. The information from residents about the use of home remedies and the social and cultural role they play in immigrants' lives was translated by CHWs into new interven-tions aimed at addressing the multiple dimensions of asthma (Corburn 2005). Since community and experiential knowledge can ensure interventions are contextually and culturally relevant, healthy twenty-first century planning must learn from and with local experts.

Planning and public health for the twenty-first century

This chapter has aimed to both critically review the histories of city planning and public health and, by drawing lessons from this review, suggest strategies to reconnect the fields to confront twenty-first century challenges of promoting greater urban health equity. The contemporary challenges for reconnecting the fields are daunting – global spread of disease, transboundary environmental pollution, burgeoning urban and slum populations, and increasing health disparities mirroring widening class inequalities. As momentum for the reconnection effort builds – as reflected in recent journal issues, conferences, government, and foundation efforts – the lessons from each field's historic missteps ought to be given closer scrutiny.

The recommendations offered here should also be viewed in a comparative perspective, since they reflect experiments aimed at 'healthy urban planning' from around the world. For instance, the WHO's City Action Group on Healthy Urban Planning[2] and the United Kingdom Office of the Deputy Prime Minister's Creating Sustainable Communities initiative[3] are both principally focused on how to reverse social exclusion and inequality more generally through the design of new collaborative governance schemes, state regulations, and building non-governmental capacity. In the United Kingdom, London and Merseyside are using HIA to address planning and development decisions (Barnes and Scott-Samuel 2002). Efforts to upgrade slums in developing countries, including strategies for achieving the Millennium Development Goals, explicitly call for the inclusion of local knowledge and integrating urban planning with health equity (WHO/UN-HABITAT 2010). Finally, one of the most successful campaigns to reduce AIDS in Haiti, the poorest country with the highest rate of HIV infection, was designed around networks of CHWs (Farmer 1999).

Contemporary efforts to reconnect planning and public health can learn from the past to understand how current trends gained resonance and what alternative futures are possible. Alternative paradigms can be both practical and socially just, as the examples here suggest. However, since many of the recommendations are offered as frameworks, not specific guidance, more work needs to be done to evaluate which practices might work best in specific cultural and political contexts. Yet, as efforts to reconnect urban planning and public health move forward, a historic perspective is necessary to critically re-engage with city planning as a structural determinant of health.

Notes

1 El Puente's work can be viewed online at www.elpuente.us
2 WHO's City Action Group on Healthy Urban Planning can be viewed at www.euro.who.int/document/e82657.pdf
3 More information on UK Office of the Deputy Prime Minister's 'Creating Sustainable Communities Initiative' can be viewed at www.communities.gov.uk/publications/communities/sustainablecommunitiesbuilding

References

American Public Health Association (APHA) Committee on the Hygiene of Housing (1948) *Planning the Neighborhood: Standards for Healthful Housing*, Chicago: Public Administration Service.

Barnes, R. and Scott-Samuel, A. (2002) 'Health impact assessment and inequalities', *Pan American Journal of Public Health*, 11 (5/6): 449–53.

Barton, H., Grant, M., Mitcham, C., and Tsourou, C. (2009) 'Healthy urban planning in European cities', *Health Promotion International*, 24: i91–9.

Brown, B. and Campbell, R. (2005) *Smoothing the Path from Prison to Home*, New York: Vera Institute of Justice. Online, available at: www.vera.org/publication_pdf/319_590.pdf (accessed 23 February 2009).

Chadwick, E. (1842) *Report on the Sanitary Condition of the Labouring Population and on the Means of its Improvement*, London, May 1842. Online, available at: www.deltaomega.org/ChadwickClassic.pdf (accessed 22 August 2011).

Corburn, J. (2005) *Street Science: Community Knowledge and Environmental Health Justice*, Cambridge, MA: MIT Press.

Corburn, J. (2009) *Toward the Healthy City: People, Places and the Politics of Planning*, Cambridge, MA: MIT Press.

Du Bois, W.E.B. (1906) *The Health and Physique of the Negro American: Report of a Social Study Made under the Direction of Atlanta University*. Online, available at: http://www.archive.org/details/healthphysiqueof00dubo (accessed 23 July 2011).

Duffy, J. (1990) *The Sanitarians: A History of American Public Health*, Chicago: University of Illinois Press.

Duhl, L.J. and Sanchez, A.K. (1999) *Healthy Cities and the City Planning Process*. Online, available at: www.who.dk/document/e67843.pdf (accessed 11 November 2007).

Fairfield, J.D. (1994) 'The scientific management of urban space: professional city planning and the legacy of progressive reform', *Journal of Urban History*, 20: 179–204.

Farmer, P. (1999) *Infections and Inequalities: The Modern Plagues*, Berkeley, CA: University of California Press.

Freudenberg, N., Daniels, J., Crum, M., Perkins, T., and Richie, B.E. (2005) 'Coming home from jail: the social and health consequences of community reentry for women, male adolescents, and their families and communities', *American Journal of Public Health*, 95 (10): 1725–36.

Geiger, J. (2005) 'The unsteady march', *Perspectives in Biology and Medicine*, 48 (1): 1–9.

Gross, J., LeRoy, G., and Janis-Aparicio, M. (2002) *Community Benefit Agreements: Making Development Projects Accountable*, Washington, D.C.: Good Jobs First and the California Public Subsidies Project.

Hull House Residents (1895) *Hull House Maps and Papers*, New York: Thomas Y. Crowell & Co.

Krieger, N. (2011) *Epidemiology and the People's Health: Theory and Context*, New York: Oxford University Press.

Ledogar, R., Penchaszadeh, A., and Garden-Acosta, L. (2000) 'Asthma and Latino cultures: different prevalence reported among groups sharing the same environment', *American Journal of Public Health*, 90: 929–35.

Marsh, B. (1908) 'City planning in justice to the working population', *Charities and the Commons*, 19: 1514–18.

Melosi, M. (2000) *The Sanitary City: Urban Infrastructure in America from Colonial Times to the Present*, Baltimore, MD: Johns Hopkins University Press.

Olmsted Jr., F.L. (1910) 'City planning: an introductory address', *American Civic Association*, 2 (4): 1–30.

Peterson, J. (1979) 'The impact of sanitary reform upon American urban planning, 1840–1890', *Journal of Social History*, 13: 83–103.

Peterson, J. (2003) *The Birth of City Planning in the United States, 1840–1917*, Baltimore, MD: Johns Hopkins University Press.

Rich, J.D., Wakeman, S.E., and Dickman, S.L. (2011) 'Medicine and the epidemic of incarceration in the United States', *New England Journal of Medicine*, 364 (22): 2081–3.

Susser, M. and Stein, Z. (2009) *Eras in Epidemiology: The Evolution of Ideas*, Oxford: Oxford University Press.

Tarr, J.A. (1996) *The Search for the Ultimate Sink: Urban Pollution in Historical Perspective*, Akron, OH: University of Akron Press.

United Nations Department of Economic and Social Affairs (UN DESA) (2012) *World Urbanization Prospects, the 2011 Revision*. Online, available at: http://esa.un.org/unpd/wup/index.htm (accessed 21 July 2012).

World Health Organization (WHO)/ United Nations Human Settlements Programme (UN-HABITAT) (2010) *Hidden Cities: Unmasking and Overcoming Health Inequities in Urban Settings*, Kobe: World Health Organization Centre for Health Development. Online, available at: http://www.hiddencities.org/report.html (accessed 16 January 2011).

9

THE 100% CONDOM USE PROGRAMME

A structural intervention to prevent HIV and sexually transmitted infections in Asia

Wiwat Rojanapithayakorn and Richard Steen

The 100% Condom Use Programmes (100% CUP) have been credited with reversing the course of rapidly expanding generalized HIV epidemics in several Asian countries (Ruxrungtham *et al.* 2004; WHO SEARO 2007). In others, they have interrupted transmission in commercial sex networks before HIV could extend substantially into the general population. These successes followed a structural approach to addressing overlapping HIV and sexually transmitted infection (STI) epidemics that progressed from analysis of transmission dynamics and underlying structural factors to implementation of multi-sectoral interventions at a national scale to change them.

The 100% CUP is an intervention to prevent sexual transmission of HIV in the general population by ensuring high levels of condom use among sex workers and their clients. The structural nature of 100% CUP is embodied in a simple premise – that of shifting responsibility for condom use from individuals (sex workers and clients) to the establishments or venues where sex work takes place. By ensuring condom use in sex work, it was argued, fewer sex workers would become infected, and downstream transmission from male clients of sex workers to their regular and casual partners would be interrupted, removing the major driver of HIV/STI epidemic growth.

In Thailand, such fundamental structural change in the organization of sex work benefited from high-level political support from the start (Rojanapithayakorn 2006). The programme has gone well beyond a change in public health policy, however. Implementation has emphasized multi-sectoral coordination to address structural factors in sex work settings and to promote enabling environments for prevention. It also included a number of direct interventions – from STI services to free condom supply – that were seen as critical to achieving desired outcomes.

While the basic premise behind 100% CUP may be simple, sex work itself is not. The organization of sex work and the environment in which it takes place change constantly, posing multiple challenges to sex workers and to programmes seeking to improve health and social conditions. Sex workers are highly mobile and provide services under different arrangements that change over time. Critically, legal status, criminalization, and international pressure related to human trafficking are factors that often act at a level above the health sector, and may hinder public health efforts by driving sex workers 'underground' into more vulnerable situations and away from health services. Cambodia's experience with rebuilding 100% CUP in the face of such macro-level environmental factors illustrates some of these ongoing structural challenges. The experiences of China, Mongolia, and Vietnam extend such insights, and highlight the importance of scale as a structural determinant when intervening in sex work.

This paper focuses on several aspects of 100% CUP as a structural intervention – first, as an initial public health response to the early conditions of low condom use and rapid HIV/STI transmission; second, as an adaptable strategy to variable public infrastructures and changing conditions of sex work; and third, as a feasible model for national scale-up. Along the way, we consider obstacles and challenges to the programme, including some that are also faced by interventions in sex work in other settings, particularly with regard to the environments where sex work takes place (Rekart 2005).

Early conditions and initial response: Thailand

At the beginning of Thailand's HIV epidemic in 1984, few HIV cases were found among female sex workers. However, an abrupt increase was observed in 1989, when 33 per cent of sex workers were found to be infected in Rayong, an eastern province of Thailand. Soon after, similar rates were detected among sex workers in northern provinces (Weniger et al. 1991). These findings created serious concerns among policy-makers and public health experts.

Sex work in Thailand was mainly organized in a range of establishments such as brothels, massage parlours, tea houses, low-class hotels, bars, nightclubs, etc. There were about 100,000 sex workers in the country; many Thai men frequented sex establishments regularly; and the majority of them did not use condoms (Boonchalaksi and Guest 1994). The fear was that HIV would spread rapidly from male clients to the general population. As predicted, sexual transmission of HIV in Thailand was rapidly increasing among sex workers in all regions of the country, and among STI clinic attendees (the majority of whom contracted the diseases from sex workers) as well as army recruits. Up to 140,000 new cases of HIV infection occurred per year during the early 1990s (UNDP 2004).

Since the beginning of the epidemic, interventions to prevent and control HIV were limited to information and education, treatment services for STIs, and general condom promotion (Department of Communicable Disease Control 1989). However, such interventions proved incapable of controlling Thailand's rapidly growing HIV epidemic. Education programmes among the most at-risk populations and the general public were unable to reduce risk behaviours; high coverage of STI services failed to control the high incidence of STIs; and condom promotion for the target groups and the general population did not achieve significant levels of condom use. Recognizing the limitations of such individual-based interventions, a structural approach to ensuring universal condom use in sex work was developed and piloted (Rojanapithayakorn 1991).

The 100% CUP was started in November 1989 in Ratchaburi province in central Thailand (Rojanapithayakorn and Hanenberg 1996). Ratchaburi province was selected because local government authorities had a good understanding of the HIV/AIDS problem and were willing to pilot the approach. Strong policy support from the provincial governor facilitated collaboration among various sectors within the province.

Measurable progress, including a rise in condom use to over 90 per cent, was seen after a few months of implementation, and STI prevalence among sex workers soon dropped to very low levels (Rojanapithayakorn and Hanenberg 1996). Such findings led to the expansion of the approach to nearby provinces where similar results were quickly demonstrated. Recognizing this, the Thai National AIDS Committee (NAC), chaired by the prime minister, agreed in August 1991 to implement the programme nationwide (Rojanapithayakorn 1991). With the endorsement of the NAC, the programme received full support from the Ministry of Health and the Prime Minister's Office (PMO). Provincial health departments were responsible for day-to-day programme implementation activities while the PMO's inspector generals were assigned to manage the overall activities of provincial implementation. Nationwide coverage of the 100% CUP was achieved in April 1992, and the programme has remained a major HIV prevention strategy of the country until today.

Principles and strategies

The 100% CUP aimed to change the sex work environment by enabling sex workers in all sex establishments to refuse sex services to customers who did not agree to use condoms. By monopolizing the sex business around universal condom use, customers could no longer control decision-making about using condoms. Local authorities and owners of sex businesses were responsible for promoting and maintaining such an enabling environment (Rojanapithayakorn 1991). The implementation approach involved: (1) cooperation of local key players (government authorities, owners of sex establishments, and sex workers) to require condom use in all sexual encounters; (2) agreement on universal condom use, i.e. if a customer refused to use a condom, there would be no sex service provided (no condom – no sex); (3) universal coverage of sex establishments (all places and all types) so that customers would not be able to purchase sex services anywhere without using condoms; and (4) sanctions for non-cooperative establishments (but never for sex workers).

Implementation steps included: (1) organizing meetings of provincial HIV/AIDS committees to raise awareness of the threat of the HIV/AIDS epidemic, obtain consensus and agreement to implement 100% CUP, and develop a work plan for its implementation; (2) holding meetings between the HIV/AIDS committee, owners of all sex establishments, and representative sex workers to obtain cooperation in implementing the programme; (3) educating sex workers about the programme; (4) monitoring to ensure that the policy was adhered to by all sex establishments; (5) providing logistical support for the programme (condoms, water-soluble lubricants, STI services, and educational materials) by provincial AIDS/STI units and the regional STI centres; and (6) monitoring and evaluation of programme outcomes (Rojanapithayakorn 1991).

To ensure compliance, a sanctions policy was endorsed by all sectors. Responsibility for enforcing condom use was on the establishment, which could be closed if non-compliant (although this was rarely done).

The main sectors involved in the programme included: (1) health, responsible for condom supply; STI services for sex workers and clients; health education and information for target groups; data collection from STI patients on condom use; and reporting non-compliant sex establishments to monitoring working groups; (2) local administration, such as the governor's office and the police, coordinating between all sectors and participating in monitoring working groups to identify and manage sex establishments; and (3) sex business owners, managers, and sex workers, responsible for ensuring safer sex practices through universal condom use in all sexual encounters.

Management of non-cooperative sex establishments was an important component of this structural intervention. The objectives of this 'sanction' management were to make the sex business sector aware of the methods used to monitor and verify the use of condoms in sex work, and to motivate them to ensure a high level of condom use. This was similar to sanctions for failing to follow compulsory seat-belt use laws or for smoking in prohibited public places. Sanctions against non-cooperative establishments included regular warnings, temporary or permanent closure, or withdrawal of business permits.

Monitoring condom use

A local coordinating committee was established to monitor programme implementation (Rojanapithayakorn 1991). Members included representatives from all participating sectors, including sex establishments. Monthly meetings were conducted to gather relevant information to be reported to the provincial governor, who chaired the Provincial AIDS Committee. The monitoring process included activities to verify the use of condoms in sex establishments, and evaluation of programme outcomes and impact.

Several methods were proposed to monitor condom use in the 100% CUP (Rojanapithayakorn 1991). These included: (1) interviewing all men receiving services at government STI clinics about the use of condoms with sex workers; (2) obtaining condom use information from the contract tracing system within the STI control programme (i.e. if a tourist came to the province, had unprotected sex with a sex worker, and subsequently sought STI treatment outside the province, the contract tracing system would relay information about the entertainment establishment where condoms were reportedly not used); (3) conducting mystery shopping (volunteers who pretended to be customers, insisted on not using a condom, and noted the sex worker's response); (4) testing sex workers for STIs during routine health checkups; and (5) checking records on the number of condoms distributed from the STI control programme to sex establishments.

The first and the second methods were recommended as appropriate, economical and unbiased approaches. These methods required a well-functioning STI service system, which was already in place in all provinces of Thailand. Routine checkups of sex workers were not considered reliable for condom use verification as sex workers could contract infection from a regular partner despite universal condom use with clients. A more reliable method for monitoring condom use involved the use of routine case reports and interviews with male STI clients. Since most STI patients reported recent sex work contact, male STI trends could be analyzed as a proxy for condom use in commercial sex. Patient interviews would thus serve to identify non-compliant sex work venues.

Evaluating programme effectiveness

The effectiveness of the programme depended on achieving high levels of condom use in all sex establishments. To measure success, the following indicators were used:

1   STI incidence and trends obtained from routine monthly reports from all government STI clinics;

2   prevalence of HIV infection in different target populations, based on data from routine annual sentinel surveillance;
3   behavioural surveys on attitude and practice relating to condom use, which was determined through interviews with sex workers during annual sentinel surveillance; and
4   numbers of condoms supplied to sex business sector and surveys to determine percentage of condom use in sex workers, based on condom procurement and supply records of the national STI programme.

Impact of 100% CUP in Thailand

With the programme, condom use rates in sex work began to increase nationally, from 14 per cent in early 1989 to over 90 per cent from June 1992; and steadily increasing to over 97 per cent by 2000. Consequently, the rates of curable STIs fell by over 95 per cent during the 1990s and HIV prevalence declined in most population groups (Chitwarakorn 1998; Hanenberg et al. 1994). HIV prevalence in sex workers has gradually declined from a peak of 33.2 per cent in 1994 to 2.8 per cent in 2010, with a corresponding decline in male STI clinic attendees from 8.6 per cent to 1.1 per cent and in army recruits from 4.0 per cent to 0.5 per cent (Bureau of Epidemiology 2011b).

By 1996, estimates suggested that more than 2 million HIV infections were prevented in Thailand (Robinson et al. 1996). By 2004, an estimated 5.7 million HIV infections had been averted; this figure not only includes sex workers and their clients but also averted secondary infections, which include far larger numbers of people at lower risk (Thai Working Group on HIV/AIDS Projection 2001). The decline of STI incidence has continued (Figure 9.1) and HIV prevalence remains low even among lower-risk populations, such as pregnant women attending antenatal clinics (ANC), army recruits, and blood donors (Figure 9.2) (Bureau of Epidemiology 2011a, 2011b), prompting national and international recognition (Boonchalaksi et al. 1998; Chamratrithirong et al. 1998; UNAIDS and Ministry of Public Health – Thailand 2000).

Beyond increased condom use and the decline in HIV/STIs, other social benefits can be attributed to de facto decriminalization of sex work. Official acceptance of 100% CUP implied a degree of recognition of sex work in society. Although sex work remains illegal in Thailand, authorities largely accept its existence as long as public health is not jeopardized. The beneficiaries of the programme include:

1   sex workers, who can earn a high level of income with very low risk of acquiring STIs or HIV, and whose work was decriminalized by the programme;
2   clients of sex workers, who have lower HIV/STI risk;
3   sex business owners, who can maintain or increase income at the same level of business;
4   the health sector, which benefits from lower workload related to HIV and STIs;
5   local authorities, who can successfully maintain low HIV/STI prevalence in the population.

Sex workers themselves are key to the success of the programme. They are empowered to refuse unsafe sex and HIV risk, and have increasingly taken a larger role in programme implementation, particularly as sex work evolves to include venues and arrangements

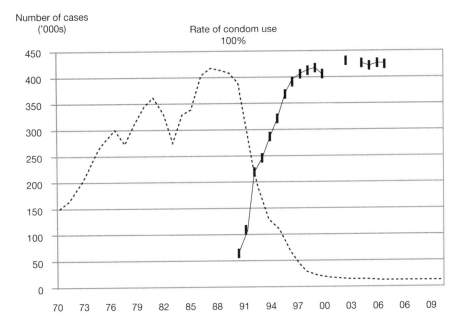

Figure 9.1 Number of STI cases and condom use rate in sex establishments, Thailand, 1970–2009

Source: Ministry of Public Health, Thailand: (1) STD Division for STI incidence data (2) Bureau of Epidemiology for condom use rate (2012)

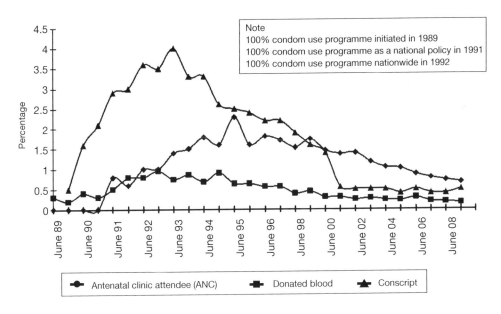

Figure 9.2 HIV prevalence among pregnant women, male conscripts, and blood donations, Thailand, 1989–2009

Source: data originally taken from Bureau of Epidemiology 2011a; 2011b

Note: switching from biannually (June and December) to annually (June) since 1995

outside fixed establishments. Most important, the programme promotes multi-sectoral collaboration beyond just the health sector – particularly local administrations, police, and sex businesses – to support sex workers, address structural factors where sex work takes place, and ensure enabling environments for HIV and STI prevention.

The economic returns from the programme, resulting from an estimated 5 million infections averted from 1989 to 2004 alone, are considerable. Condom use has become an accepted means of HIV prevention, and 100% CUP an integral part of Thailand's AIDS prevention and control programme (UNDP 2004).

The challenge of changing structural conditions: Cambodia

The success of 100% CUP in Thailand can be attributed not only to shifting responsibility for condom use from individual sex workers and clients to sex work establishments, but also depended to a large degree on multi-sectoral efforts to create an enabling environment for prevention. In practice, these changes, together with de facto decriminalization of sex work in Thai society, contributed to reducing social marginalization of sex workers and removing structural barriers to health and social services. Cambodia provides an example of what can happen when, following implementation of similar structural interventions, the enabling environment is abruptly removed.

In the mid-1990s, Cambodia, like Thailand a few years earlier, was facing one of the fastest growing HIV epidemics in Asia (Ryan *et al.* 1998). Yet, within five years after the introduction of the 100% CUP, it had become one of the few countries to have reversed its HIV epidemic. HIV prevalence declined from a high of 3 per cent in 1997 to 1.9 per cent in 2003 (NCHADS 2011b). HIV incidence and prevalence have continued to decline among sex workers, male risk groups, and antenatal women, and mortality has stabilized. In recognition of these efforts, Cambodia was awarded a Millennium Development Goal award for outstanding national leadership, commitment, and progress towards Goal 6, particularly in halting and reversing the spread of HIV (UNAIDS 2011).

Early conditions and response

Cambodia confronted HIV under extremely vulnerable conditions in the early 1990s as the country emerged from instability. Rapid growth of HIV was fuelled by unprotected sex work (less than 20 per cent consistent condom use in 1996) and poorly controlled STI epidemics (Ryan *et al.* 1998). These included chancroid and other ulcerative STIs, potent cofactors that had facilitated rapid HIV transmission in neighbouring Thailand a few years earlier.

The 100% CUP was announced in 1998, piloted in Sihanoukville that same year, and consolidated nationwide from 2000 to 2001. As in Thailand, the policy ensured high-level support, programmatic coordination, and promotion of an enabling environment through local condom-use working groups and monitoring teams. Increased investment in prevention services was documented over the period 2001–2004 (Sopheab *et al.* 2008). Within a few years, the 100% CUP had increased condom use in direct (brothel-based) sex work settings to high levels, resulting in measurable reductions in several common STIs as well as HIV. These reductions were seen in male bridging populations and pregnant women in addition to direct and indirect sex workers (NCHADS 2011b).

Changing structural conditions

Yet, as in other countries in the region, the context of sex work in Cambodia has been changing since the early successes of a decade ago (Sopheab *et al.* 2008). Sex work has progressively moved from brothels (70 per cent of sex workers in the late 1990s) to 'indirect' settings (90 per cent of 'entertainment workers' today) (NCHADS 2011b). These include massage parlours, karaoke venues, beer gardens, and restaurants where sex is negotiated but does not take place on site (Kim *et al.* 2005). Second, due in part to the recent economic recession, the number of women selling sex is estimated to have increased threefold over the past ten years. Figure 9.3 illustrates the effect of these trends on the context of sex work in Cambodia.

Third, the 'transition' to indirect sex work was accelerated in early 2008 with the introduction by the Interior Ministry of a Law on Suppression of Human Trafficking and Sexual Exploitation (LSHTSE), and subsequent forced closure of most brothels. The consequences of the law included measurable effects on public health programmes (Pearshouse 2008). Sex workers were arrested or driven underground to avoid arrest, increasing their vulnerability to exploitation and violence. This 'disabling environment' also reduced sex workers' access to services (Busza 2006). During this period, reports indicated a rapid decline in STI clinic attendance by direct sex workers and increasing male STI case reports (NCHADS 2011b).

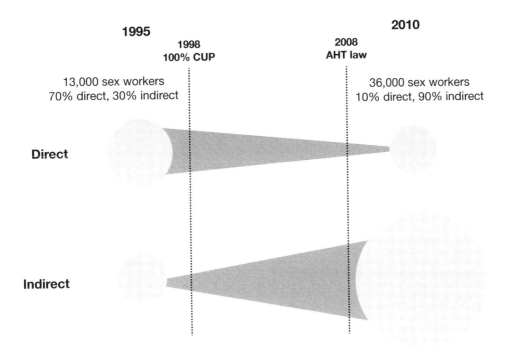

Figure 9.3 Changing patterns and size of sex work in Cambodia

Source: WHO Western Pacific Regional Office (forthcoming), reproduced with permission

121

Evolving response

Facing new challenges, the Cambodian government and its partners (the sex business sector and non-governmental organizations) have enacted a number of innovative responses to reconstruct an enabling environment for prevention, to increase outreach contacts, and promote clinic attendance for those engaged in sex work. To reflect the changing nature and composition of sex work in the new environment, the term 'entertainment worker' (EW) was adopted.

The first challenge is to re-establish working arrangements that have been disrupted by the LSHTSE, closure of brothels, and collapse of 100% CUP coordination committees. New multi-sectoral partnerships are being promoted to accomplish this. These partnerships include EWs, establishment owners/managers, police and local authorities, as well as representatives from anti-trafficking and drug enforcement units. Their aim is to find ways to limit abuses related to trafficking and drug use, while supporting and facilitating public health objectives and programmes in sex work settings.

Second, the new focus on EWs presents challenges for outreach efforts, which must be reorganized to reach a growing number of indirect establishments as well as freelance workers. Since clinic attendance is now entirely voluntary and self-motivated (rather than organized through brothels), efforts are being made to increase both the 'push' and 'pull' sides of promoting checkups. As part of the 'push' strategy, peer workers are using new approaches to attract EWs to attend clinics. A large number of peer workers are recruited and trained with a target of one peer worker for every ten EWs. Innovative approaches are also being tested, including 'smart girl' campaigns to increase the social status of EWs who use condoms, attend clinic checkups, and are actively involved in prevention efforts.

On the 'pull' side, clinical services for EWs are being expanded and efforts made to make them more relevant to their needs. The Continuum of Prevention to Care and Treatment (CoPCT) approach envisions providing a broad range of health and social services, from reproductive health (family planning, pregnancy, and abortion services) to voluntary counselling and testing (VCT), antiretroviral therapy (ART), drug use prevention, and other social services (NCHADS 2011a).

The Cambodian experience illustrates the highly dynamic nature of sex work environments, and how factors outside the sphere of public health programmes can undermine and reverse public health gains. It also provides an example of how the focus of structural interventions can be widened, leading to greater adaptability and responsiveness of programmes to changing conditions.

The challenge of scale: China

To be effective, prevention interventions must reach coverage thresholds whereby disease transmission is interrupted (Jamison *et al.* 2006). Achieving sufficient coverage and scale can thus be considered an important structural challenge that is influenced by factors such as migration, population mobility, and the feasibility of scaling up the interventions themselves (Lau *et al.* 2008).

By conservative estimates, there are 2.5 million female sex workers in China (NCAIDS 2006). Highly mobile, they work in direct and indirect venues and also as freelancers, often under difficult conditions (Wang *et al.* 2009, 2010; Yi *et al.* 2010). Sex work remains illegal in China, a policy that is enforced by periodic police crackdowns and incarceration (Tucker *et al.* 2010).

HIV began spreading quickly through networks of injecting drug users (IDU) in several southern provinces in the late 1990s. Conditions were already ripe for sexual transmission. Following economic liberalization (Open Door policy) in the 1980s, population mobility and migration increased markedly, stimulating a rapid increase in commercial sex. By the time HIV began spreading among IDUs in Yunnan and neighbouring provinces, conditions – including low condom use and high rates of other STIs – were conducive for rapid heterosexual transmission through overlapping commercial sex networks (Hong and Li 2009).

Recognizing the potential for rapid HIV spread, China quickly took action to strengthen targeted interventions among high-risk populations. Beginning in the late 1990s, interventions to promote condom use in sex work and reduce unsafe injecting behaviours were actively promoted and evaluated. During 2001–2003, 100% CUP was piloted in several counties and districts in Hubei, Jiangsu, Hainan, Hunan, Guangxi, and other provinces (WHO WPRO 2004). These early pilots led to rapid increases in condom use and declining STI rates among sex workers. Nationwide implementation began in 2004. Figure 9.4 illustrates the progressive development and extension of China's response, from pilots to policy to large-scale interventions, with contributions from national government and international partners.

China adopted a combined approach of government and partners to scale up HIV prevention programmes in sex work for high coverage. Following high-level decrees

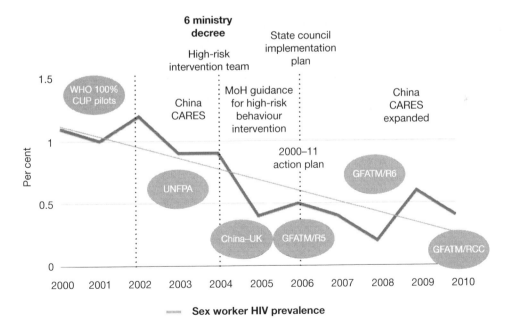

Figure 9.4 Policy and programme roll-out and sex worker HIV trends in China

Source: WHO Western Pacific Regional Office (forthcoming), reproduced with permission.

and related programme guidance between 2004 and 2006, sex worker interventions advanced from individual regional projects to government responsibility across all counties and districts of China (NCAIDS 2011). Basic outreach and services were provided from the Chinese Center for Disease Control and Prevention (CDC) platform of high-risk behaviour intervention teams. This has resulted in high coverage of entertainment establishments across the country. HIV surveillance is conducted annually through these establishments, providing important data for monitoring trends in condom use, HIV, and syphilis.

Despite wide coverage, there is concern that some sex workers of lower socio-economic status and higher risk may be missed by current outreach efforts. To identify and reach more sex workers in settings outside identified establishments, outreach and peer interventions are being strengthened. CDC is also working with family planning and STI clinics in several areas to improve referrals and access to reproductive health and STI services.

China managed at an early stage to shut down HIV transmission through known sex work networks despite high population mobility. Core 100% CUP and related interventions have raised condom use to high levels among large numbers of sex workers and appear to have kept HIV at very low levels among sex workers and clients. Implementation of the 100% CUP, initially in several key provinces, then as national policy, introduced important structural changes, which likely contributed to China's success in slowing sexual transmission. Furthermore, an intervention model with clear components – multi-sectoral coordination, outreach, condom distribution, and HIV/STI screening – proved replicable on a national scale.

Adaptation and challenges

Experiences from other Asian countries broaden the understanding of structural factors in sex work, support effectiveness of 100% CUP as a structural intervention, and highlight the need for flexibility in adapting to different conditions.

Mongolia scaled up 100% CUP from a provincial pilot to nationwide coverage between 2002 and 2007. Reported condom use by sex workers with their last client increased to over 90 per cent, syphilis prevalence has declined, and HIV prevalence among sex workers has remained at 0 per cent in second-generation surveillance surveys. Following initial programme successes, however, conditions continue to change, creating new vulnerabilities for sex workers and greater transmission risk. Increased mining and road construction have stimulated demand for sex work, while limited economic opportunities in recent years have driven more women into sex work. High mobility of sex workers and their informal and changing work settings complicate outreach and follow-up. In addition, several factors have weakened implementation of programmes. High turnover of police and local authorities – who require continuous training – complicates local work for a supportive enabling environment. Furthermore, in many areas, there are few non-governmental organizations that are able to assist with community-based outreach work. As in other countries, Mongolia is seeking solutions to these evolving challenges (WHO WPRO 2006a).

Vietnam incorporated 100% CUP into its national harm reduction strategy and has reported rising condom use in sex work from low levels to above 90 per cent in select provinces (National Committee for AIDS, Drugs, and Prostitution Prevention and Control 2010). Components of an effective response in Vietnam included clear policy, high-level political endorsement, and sustained implementation support through multiple channels. A comprehensive harm reduction approach to drug use and sex work has proven to be highly synergistic in an epidemic with overlapping injecting and sexual risk behaviours.

Vietnam has taken a pragmatic approach to implementing direct interventions and services (National Committee for AIDS, Drugs, and Prostitution Prevention and Control 2010). To improve outreach, 'peer educators' are selected from among entertainment establishment (EE) owner/managers as well as current and former sex workers. This has reportedly resulted in strong and stable outreach, since EE managers are older and less mobile than young sex workers. Multiple approaches are also used to improve sex workers' access to direct interventions. These include free condom distribution to those at highest risk – such as street-based sex workers – especially in early phases before condom use becomes normative. At the same time, condom social marketing is increasingly targeting non-traditional outlets where sex work takes place or is negotiated. Efforts are also made to bring STI services closer to sex workers, by using a mix of fixed and mobile teams, with coordination between clinic staff and EE owners.

Evidence from multiple causes of declining HIV and STI transmission in sex work suggest that these changes are having an overall impact on HIV/STI transmission in Vietnam. However, national trends can conceal large regional variation. Bio-behavioural surveys and other data reveal significant variability by province, in type of sex work, and proportion of drug-using sex workers, as well as in condom use and STI outcomes (Le *et al.* 2010; Nemoto *et al.* 2008; Tuan *et al.* 2007). Variability has also been seen in other countries where better outcomes have been reported in areas of strong programme implementation backed by high-level political support.

Discussion

Accumulated experience with 100% CUP across countries and over time demonstrates its feasibility, replicability, and potential for substantial public health benefit. Thailand and Cambodia achieved national coverage and averted millions of HIV infections. China and Mongolia, starting with much smaller HIV epidemics, have also reached national scale and succeeded in decreasing or stabilizing HIV at low levels among sex workers (WHO WPRO 2004). Myanmar and Vietnam have documented strong implementation in some areas with significant but sub-national coverage (WHO SEARO 2007; WHO WPRO 2004). The Philippines has adapted 100% CUP as policy but programme coverage remains low (WHO WPRO 2006b). These experiences illustrate how structural conditions of sex work influence risk and vulnerability, and highlight important factors for a successful response.

The 100% CUP has facilitated substantial structural change affecting several key determinants of risk and disease transmission under heterogeneous and changing conditions in sex work environments. First and fundamentally, 100% CUP has transformed the organization of sex work and the basic ground rules governing its practice. Condom use has changed from being a negotiated detail – usually under conditions of unequal power – between sex worker and client, to a prerequisite to entering into commercial sex transactions. The result has been rapid increases in condom use, from low levels to over 90 per cent in most countries, verified by declining HIV and STI prevalence.

Less overt but no less important, the de facto decriminalization of sex work that accompanied 100% CUP implementation in several countries has resulted in more enabling conditions for risk reduction in sex work settings. With high-level political support for the programme, official and law enforcement positions toward sex work changed in many places from suppression of the business to support for public health objectives and facilitation of sex workers' access to services. The importance and limitations of this change are well-illustrated by the experience of Cambodia, where subsequent high-level political decisions culminating in anti-trafficking legislation disrupted the collaboration between public health authorities and sex businesses, and exacerbated structural conditions, risk, and marginalization of sex workers.

Third, the involvement of sex workers themselves as partners in public health programmes has strengthened the response and further legitimized their role. This was particularly important in settings where sex work is loosely structured outside fixed establishments. Since community involvement itself is a recognized structural intervention in public health and HIV/STI prevention, more research and innovation are needed to determine factors for success and replicable models. One study in the Dominican Republic demonstrated better outcomes when community empowerment was combined with policy change and other structural components of 100% CUP (Kerrigan et al. 2006) (see Chapter 15, Kerrigan et al., in this volume).

Fourth, to the extent that scale is a structural factor, 100% CUP has proven to be a feasible approach to achieving high coverage and impact. The examples of China and Mongolia show that national scale-up is feasible even with limited resources. The 100% CUP is a low-cost programme built largely on existing public health services and infrastructure, with high economic return in terms of averted morbidity and mortality. Essential activities are largely integrated into routine tasks of responsible sectors. This contrasts with other models where parallel structures are set up requiring large government investment and donor support.

100% CUP has proven feasible, effective, and sustainable in a range of sex work settings – from direct sex establishments in Thailand and Cambodia to indirect venues in China, Thailand, and Vietnam, and freelance sex work in Mongolia. During two decades of 100% CUP in Thailand, the intensity of programme efforts has decreased while programme impact has been maintained. Condom use has become a norm in sex work similar to use of seat belts in many countries.

Challenges remain, however, and continued monitoring of the programme is needed to ensure high levels of coverage and sustained positive outcomes in changing sex work environments. Sex work continues to evolve and remains dynamic in terms of patterns and mobility. Programme coverage should extend to unreached populations, including male sex workers and sex services such as gay clubs and bars. Innovation and adaptation are critical to address changing environments, reach those in need, and provide essential services.

Finally, the underlying epidemiologic analysis behind 100% CUP has been validated by experience in half a dozen countries. Not only does increasing condom use in sex work reduce risk and disease burden for sex workers themselves, but – as demonstrated in several countries by triangulating data from different populations – substantial benefits accrue along the chain of infection, including to clients and their lower-risk partners.

References

Boonchalaksi, W. and Guest, P. (1994) *Prostitution in Thailand*, Nakhon Pathom: Institute of Population Research, Mahidol University.

Boonchalaksi, W., Chamratrithirong, A, and Guest, P. (1998) *100 Percent Condom Programme and the Decline of Sexually Transmitted Diseases (STDs) in Thailand*, A Report of the Institute for Population and Social Research, Mahidol University, 1998.

Bureau of Epidemiology, Thailand (2010) *Fact Sheet on the Surveillance of HIV, STI and Risk Behaviours among Service Workers Year 2010* (in Thai), Nonthabiru: Ministry of Public Health, Thailand.

Bureau of Epidemiology, Thailand (2011a) *HIV–1 Prevalence in Royal Thai Army Recruits by Province of Residence*. Online, available at: http://www.boe.moph.go.th/files/report/20100901_93131371.pdf (accessed 21 May 2011).

Bureau of Epidemiology, Thailand (2011b) *Results of the Sentinel Surveillance of HIV in Thailand, Round 1–Round 28 (1989–2010)*. Online, available at: http://www.boe.moph.go.th/files/report/20110407_61273173.pdf (accessed 21 May 2011).

Bureau of Epidemiology, Ministry of Public Health, Thailand (2012) *The Results of Behavioral Surveillance*. Online, available at: http://www.gfaidsboe.com/results%20of%20bss.php (accessed 23 May 2012).

Busza, J. (2006) 'Having the rug pulled from under your feet: one project's experience of the US policy reversal on sex work', *Health Policy Plan*, 21: 329–32.

Chamratrithirong, A., Thongthai, V., Boonchalaksi, W., Guest, P., Kanchanachitra, C., and Varangrat, A. (1998) *The Success of the 100% Condom Promotion Programme in Thailand: Survey Results of the Evaluation of the 100% Condom Promotion Programme*. IPSR Publication No. 238, Nakhon Pathom, Thailand: Institute for Population and Social Research, Mahidol University.

Chitwarakorn, A. (1998) 'Sexually transmitted diseases in Thailand', in T. Brown, R. Chan, D. Mugrditchian, B. Mulhall, D. Plummer, and W. Sittitrai (eds) *Sexually Transmitted Diseases in Asia and the Pacific*, Armidale, NSW, Australia: Venereology Publishing.

Department of Communicable Disease Control, Ministry of Public Health (1989) *National Medium Term Programme for the Prevention and Control of AIDS in Thailand, 1989–1991*, Bangkok: Ministry of Public Health.

Hanenberg, R.S., Socal, D.C., Rojanapithayakorn, W., and Kunasol, P. (1994) 'Impact of Thailand's HIV-control programme as indicated by the decline of sexually transmitted diseases', *The Lancet*, 344 (8917): 243–5.

Hong, Y. and Li, X. (2009) 'Behavioral studies of female sex workers in China: a literature review and recommendation for future research', *AIDS and Behavior*, 13: 603–13.

Jamison, D.T., Breman, J.G., Measham, A.R., Alleyne, G., Claeson, M., Evans, D.B., Jha, P., Mills, A., and Musgrove, P. (eds) (2006) 'Cost-effective strategies for the excess burden of disease in developing countries', in *Priorities in Health*, New York: Oxford University Press.

Joint United Nations Programme on HIV/AIDS (UNAIDS), Ministry of Public Health – Thailand (2000) *Evaluation of the 100% Condom Programme in Thailand, UNAIDS Case Study*, Geneva: Joint United Nations Programme on HIV/AIDS.

Joint United Nations Programme on HIV/AIDS (UNAIDS) (2011) *Cambodia Takes MDG Prize for Excellence in its AIDS Response*. Online, available at: http://unaidstoday.org/?p=848 (accessed 27 September 2011).

Kerrigan, D., Moreno, L., Rosario, S., Gomez, B., Jerez, H., Barrington, C., Weiss, E., and Sweat, M. (2006) 'Environmental–structural interventions to reduce HIV/STI risk among female sex workers in the Dominican Republic', *American Journal of Public Health*, 96: 120–5.

Kim, A.A., Sun, L.P., Chhorvann, C., Lindan, C., Van Griensven, F., Kilmarx, P.H., Sirivongrangson, P., Louie, J.K., Leng, H.B., and Page-Shafer, K. (2005) 'High prevalence of HIV and sexually transmitted infections among indirect sex workers in Cambodia', *Sexually Transmitted Diseases*, 32 (12): 745–51.

Lau, J.T., Choi, K.C., Tsui, H.Y., Zhang, L., Zhang, J., Lan, Y., Zhang, Y., Wang, N., Cheng, F., and Gu, J. (2008) 'Changes in HIV-related behaviours over time and associations with rates of HIV-related services coverage among female sex workers in Sichuan, China', *Sexually Transmitted Infections*, 84 (3): 212–16.

Le, M.N., D'Onofrio, C.N., and Rogers, J.D. (2010) 'HIV risk behaviors among three classes of female sex workers in Vietnam', *Journal of Sex Research*, 47 (1): 38–48.

National Center for AIDS/STD Control and Prevention, China CDC (NCAIDS) (2006) *Update on the HIV/AIDS Epidemic and Response in China*, Beijing: Ministry of Health, People's Republic of China.

National Center for AIDS/STD Control and Prevention, China CDC (NCAIDS) (2011) *Policies and Laws*. Online, available at: http://www.chinaaids.cn/n443289/n443295/n447114/index.html (accessed 30 September 2011).

National Center for HIV/AIDS, Dermatology, and STIs (NCHADS) (2011a) *Standard Operating Procedures for Continuum of Prevention to Care and Treatment for Women Entertainment Workers in Cambodia*. Online, available at: http://www.nchads.org/index.php?id=21 (accessed 30 September 2011).

National Center for HIV/AIDS, Dermatology, and STIs (NCHADS) (2011b) *Statistical Reports*. Online, available at: http://www.nchads.org/index.php?lang=en (accessed 30 September 2011).

National Committee for AIDS, Drugs, and Prostitution Prevention and Control – Viet Nam (2010) *The Fourth Country Report on Following Up the Implementation to the Declaration of Commitment on HIV and AIDS*, Hanoi: National Committee for AIDS, Drugs, and Prostitution Prevention and Control.

Nemoto, T., Iwamoto, M., Colby, D., Witt, S., Pishori, A., Le, M.N., Vinh, D.T., and Giang, L.T. (2008) 'HIV-related risk behaviors among female sex workers in Ho Chi Minh City, Vietnam', *AIDS Education and Prevention*, 20 (5): 435–53.

Pearshouse, R. (2008) 'Cambodia: human trafficking legislation threatens HIV response', *HIV/AIDS Policy Law Review*, 13: 21–2.

Rekart, M.L. (2005) 'Sex-work harm reduction', *The Lancet*, 366: 2123–34.

Robinson, N.J., Silarug, N., Surasiengsunk, S., Auvert, B., and Hanenberg, R. (1996) 'Two million HIV infections prevented in Thailand: estimate of the impact of increased condom use'. Paper presented at XI International Conference on AIDS, Vancouver, July 1996 (Abstract MoC904).

Rojanapithayakorn, W. (1991) *100% Condom Policy: Measures for AIDS Control in Thailand* (in Thai), Bangkok: Roen-kaew Printing.

Rojanapithayakorn, W. (2006) 'The 100% condom use programme in Asia', *Reproductive Health Matters*, 14: 41–52.

Rojanapithayakorn, W. and Hanenberg, R. (1996) 'The 100% condom program in Thailand', *AIDS*, 10: 1–7.

Ruxrungtham, K., Brown. T., and Phanuphak, P. (2004) 'HIV/AIDS in Asia', *The Lancet*, 364 (9428): 69–82.

Ryan, C.A., Vathiny, O.V., Gorbach, P.M., Leng, H.B., Berlioz-Arthaud, A., Whittington, W.L., and Holmes, K.K. (1998) 'Cambodia: explosive spread of HIV–1 and sexually transmitted diseases', *The Lancet*, 351: 1175.

Sopheab, H., Morineau, G., Neal, J.J., Saphonn, V., and Fylkesnes, K. (2008) 'Sustained high preva- lence of sexually transmitted infections among female sex workers in Cambodia: high turnover seriously challenges the 100% Condom Use Programme', *BMC Infectious Diseases*, 8: 167.

Sexually Transmitted Disease Division, Department of Disease Control, Ministry of Public Health of Thailand (n.d.) Annual reports on sexually transmitted infection situation, 1970–2009. Unpublished data.

Thai Working Group on HIV/AIDS Projection (2001) *Projections for HIV/AIDS in Thailand: 2000–2020*, Bangkok: Ministry of Public Health.

Tuan, N.A., Fylkesnes, K., Thang, B.D., Hien, N.T., Long, N.T., Kinh, N.V., Thang, P.H., Manh, P.D., and O'Farrell, N.O. (2007) 'Human immunodeficiency virus (HIV) infection patterns and risk behaviours in different population groups and provinces in Viet Nam', *Bulletin of the World Health Organization*, 85 (1): 35–41.

Tucker, J., Ren, X., and Sapio, F. (2010) 'Incarcerated sex workers and HIV prevention in China: social suffering and social justice countermeasures', *Social Science & Medicine*, 70 (1): 121–9.

United Nations Development Programme (UNDP) (2004) *Thailand's Response to HIV/AIDS: Progress and Challenges*, Bangkok: United Nations Development Programme.

Wang, H., Chen, R.Y., Ding, G., Ma, Y., Jiao, J.H., Wu, Z., Sharp, G.B., and Wang, N. (2009) 'Prevalence and predictors of HIV infection among female sex workers in Kaiyuan City, Yunnan Province, China', *International Journal of Infectious Diseases*, 13 (2): 162–9.

Wang, H., Chen, R.Y., Sharp, G.B., Brown, K., Smith, K., Ding, G., Jin, X., Xu, J., Dong, R., and Wang, N. (2010) 'Mobility, risk behavior and HIV/STI rates among female sex workers in Kaiyuan City, Yunnan Province, China', *BMC Infectious Diseases*, 10: 198.

Weniger, B.G., Limpakarnjanarat, K., Ungchusak, K., Thanpresertsuk, S., Choopanya, K., Vanichseni, S., Uneklabh, T., Thongcharoen, P., and Wasi, C. (1991) 'The epidemiology of HIV infection and AIDS in Thailand', *AIDS*, 5 (Suppl. 2): S71–85.

World Health Organization South-East Asia Regional Office (WHO SEARO) (2007) *HIV/AIDS in the South-East Asia Region*, New Delhi: World Health Organization.

World Health Organization Western Pacific Regional Office (WHO WPRO) (2004) *Experiences of 100% Condom Use Programme in Selected Countries of Asia*, Manila: World Health Organization.

World Health Organization Western Pacific Regional Office (WHO WPRO) (2006a) *100% Condom Use Programme: Experience from Mongolia*, Manila: World Health Organization.

World Health Organization Western Pacific Regional Office (WHO WPRO) (2006b) *Joint UNFPA/WHO Meeting on 100% Condom Use Programme*, Manila: World Health Organization.

World Health Organization Western Pacific Regional Office (WHO WPRO) (forthcoming) *The Next Generation HIV/STI Programming with Sex Workers: Priority Health Sector Interventions for Asia and the Pacific*, Manila: World Health Organization.

Yi, H., Mantell, J.E., Wu, R., Lu, Z., Zeng, J., and Wan, Y. (2010) 'A profile of HIV risk factors in the context of sex work environments among migrant female sex workers in Beijing, China', *Psychology, Health & Medicine*, 15 (2): 172–87.

10

THE SONAGACHI/DURBAR PROGRAMME

A prototype of a community-led structural intervention for HIV prevention

Dallas Swendeman and Smarajit Jana[1]

Introduction

The Sonagachi Project was initiated in 1992 as a sexually transmitted disease (STD)/ HIV risk appraisal and intervention programme targeting sex workers in Kolkata, India. Over the past 20 years, it has evolved into Durbar, a community-led structural intervention (CLSI) programme serving more than 60,000 sex workers, family members, and allies who own and operate multiple projects under the Durbar organizational umbrella. Durbar has become a global model for effective STD/HIV prevention, community mobilization, and empowerment with sex workers (Blankenship *et al.* 2006; Shahmanesh *et al.* 2008; Swendeman *et al.* 2009) that has been recognized by the World Health Organization (WHO) (UNAIDS 2000) and the Gates Foundation's scale-up of HIV prevention in India under Project Avahan (Piot 2010). In this chapter we describe the evolution of Durbar from a typical STD/HIV public health intervention known as SHIP (STD/HIV Intervention Programme) into a CLSI characterized by community mobilization and ownership development. In addition, to inform replications of CLSI, we synthesize three generalizable stages of CLSI development (participation, partnership, and ownership), which incrementally build community capacities to lead and sustain interventions over time.

Community-led structural interventions

CLSIs are most broadly defined as community-level interventions that mobilize communities to identify and intervene upon structural factors driving vulnerability to disease (Jana *et al.* 2004). CLSIs encompass a range of participatory approaches in public health such as community organizing, community development, community and capacity building, conflict-oriented social action, and empowerment (Minkler *et al.* 2008). CLSIs are inherently ecological and emphasize the interplay between structure and agency, that is, reshaping opportunity structures through structural interventions while building individual and community agency through empowerment processes. CLSIs include 'social' interventions in which interpersonal norms and behaviours are targeted through organizational policies in settings where risk is produced (Blankenship *et al.* 2006), as well as interventions that reflect community priorities and target more distal or structural factors that drive vulnerability to multiple and intersecting diseases and social problems (Jana *et al.* 2004).

Community-based interventions such as CLSIs are ideally initiated and led by the community (Laverack and Labonte 2000; Minkler *et al.* 2008). However, this is often not feasible in a meaningful way when affected communities are marginalized and lack the resources, capacities, skills, and consciousness to design and implement effective interventions. For example, sex workers in India typically come from impoverished backgrounds, with little to no education, and live and work under conditions of uncertainty due to constant threats from police, criminal mafias, and other power-brokers (such as madams, pimps, and landlords). As a result of social and economic marginalization, public health interventions in at-risk communities are typically initiated and implemented by external change agents. This has been a source of criticism, particularly when empowerment and community-led action are programme priorities (Laverack and Labonte 2000). Persistent challenges in community-based interventions rest not only in how to resolve tensions between community-driven and externally-driven priorities and capacities, but also in creating enabling environments that foster community-led involvement at multiple levels (Jana *et al.* 2004). Furthermore, marginalized and oppressed communities, such as sex workers, often lack the 'critical consciousness' to not be resigned to fatalistic conceptions of their circumstances, to recognize structural factors driving their risk, and to envision alternative futures and pathways for change (Freire 1970). Over the past 20 years, Durbar has successfully resolved these tensions (e.g. Cornish and Ghosh 2007), which we aim to illustrate in this chapter. Similarly, replicating and scaling up CLSIs can be particularly challenging due to tensions between the goals of reproducing effective intervention components versus reproducing processes that support community mobilization and capacity building to participate in, lead, own, and sustain interventions. Therefore, this chapter also aims to demonstrate how community mobilization and capacities can be built over time, with support from public health professionals, through community[2] participation in implementing essential public health interventions, partnership in intervention planning and decision-making, and eventually ownership to sustain interventions.

Background

Kolkata (formerly Calcutta) is a large city of 4 million residents, the capital of the state of West Bengal, and the largest urban area in north-east India (Census of India 2011). It is the original seat of British colonial rule in India and, until Indian independence, was the second largest city in the British Empire after London. Kolkata is typical of most cities in the world today, with substantial social dislocation from migration associated with industrialization, warfare, modernization, and educational opportunities (Sheth 1967). Migrant workers, truck drivers, drug traders, college students and unknown proportions of most other classes of men in Kolkata have participated in a brothel-based sex work economy that has been operating for centuries. In fact, Durbar is not the first structural intervention for sexually transmitted diseases in Kolkata. In 1868, STD outbreaks (notably syphilis) among British soldiers, officers, and traders returning from

India, and consequently their wives and sex partners in Britain, led Parliament to pass the Indian Contagious Disease Act (UNAIDS 2000). Like similar interventions in cities across the world during the late nineteenth and early twentieth centuries, the focus was on police suppression of open sex work in relatively normalized entertainment venues, which drove sex work underground (Reckless 1933). While this limited access to sex work, it was not sustained and resulted in further entrenching the stigmatization and marginalization of sex workers (Scambler and Paoli 2008).

In 1991, HIV was positioned to spread quickly throughout India, entering the country through the well-known drug trafficking route from the Golden Triangle in Southeast Asia through north-east India, including West Bengal and Kolkata. Sex workers in Kolkata were at a high potential risk, since their customers included truck drivers and other migrant workers who are often core transmitters in India and around the world (Pandey *et al.* 2008). HIV surveillance among sex workers in other major Indian cities, low rates of condom use, and high STD rates led to estimates that 85 per cent of Kolkata's sex workers could become HIV infected within five to ten years (UNAIDS 2000). Experience also demonstrated that access to sex workers, particularly in brothel-based red light areas, was not easily granted by local powerbrokers fearing disruption in local sex work economies.

Sex work in India is primarily controlled by a nexus of local criminals and law enforcement agencies. Sex work and sex workers are considered immoral and face stigma and discrimination from individuals and institutions. The children of sex workers are equally discriminated against and often barred from attending schools. The law that regulates the sex trade directly or indirectly criminalizes sex work and sex workers, which further reduces their social and political power for negotiation. The social and structural environment of the sex trade and its ambiguous regulatory mechanisms create a condition of persistent insecurity for sex workers and their families. An individual sex worker must engage in a perpetual struggle to negotiate her work through dealings with multiple visible and invisible powerbrokers in her day-to-day practices, including police harassment and extortion of money by local criminals. The economic and social insecurity faced by sex workers results in a daily battle to feed, house, and educate their families. The possible risk of acquiring HIV infection and then AIDS many years later is rarely a priority issue to a sex worker. As a result, sex workers often have little interest in intervention programmes even if services are delivered to their doorsteps.

Programme initiation

The STD/HIV Intervention Programme

Under this backdrop the STD/HIV Intervention Programme (SHIP) was initiated in 1992 in Sonagachi, one of the oldest and largest red light districts in Kolkata. The programme was established through the National AIDS Control Organization (NACO), the nodal agency for development of HIV policy and programmes in India, with technical assistance from the World Health Organization. Dr Smarajit Jana, a physician at the All India Institute of Hygiene and Public Health in Kolkata with prior experience working in occupational health and safety, was asked to lead the programme. SHIP's mission and action plan seemed simple; to prevent HIV and STD among sex workers through condom promotion, peer health education, and local STD treatment clinics. To gain access to sex workers and negotiate deals with power-brokers such as politicians, police, and brothel owners, Dr Jana and his small team of educated professionals framed HIV risk as an occupational hazard with clear economic consequences. A pragmatic message was communicated: if sex workers became HIV infected and the red light areas became associated with AIDS, business would be lost. Notably, male clients of sex workers were made off-limits to the programme but access to sex workers was granted. The SHIP team established a local sexual health clinic, hired a small group of about a dozen sex worker peer health educators, and distributed condoms.

In 1992, SHIP, and most public health researchers and practitioners, intervened with sex workers to prevent HIV infection by encouraging condom use. The common underlying but insufficient assumption was based on a rational actor model of behaviour (Sen 1977) – that sex workers and other at-risk individuals and communities would act in their self interest by using condoms and seeking STD treatment when made aware of STD risks, routes of transmission, benefits and availability of condoms, and STD treatment. By contrast, the sex workers were typically more concerned about daily survival for themselves and their families as opposed to long-term uncertainties associated with HIV and AIDS. Since condom use was not normative at that time, sex workers antici-pated that clients would refuse condom use or take their business to other sex workers, perhaps with violent consequences for the sex workers enacted by clients or powerbro-kers such as madams, landlords, neighbourhood 'goons', babus (dependent male part-ners), or police. STD testing and treatment were available at government hospitals but were not acceptable or accessible to sex workers due to stigma, legal concerns, and logis-tical barriers such as travel time and treatment costs. Given this reality, few sex workers were empowered to use condoms or to seek and complete treatment for STDs with any consistency. Thus, the major challenges at programme initiation for SHIP were to reach out to the community and improve engagement with HIV-related services. However, what was relevant to HIV programme implementers at that point in time (i.e. condom use and STD treatment) was not important to sex workers. It was evident that the primary challenge for the public health team was how to mobilize the sex worker community to engage in HIV prevention activities and also influence the outcomes of HIV programming.

Responding to the perceived needs of the community

It is essential to address the needs of the community to facilitate a process of action and social change for improving health (Minkler *et al.* 2008). Although SHIP's emphasis was on the sexual health needs of sex workers, it also attempted to respond to the general needs of the community. Experience across the globe demonstrates that communities mobilize based on their perceived needs and then come together to address common interests or threats. Common examples include villager-led water harvesting in Maharashtra and microfinance programmes in India, as well the lesbian, gay, bisexual and transgender (LGBT) community's response to HIV/AIDS in the early days of the epidemic in the United States in which large numbers of community members mobi-lized action around their everyday needs (e.g. lack of resources for basic survival or deaths of friends and family members). Unfortunately, this is not typically the case for many groups vulnerable to HIV infection. HIV often remains a peripheral issue to sex workers and other at-risk groups compared to other more proximal priorities and challenges in their daily lives.

In 1992, the need for basic health care was a priority for the sex worker community in Kolkata. Although private practitioners offered care in the red light areas, the costs were often exorbitant and unaffordable to the majority of sex workers. Education for children was, and continues to be, another pressing community need. Being mostly illiterate, sex workers wanted their children to be educated and have more opportunities than they had. Yet, when SHIP began, sex workers' children were denied admission to schools if their mothers' profession was known; if discovered, their children experienced stigma and discrimination from peers, teachers, administrators, and other parents. More broadly, and to this day, social and economic security has been a persistent priority for the sex worker community. Frequent police raids have upset the very base of the sex industry. Social stigma have marginalized sex workers and their children in every sense. In addition, exploitation and threats of violence by madams, pimps, moneylenders, and local powerbrokers has undermined the economic security of sex workers. Together, these issues have evoked persistent feelings of insecurity among sex workers, often making HIV a low priority. Within a year of intervention initiation, SHIP learned that it would have to implement different strategies to engage sex workers in HIV prevention and build widespread support for condom use norms and engagement in STD treatment.

Participation

The SHIP team understood the need for worker participation in occupational health interventions. The socio-political context of India and West Bengal also primed the project for a participatory approach based on its vibrant history of social justice and civil rights movements (Ray and Korteweg 1999). Thus, the SHIP team sought the participation of civil society, government, and medical organizations to leverage existing resources for personnel, office and clinic space, and STD testing and treatment. Perhaps most important, the team also sought the participation of sex workers to hire and train as peer educators community health workers (CHW) who could create a bridge between the project and the community. Over the first two years of the project, the CHW roles for sex workers were diversified into clinic assistants, social promoters for condoms who sold condoms for a nominal fee in brothels, and peer educators who worked in clinics and conducted outreach on the streets and home visits in the brothels. Different coloured lab coats demarcated their various roles and afforded them access and status as project staff, serving to inspire the broader community of sex workers that it was possible to achieve respect from mainstream actors (e.g. SHIP and its professional staff) despite their perceived 'fallen' status. The CHWs also functioned, informally, as the face and voice of the sex worker community in project activities.[3]

Mobilizing community via a new identity

What happened in Sonagachi is quite revealing. Being pressed by the varied needs and demands of the community members, the SHIP team felt the necessity to reconcile the project's aims with the priority needs expressed by the community. The SHIP team realized that the larger community of sex workers should have an official forum to formalize the reciprocal exchange of information, ideas, and guidance on programme implementation and development that the peer CHWs had been fulfilling informally up to that point. A series of community forums with sex workers resulted in further advancements of community participation and community mobilization. The process of negotiation between SHIP and community members reached the consensus that SHIP could not address all the issues and challenges linked to sex work. The sex workers would thus have to mobilize themselves, with moral and technical support from SHIP, in their fights for rights and social justice.

In response, a few enlightened peer CHWs from SHIP started mobilizing their friends and colleagues on the issue of police raids and harassment, which was not an easy task despite being a common threat faced by sex workers on a regular basis. Sex workers believed that they were 'immoral human beings' and could not share equal rights and dignity like other citizens of the country.

It was, therefore, necessary to undertake the significant challenges of building sex workers' self-esteem, helping them develop a positive and future-oriented approach toward life and occupation, and enabling them to raise their voices against injustices. This was a formidable task among sex workers who had been forced to live at the margins of the society for generations. It required a process to re-establish faith in themselves, followed by building dreams and aspirations to stand against the ongoing injustices they faced. A few members of the sex worker community began questioning their socially imposed identity as bad or fallen women. It was not just discarding the term prostitute, which they considered demeaning and abusive in nature, but deconstructing the phenomenon of prostitution and reconstructing their social identity by questioning existing social values, norms, and practices. More sex workers began engaging in this process of critical reflection (Freire 1970), questioning anything and everything in and around their life and occupation. Sex workers and SHIP staff members jointly engaged in this interactive process, which helped the community construct a new social identity as a 'sex worker' and established its moral and social justification as a valid occupation. They argued that they do not do any social harm, do not use coercive tactics or physical force, nor bribe. Rather, they provide a service for which they took a payment that is justifiable in a market economy.

This discourse ignited the imagination of the community members, and in the process they carved a new social and political identity that proved to be the most critical element of their community mobilization (Ghose et al. 2008). Articulation of a moral stand appears to be the prerequisite condition for initiation of any new positive social action. This transformative process not only strengthened the sex workers' self-esteem but also built their new vision and aspirations. Questioning one's own value and belief system is not an easy proposition. Interestingly, this questioning and consciousness raising process was not built or created through any formal capacity building programme; rather, it followed from an organic and non-formal pedagogical communication. Slowly but steadily, more and more sex workers became engaged in the process.

Building self-esteem and confidence among sex workers is still continuing in Sonagachi, where old community members engage newcomers in the discourse and process of deconstructing and rebuilding a positive identity in what could be called a process of 'conscientization' (Freire 1970).

Partnering with a mobilizing community

The Durbar Mahila Samanwaya Committee

The sex workers' forum and emerging collective was formalized and officially registered with the government in July of 1995 as the Durbar Mahila Samanwaya Committee (DMSC), which generally translates as the enduring women's cooperative committee. DMSC comprises a lead committee in Kolkata and branch committees in local red light areas (currently totalling 51), each having four officers (president, vice-president, secretary, treasurer) elected for two-year terms by local DMSC members with two-term limits, paid by DMSC (from membership fees and donor resources). This democratic process ensures a constant flow of new leadership opportunities and resistance to entrenchment of individuals in the organization at the expense of broader community involvement. Separately, sex workers can work as programme staff, but not while holding a position as a DMSC official. The highest skilled sex worker staff are promoted through the programme ranks as supervisors, coordinators, and eventually programme directors, often while improving their literacy skills.[4]

During the partnering phase of the CLSI, DMSC functioned as a community advisory board and community partner to SHIP. DMSC also intervened in crisis management for the sex worker community and worked as community organizers to build solidarity among sex workers, form a media savvy political voting bloc to leverage advocacy with powerbrokers at local and national levels, and lead a rights-based social movement. These examples of CLSI activities continue to be core functions of DMSC today. While these are clear examples of community-led activities, in the partnering phase they were more heavily supported by or implemented in partnership with SHIP. For example, advocacy efforts were, and continue to be, conducted with representatives from both SHIP and DMSC, with the status and power of DMSC supported by their political voting bloc and media exposure that they were able to generate.

Continuing to respond to the community's perceived needs

Inspired by a new vision and aspiration, DMSC engaged in a series of activities to address police violence. These included advocacy, negotiation, and network building, and were met with mixed success. In carrying out these activities initially, DMSC began to recognize that it was not the behaviour of the individual police officer but the regulating mechanism of the sex trade that made sex workers vulnerable to police abuse. Law enforcement agencies were empowered to indiscriminately raid, harass, and physically abuse sex workers through both their marginalized status and provisions of the Immoral Traffic Prevention Act (ITPA), which does not criminalize sex work but rather anyone who receives money from an exchange of money and sex between two individuals, as well as involvement of minors.

Slowly but steadily, DMSC members started to identify the underlying causes of sex workers' vulnerability not only to HIV/AIDS, but also to other social problems like violence, discrimination, and stigmatization. The community began to comprehend that its lack of access to official institutions and identification documents (e.g. voter registration, citizenship, rent receipts, bank accounts, insurance schemes) were all linked to its marginalized social and political status. This again was associated with sex workers' occupational status, which was neither legal nor illegal in the country. As a result, DMSC began making efforts to increase the sex worker community's access to banking, education, and official forms of identification while raising their voices against identified structural barriers such as laws, policies, and even administrative practices.

The political struggle experienced by DMSC went hand in hand with the development of ownership over the process and product of the HIV intervention, along with the movement to become recognized as workers, repeal the ITPA (that results in criminalization of family members who receive money from sex workers), and eliminate police abuses. Three years after the initiation of SHIP in 1992, sex workers in the community rallied behind the charter of DMSC's demands and formed the rank and file of the organization by participating in steering committees for community-prioritized projects and in social movement-style activities such as street rallies, engagement with the local intelligentsia, and generation of news media coverage. These activities raised sex workers' levels of consciousness, improved the leadership skills within DMSC to deal with policymakers and powerbrokers, contributed to organizational strength, and increased DMSC's and sex workers' sense of social respectability. DMSC also demonstrated social responsibility and accountability in addressing many other social issues and challenges such as domestic violence, dowry practices, child marriage, and sex work trafficking through establishment of self-regulatory boards, which has improved their image as a respectable civil society organization within India.

Usha multi-purpose cooperative society

One month after DMSC officially registered with the state of West Bengal in 1995, the organization was able to form the Usha micro-banking cooperative, with significant support from the SHIP team. DMSC had to lobby the state government in order to alter the existing cooperative laws to enable official registry as a sex worker cooperative rather than a generic housewife cooperative. Since its inception, Usha has provided savings and lending services for sex workers, underwritten condom social marketing activities (i.e. sale of condoms by sex workers for a nominal fee to other sex workers and clients), supported day care and schools for children, and created other economic alternatives for elderly sex workers or those who want to opt out of the profession. Sex workers have participated in Usha activities as home-visiting 'daily-collector' banking representatives who go door-to-door in the brothels, encourage workers to start daily or weekly savings plans, follow up daily to support workers in adhering to those plans, and report account balances at each visit. A message has been communicated that even seemingly trivial deposits add up over time to build a nest egg of significant savings.

Notably, the focus of microfinance in this context is not primarily on creating alternatives to sex work, but rather to enable sex workers to safely save their money and borrow from savings when needed. Sex workers are the financial drivers of the sex work communities and are seen as a source of money by various other community actors, including madams, landlords, babus, and police. Stigma, lack of education, and lack of documentation all limit access to traditional banking and result in dependence on the informal financial sector of corrupt moneylenders. Prior to Usha, sex workers would typically hide their savings in their rooms. Particularly after busy Puja/festival seasons, sex workers could expect larger sums of cash to be confiscated by mafia/hoodlums and police in raids executed under the pretence of rescue missions. By creating safe savings and lending opportunities, Usha has functioned to reduce sex workers' exposure to theft, violence, and reliance on moneylenders, exploitative madams, or pimps from whom sex workers had typically borrowed money at extremely high interest and at risk of debt bondage. When a sex worker needs to borrow money from Usha, typically to pay for children's schooling or for medical treatment, they actually borrow from and repay their own savings accounts, after careful counselling and problem solving with the cooperative's representatives.

The Usha model ultimately encourages long-term financial security for retirement by leveraging savings for the purchase of property and other resources needed for small businesses (e.g. taxis with husbands or sons; farmland in villages with family members), again with careful counselling and approval by the Usha cooperative. Early attempts by SHIP and DMSC at more traditional microfinance strategies, such as job training and craft industries, were met with failure due to lack of real alternative work opportunities and low demand for craft products, a disempowering and not uncommon result of similar programmes (Brett 2006). As a result, the community prioritized the limited alternative employment opportunities available, such as repair work (electrical, mobile phone, plumbers, etc.) and beauty services, to prevent their children from entering sex work as they transitioned to adulthood, or to support older sex workers who could no longer sustain themselves via sex work.

Transforming economic incentives and power relations

Usha and the sex workers' participation brought about a radical realignment of the control of resources and economic choices in the community by reducing the ease with which they had previously been robbed, extorted, or forced into debt bondage. This, in conjunction with SHIP's advocacy and DMSC's social movement activities, set the stage to reposition the power relations in the community. With the economic incentive for thefts, raids, and usurious lending reduced through Usha's work and the carrot-and-stick advocacy strategies employed by DMSC and SHIP, the sex workers successfully transformed their relationships with police, madams, partners, and others to be less coercive and more supportive and cooperative. DMSC led dramatic social action 'naming and shaming' (e.g. Alinsky 1969), street protests against police abuses, and threateningly violent protests and crisis interventions against criminal abusers.

Simultaneously, SHIP, DMSC, Usha, and their staff gained the support of allied political elites to encourage change in policing policy to be consistent with the law (sex work is not illegal in India), take appropriate disciplinary action, and prosecute criminal abusers. These actions typically included organizing meetings between sex workers and police to air and address grievances, and over time, to build trust and cooperative relationships to address real criminal activities in their communities. In addition, in 2000, DMSC established self-regulatory boards to monitor and interview all new sex workers in the red light areas and prevent trafficked and underage women from working in the brothels covered by the programme. This has resulted in a significant reduction in the number of underage girls working in the brothels, reduced the vulnerability to police raids to rescue minors, and potentially improved empowerment at the community level by removing the most disempowered from the brothels, thereby raising the bar for negotiating power. More recently, in the past five years, one of the most effective strategies implemented has been legal interventions in which civil lawsuits are filed against police, landlords, or abusive babus. Durbar currently employs two full-time lawyers to advocate for the rights of sex workers in the local courts and on the national stage.

Transforming the status quo and ideological structure for decision-making

While SHIP and Usha currently mobilize financial resources, DMSC mobilizes the social resources in the community in its role as a social movement organization (Ghose *et al.* 2008). In DMSC's advocacy with powerbrokers and community mobilization, a simple 'master frame' is utilized: 'Sex work is real work and we demand workers' rights.' While this is well-matched to West Bengal's political environment, which is dominated by a history of Marxist-based politics and situated in the world's largest democracy, it also has implications for motivating individual- and community-level changes. Social justice and rights-based frameworks may be particularly encouraging for social movements (Benford and Snow 2000). Similarly, the status quo, framing of choices, and perceived fairness in negotiated decision-making experiments have been consistently found to influence individual decision-making (Kahneman 1994; Latimer *et al.* 2007). In Durbar's case, a positively framed 'sex worker' identity was associated with a constellation of behaviours, specifically condom use, STD treatment, and solidarity with fellow workers (Ghose *et al.* 2008). Thus, the status quo was transformed from no condom use to condom use, which was then reinforced by rights-based framing and identity-based self-affirmation processes in decision-making and behaviours.

These reframing efforts were the result of the engagement and dialogue with socio-cultural intelligentsia (artists, writers, musicians, journalists) in Kolkata. Durbar now broadly diffuses these frames and identity processes through daily interactions with sex workers and clients, street rallies and protest marches, and by organizing regular cultural programmes (film, theatre, music, and dance performances), local and national conferences, and 'Mela' festivals that draw thousands of sex workers from throughout West Bengal, India, and the world.

Replicating the community-led partner strategy for multiple affinity groups

The structures, processes, and strategies pioneered by Durbar for sex workers have subsequently been replicated by the organization for a plethora of interest groups in the broader sex worker community (and more recently in the unorganized labour sectors of domestic, entertainment, and construction workers) to identify priority needs and organize and mobilize action toward meeting those needs. For each of these affinity groups, a community association is formed based on a shared identity and priorities for action to mobilize around, using the democratic leadership structure modelled by DMSC. In keeping with the dynamic established between SHIP and the sex worker community that recognized the limits of SHIP's scope of work, DMSC has created or spun off multiple sub-organizations, community associations, and projects that harness energies from different segments of the community to express and address their diverse needs, such as the Komol Gandhar performance troupe of sex workers and their children; the Positive Hotline and Kolkata Network of HIV Positives (now independent of Durbar); the Sathi Sangathan babu (male partners) collective; and anti-trafficking self-regulatory boards (SRB). This also has important implications for leadership development of sex workers and members of the specific interest or affinity groups (e.g.

children, partners), as each of the sub-organizations has elected leadership positions that rotate periodically, creating more opportunities for involvement and individual development.

Ownership development to sustain interventions

In April 1999, DMSC and Usha formed a non-governmental organization (NGO), the Society for Human Development and Social Action, to officially take over the implementation and management of the project from the public health institute and the collaborating organizations that originally initiated the project. This NGO, now called Durbar, is made up of sex workers, project staff and other workers formerly associated with the collaborating government, NGOs, and community-based organization (CBO) partners. The goal of Durbar is to further enable the sex worker community to run and sustain projects without dependence on external change agents and resources. SHIP transitioned from being the lead organization to one of many programmes under the Durbar organizational umbrella. The organizational transition also coincided with a leadership change. The original leader of SHIP took another position at a large international NGO and was replaced by a representative from the sex worker community – a sex worker's son.

The next major transition occurred in December 2005, when a DMSC sex worker leader was officially appointed as the new Executive Director of Durbar. Notably, the transition had been planned several years earlier, but it was recognized that more education and training was needed to build the capacities of the community leader to function effectively and meaningfully in the executive role, and not simply be a figurehead. This organizational and leadership transition represented the culmination of the project to become led by community members at the highest level of executive leadership. However, a CLSI that consists solely of an executive from the community, or ownership by a CBO, as symbolic figureheads, does not necessarily result in opportunities for broader community participation. True ownership development necessitates the development of opportunities for the broader community to have control over the process and product of intervention programmes, specifically by prioritizing community ownership of programme design and implementation through management structures, resources (e.g. direct negotiation with funders), and user-friendly capacity building and monitoring and evaluation tools and results.

Repositioning Durbar as mainstream organization

DMSC's inception less than three years after initiating SHIP, followed by the rapid development toward programme ownership over seven years, is remarkable. DMSC has expanded its vision and aspirations over time, shifted short- and medium-term goals, and thereby constantly expands the horizon of community-led activities. This is one of the most unique examples of how one of the most marginalized occupations globally has succeeded in expanding the scope of a narrow, vertical HIV intervention programme into a comprehensive development programme following CLSI approaches. It moved from a health promotion project to a development programme.

Durbar has further broadened its societal stake by going beyond the immediate needs and interests of the sex worker community. Over the past two years, Durbar has played a leadership role in championing causes of unorganized and unrepresented labour in West Bengal as well as in India. Durbar is linking with and supporting other disenfranchised communities in India, such as other unorganized labour sectors (e.g. entertainers, domestic and construction workers) and tribal communities with the objective of developing a wider societal network. In the process, Durbar is repositioning itself within the broader societal structure. Through this process, slowly but steadily, Durbar can 'fudge' the age-old and sharp socio-cultural demarcation between the mainstream and the stigmatized sex worker communities. CLSI-based strategies could be considered one of the most successful approaches to community development and its gain could be measured on the findings of the pre-poll campaign held in India in 2011. A total of 63 per cent of candidates (out of 563 candidates running for assembly election) added their signatures in support of the Durbar charter of demands, which included repeal of the ITPA and recognition of their work and their SRBs.

Conclusion

Durbar's remarkable example may suggest that CLSIs are only possible in a narrow range of settings that have relatively supportive social and political climates. However, the Durbar example should really be seen to represent what is possible, rather than improbable, for public health interventions with marginalized communities through an incremental development of community-led activities over several stages. The first stage of CLSIs, participation, is typically initiated by outside change agents who mobilize external political and fiscal support for new endeavours, typically with funding earmarked for more traditional public health intervention strategies and goals. This initial phase focuses on framing the problem and project to gain community entry and participation, appraising community risks and assets, providing essential services consistent with funding constraints, and creating opportunities for direct community participation as staff in intervention delivery. Through direct participation in and support from intervention programmes, community members can build their capacities to lead intervention activities at increasingly high levels over time. Simultaneously, the community participants and their social networks can be supported in building critical consciousness around the disease priority, their own needs, and the structural factors that link them. In the Durbar case, the public health team reframed HIV from a behavioural risk problem to an occupational health and safety issue that resulted in the identification of a different set of issues and challenges that led to building intervention strategies that addressed structural factors.

The partnership stage of CLSIs capitalizes on capacities developed during the participation stage to advance from community-led implementation to community-led programme prioritization. Supporting the establishment of a formal community association, separate from but partnered with an intervention programme, counterbalances the innate power differentials between marginalized at-risk communities, high-status intervention staff, and other stakeholders. The process also ameliorates tensions between community-driven and public health intervention priorities as the community comes to recognize the values and limitations of the public health intervention and accepts responsibility for addressing priorities beyond the scope of the intervention but with its support. In Sonagachi/Durbar, the sex worker peer CHWs, with support from SHIP, mobilized their community and formed DMSC and Usha to organize, fund, and sustain structural interventions targeting community-driven priorities such as: sex worker solidarity; secure savings and lending; children's education; expansion to new communities; trafficking prevention; rights promotion; and de-stigmatization of sex workers. These factors are linked to HIV risk, but are also so far 'upstream' that they are often beyond the scope of HIV intervention programmes.

The ownership stage of CLSIs focuses on sustaining and expanding interventions by transitioning organizational ownership to the community organization partner via executive leadership and institutional and financial homes. For example, Durbar is now the lead umbrella organization to spearhead multiple structural (and behavioural) interventions, including SHIP, which was previously the lead organization in the intervention. The ownership development that occurred over the first seven years of the CLSI enabled Durbar to continue and sustain itself even when the leaders of the public health intervention team moved on to other opportunities with larger organizations, which is typical in the field.

Most public health intervention programmes emphasize transfer of knowledge and technology to the targeted population. The basic problem behind this type of intervention is that it de-links individual behaviour from the social context, focuses on gaps between knowledge and behaviours, and ignores the fact that within a particular social context individuals may not have the agency, desire, or power to make decisions and follow through with action. Vulnerability of individuals or communities is determined by their social position, status, and their access to services and power. Therefore, the issues of health and development are not just behavioural but linked to structures and social environments. The typical top-down public health intervention does not redress the power structure that reinforces at-risk individuals' and communities' powerlessness and marginalization. It never questions the existing order of things. In the case of CLSIs, programmes are strategized and implemented in partnership with the community to address structural issues and reduce vulnerability to disease and related social problems through a process of active participation and ownership building. To address the issues of health and development, this type of intervention dares to question and change the existing power relations at all social and political levels by mobilizing and empowering the at-risk community. CLSIs ensure active participation of the community beyond being passive beneficiaries and recipients of services. They create an enabling environment to support incremental community engagement, empowerment, and sustained improvements in health, social status, and quality of life.

Notes

1   This case study is informed by the authors' direct experiences with the intervention programme over the past 20 years. Dr Smarajit Jana, MD, trained in tropical medicine and as an occupational health and safety physician, is the founder of the STD/HIV Intervention Programme (SHIP) also known as the Sonagachi Project, which evolved into the CLSI now known as Durbar. In 2000, Dr Jana left his post as Programme Director of SHIP and has since served as the Chief Advisor to Durbar. Dr Dallas Swendeman, PhD, MPH, is trained in medical anthropology and multidisciplinary community health sciences, and has been working in the evidence-based HIV prevention field since 1993. Dr Swendeman has been conducting collaborative research and evaluation projects with Durbar since 2001, which has included a quasi-experimental longitudinal replication trial, mixed-methods research involving ethnographic interviews and cross-sectional random household surveys, and participant-observational ethnographic research under a fellowship from the American Institute of Indian Studies.

2   Note that 'community' is a somewhat contested construct in public health interventions in that a community is often an amorphous and unbounded group of individuals which can be defined by geography, identity, occupation, behaviours, disease risks, and so forth, often with overlapping categorizations. Primary challenges in community mobilization work include processes of identifying, defining, and building community for collective action.

3   Over the past five years the peer CHWs have gradually stopped using the coloured lab coats. As the community organizing and mobilization work described raised the status of all sex workers in the communities they served, the peer CHWs received less personal benefit from the added status afforded to being project workers. Simultaneously, such highly visible demarcation as project staff (as something other or different than sex workers) increasingly presented barriers to engaging the broader sex worker community.

4   Currently and over the past five to ten years, DMSC membership has provided the status and protection (when dealing with police in particular) that previously only the peer CHWs had. This is one reason that the programme is currently experiencing challenges in hiring younger sex workers to work as peer CHWs. Thus, the overwhelming majority of the peer CHWs are older sex workers who are supplementing or replacing their declining incomes from sex work with project-based incomes.

References

Alinsky, S.D. (1969) *Reveille for Radicals*, Chicago: University of Chicago Press.

Benford, R.D. and Snow, D.A. (2000) 'Framing processes and social movements: An overview and assessment', *Annual Review of Sociology*, 26: 611–39.

Blankenship, K.M., Friedman, S.R., Dworkin, S., and Mantell, J.E. (2006) 'Structural interventions: concepts, challenges and opportunities for research', *Journal of Urban Health*, 83: 59–72.

Brett, J.A. (2006) 'We sacrifice and eat less: the structural complexities of microfinance participation', *Human Organization*, 65: 8–19.

Census of India (2011) *Census of India: Provisional Population Tools*. Online, available at: http://censusindia.gov.in/2011census/censusinfodashboard/index.html (accessed 4 April 2012).

Cornish, F. and Ghosh, R. (2007) 'The necessary contradictions of community-led health promotion: a case study of HIV prevention in an Indian red light district', *Social Science & Medicine*, 64: 496.

Freire, P. (1970) *Pedagogy of the Oppressed*, New York: Seabury Press.

Ghose, T., Swendeman, D., George, S., and Chowdhury, D. (2008) 'Mobilizing collective identity to reduce HIV risk among sex workers in Sonagachi, India: the boundaries, consciousness, negotiation framework', *Social Science & Medicine*, 67: 311–20.

Jana, S., Basu, I., Rotheram-Borus, M.J., and Newman, P.A. (2004) 'The Sonagachi Project: a sustainable community intervention program', *AIDS Education and Prevention*, 16: 405–14.

Joint United Nations Programme on HIV/AIDS (UNAIDS) (2000) *Female Sex Worker HIV Prevention Projects: Lessons Learnt from Papua New Guinea, India, and Bangladesh*, Geneva: Joint United Nations Programme on HIV/AIDS.

Kahneman, D. (1994) 'New challenges to the rationality assumption', *Journal of Institutional and Theoretical Economics – Zeitschrift für die gesamte Staatswissenschaft*, 150: 18–36.

Latimer, A.E., Salovey, P., and Rothman, A.J. (2007) 'The effectiveness of gain-framed messages for encouraging disease prevention behavior: is all hope lost?', *Journal of Health Communication*, 12: 645–9.

Laverack, G. and Labonte, R. (2000) 'A planning framework for community empowerment goals within health promotion', *Health Policy and Planning*, 15: 255–62.

Minkler, M., Wallerstein, N., and Wilson, N. (2008) 'Improving health through community organizing and capacity building', in B. Glanz, K. Rimer, and K. Viswanath (eds) *Health Behavior and Health Education Practice: Theory, Research, and Practice*, 4th edition, San Francisco, CA: Jossey-Bass.

Pandey, A., Benara, S.K., Roy, N., Sahu, D., Thomas, M., Joshi, D.K., Sengupta, U., Paranjape, R.S., Bhalla, A. and Prakash, A. (2008) 'Risk behaviour, sexually transmitted infections and HIV among long-distance truck drivers: a cross-sectional survey along national highways in India', *AIDS*, 22: S81–90

Piot, P. (2010) 'Setting new standards for targeted HIV prevention: the Avahan initiative in India', *Sexually Transmitted Infections*, 86: i1–2.

Ray, R. and Korteweg, A.C. (1999) 'Women's movements in the third world: identity, mobilization, and autonomy', *Annual Review of Sociology*, 25: 47–71.

Reckless, W.C. (1933) *Vice in Chicago*, Chicago, IL: University of Chicago Press.

Scambler, G. and Paoli, P. (2008) 'Health work, female sex workers and HIV/AIDS: global and local dimensions of stigma and deviance as barriers to effective interventions', *Social Science & Medicine*, 66: 1848–62.

Sen, A. (1977) 'Rational fools: a critique of the behavioral assumptions of economic theory', *Philosophy and Public Affairs*, 4: 318–44.

Shahmanesh, M., Patel, V., Mabey, D., and Cowan, F. (2008) 'Effectiveness of interventions for the prevention of HIV and other sexually transmitted infections in female sex workers in resource poor settings: a systematic review', *Tropical Medicine and International Health*, 13: 659–79.

Sheth, N.R. (1967) 'Society and industrial work in India: a case study', *Human Organization*, 26: 77–89.

Swendeman, D., Basu, I., Das, S., Jana, S. and Rotheram-Borus, M.J. (2009) 'Empowering sex workers in India to reduce vulnerability to HIV and sexually transmitted diseases', *Social Science & Medicine*, 69: 1157–66.

11

BREAKING THE LINKS

Legal and paralegal assistance to reduce health risks of police and pre-trial detention of sex workers and people who use drugs

Daniel Wolfe, Jonathan Cohen, Heather Doyle, and Tatyana Margolin

While HIV prevention literature commonly describes sex workers and drugs users as 'hard to reach' populations, law enforcement has little difficulty finding them. In a survey conducted across Eastern Europe and Central Asia, 42 per cent of sex workers reported experiencing physical violence at the hands of the police, and 36 per cent had experienced sexual violence (Crago 2009). A 2009 report from Southern Africa documented a similar pattern of frequent arrests, unlawful or otherwise, and routine police abuse that included bribery, forced labour, and rape (Crago and Arnott 2009). The situation is equally severe for people who use drugs. A recent survey of young drug-using men in Tanzania found that 90 per cent had experienced arrest by age 30 (Mbwambo 2010). In virtually all countries where injecting drug users represent the largest share of those with HIV, laws criminalizing possession of small amounts of narcotics, combined with government registries shared by law or practice with the police, place users in constant contact with the law enforcement (Shields 2009; Wolfe 2007). The term 'unapprehended felons', coined by one advocate to refer to the fear created by laws criminalizing sodomy, aptly describes the daily reality for sex workers and people who use drugs.

The uncontrolled nature of these abuses makes even the threat of police contact a threat to health, causing sex workers and people who use drugs to retreat to isolated areas, to reuse and share syringes, to decline to call an ambulance in the event of a drug overdose, to not carry condoms or syringes, and to rush sexual transactions or drug injection (Burris *et al.* 2004; Ravi *et al.* 2007; Richter 2008; Wolfe 2007). Data increasingly suggest that police abuse may be part of a 'syndemic effect' (Singer and Clair 2003), increasing HIV risk in ways similar to correlations found between HIV incidence and past experience of sexual abuse or domestic violence. A recent study, for example, estimated that elimination of police beatings in Odessa, Ukraine might reduce risk of HIV acquisition among injecting drug users by as much as 29 per cent (Strathdee *et al.* 2010). Among Canadian sex workers, prior experience of police abuses was correlated with rape, sexual violence, and displacement from areas providing condoms and other HIV prevention services (Shannon *et al.* 2009). In addition to HIV acquisition risks, contacts with law enforcement bring with them other health-endangering abuses, including confiscation of antiretroviral treatment at point of arrest, rape, beatings, and detention in facilities offering no medical treatment or protection from infection (Crago 2009; Csete and Cohen 2010; FIDA 2008; Human Rights Watch 2010; Schleifer 2006).

Human rights abuses related to law enforcement also reinforce the entrenched discrimination sex workers and people who use drugs face from health care providers, teachers, employers, and many in the general public (Tais Plus 2008; Wolfe 2007). As one sex worker describes, 'In our country, people think sex workers are the worst people in the world … No one in the community will ever share water, food, or bowls with us' (Crago and Arnott 2009: 54). Living in constant fear of conflict with criminal law has detrimental psychological and physical effects: sex workers and drug users routinely conceal their identities, often leading to depression, inadequate diagnosis, and inadequate or interrupted treatment (Alexander 1998; Wolfe 2007; Wolffers and van Beelen 2003). Drug users and sex workers consistently report overt prejudice in health care delivery as a deterrent to seeking or continuing with health services (Grover 2010; Pinkham and Shapoval 2010; Wolfe 2007). The implicit message of criminalization, upheld by the practice of police violence without accountability, is that sex workers and drug users are unworthy of protection or support.

A striking feature of many encounters between police and sex workers or people who use drugs is that they often result not in trial or incarceration, but rather in 'pleading out' of the criminal justice system by informal means such as bribes, sex, or forced labour (FIDA 2008; Hayashi *et al.* 2009; Schleifer 2006). Thus, while multiple studies have detailed the mechanisms by which prison or incarceration acts as a structural determinant of HIV and tuberculosis risk (Beyrer *et al.* 2003; Jurgens *et al.* 2009), it is important to extend this analysis to highlight the adverse health effects of *any* form of police detention, which can begin long before incarceration and occur while in handcuffs in the street, being transported to the police station in the back of a van, or held in police lock-up or a pre-trial facility.

Structural interventions can both accentuate and diminish health risk. This chapter emphasizes the ways in which some structural factors – particularly police detention, harassment, and violence – accentuate the vulnerability of drug users and sex workers who are already marginalized in almost every society. At the same, we highlight a different structural intervention – legal services to diminish health risks associated with police action and pre-trial detention – as a means to reduce health risks. Needle and syringe programmes have been among the best-documented structural interventions for HIV prevention, moving beyond a focus on individual risk and reducing risk to injecting drug users by removing regulatory and physical impediments to sterile injection equipment. We examine ways that legal and paralegal assistance can similarly remove barriers to HIV prevention and treatment, particularly those barriers resulting from police and pre-trial detention. We define pre-trial detention, as sex workers and drug users would, to begin at the moment of first police contact. Building on previous work on the effects of legal services on reduction of HIV or health harms related to pre-trial detention (Csete and Cohen 2010; Wolfe and Cohen 2010), we describe a spectrum of scenarios and services provided anywhere from before police contact to before the initiation of trial. We emphasize the role of lawyers and paralegals not in defending people in the criminal justice system, but in keeping people *out* of that system, particularly in countries where weak rule of law diminishes the likelihood of fair trial, and for populations for whom even a single day of detention can carry acute health risks.

Advocates and high-profile United Nations officials have underscored the importance of 'decriminalization' as a means to remove impediments to effective HIV prevention and treatment (Ki-Moon 2009; Sidibé 2009). For sex workers and drug users, however, police surveillance and deprivation of liberty occur regardless of the letter of the law, including in countries where sex work per se is not against the law or where governments have proclaimed drug users 'patients rather than criminals'. The adverse health impacts of these experiences, and the mechanisms we describe to successfully mitigate them, underscore the importance of attention of what might be called de facto (as opposed to *de jure*) decriminalization. For sex workers and drug users who are often the targets of campaigns against 'social evils' or to improve 'quality of life' (Barton and Sovan 2008; Human Rights Watch 2010; Wolfe 2007), conferral of criminal status and predations by the police occur independent of the courtroom or the law on the books. It is axiomatic, though often ignored, that measures to address the health consequences of police surveillance and detention must also focus on interventions to change dynamics of arrest and detention practices, rather than only on reform of the criminal code.

Scenarios and interventions

In Russia, drug users have described police aggression as '*bezpredel*' (without limits) (Sarang *et al.* 2010). From the perspective of sex workers and people who use drugs, some of the most fearsome effects of this apparently limitless police power are felt long before incarceration or even trial. Drawing on multiple published and first-hand accounts, and our experience as grant-makers working with programmes to increase access to justice for sex workers and drug users in Eastern Europe, Africa, and Asia, we have identified four key phases of detention that occur before trial or incarceration: (1) the stop/search/arrest phase, during which police stop or round up individuals or groups, ostensibly to question, search, or arrest them; (2) the transport phase, during which police detain people in vehicles such as police vans for the purpose of transporting them to the police station; (3) the lock-up phase, during which individuals who have been 'booked' are held in police cells, prior to any determination of pre-trial release or bail; (4) the pre-trial phase, in which individuals who have been denied pre-trial release or bail are held in custody to await trial.

An important feature of the apparently limitless police power faced by sex workers and people who use drugs is that violations of due process at each of these four phases of detention routinely go unnoticed and unaddressed. Thus, while a conventional legal response to police and pre-trial detention may be to secure release through claiming due-process rights (for example, that the police lacked probable cause to arrest, that the conditions to deny bail have not been met), lawyers in this context must go beyond their traditional role. Table 11.1 illustrates a variety of ways in which lawyers and paralegals have intervened from before any police contact, when fear of detention can still result in health risk, through each phase of police and pre-trial detention.

In the sections that follow, we describe legal and paralegal interventions from three illustrative settings – Kenya, Indonesia, and Ukraine – where detention without due process at different points before trial contributes to substantial health risks for sex workers and people who use drugs. After describing each of these interventions and the contexts in which they occur, we reflect on the changing role of the legal professional in environments where criminalization and weak rule of law conspire to over-detain groups already at high risk of HIV and other health problems.

Table 11.1 Legal and paralegal interventions along the continuum from prior to police contact to pre-trial detention

Phase	Interventions		
1 Pre–arrest	Lawyers/communities strengthening relations with police through joint training workshops	Lawyers/paralegals accompanying outreach workers in heavily policed areas	Lawyers/paralegals training communities to know-your-rights and laws
2 Stop/search/ arrest	Paralegals on call to respond with 'legal first aid'	Communities carrying know-your-rights cards	
3 Transport	Lawyers/paralegals beating police to the station	Communities contacting paralegals via SMS	
4 Lock-up	Paralegals visiting lock-up to post bail or document conditions	Lawyers identifying and documenting procedural violations	
5 Pre-trial	Lawyers/doctors working together to obtain a medical exam	Lawyers/doctors working together to obtain necessary medical assistance	Lawyers/doctors working together to use health conditions to secure pre-trial release

Beyond the adversarial in Kenya: building police-community partnerships

Just by having Joan around our programme, we have noted fewer violations against sex workers. Joan working with police officers and sharing legal matters has greatly improved how police officers view our work.

(Keeping Alive Societies' Hope [KASH] 2010: 5)

The city of Kisumu in the Nyanza Province of Western Kenya is the country's third largest city, with a population of just over 355,000. Kisumu literally means 'a place of barter' in the local language and remains an epicentre for trade and business. It also has become an epicentre of the country's HIV epidemic. Nyanza Province's HIV prevalence rate is 13.9 per cent, or almost twice the national rate (National AIDS Control Council 2010). Sex workers are particularly hard-hit, with a 2001 study estimating HIV prevalence among them at 75 per cent (Morison *et al.* 2001).

Many factors contribute to the high HIV prevalence. Organizations in the region struggle with the impact of criminalization on those considered to be 'most at-risk' for HIV, including men who have sex with men, sex workers, and people who inject drugs (National AIDS Control Council 2010). Community or religious leaders periodically call for 'clean-ups' of urban and peri-urban areas, resulting in crack-downs and mass arrests by the police of sex workers (*Daily Nation* 2011; KASH 2011). With sex work not criminalized in Kenya per se and absent reasonable suspicion of another crime, many of these arrests are unlawful. Police arbitrarily arrest and detain people on suspicion of sex work based on non-probative factors such as what they are wearing or where they are walking at a certain time of night. Once arrested and detained, sex workers almost always end up paying a bribe or offering free sexual services to obtain release without ever entering the police station. The cycle of arbitrary arrest and detention of sex workers is so entrenched that many sex workers pay or service police on regular schedules (FIDA 2008).

If and when sex workers are taken into police custody, they face extreme abuse including rape, beatings, intrusive body searches, and degrading treatment (FIDA 2008). Sex workers have reported being forced to perform chores at the officers' houses; if taken into police lock-up, they may be forced to wash the cells. After 24 to 48 hours, sex workers are typically released after pleading guilty and paying a fine. Rarely do they see a lawyer. A report from the Federation of Women Lawyers in Kenya noted that police themselves were unaware of a single case where an arrested sex worker pleaded not guilty and the case was heard and determined by a court. Such arrests, automatically marked as successful prosecutions, bring professional benefits to those officers who make them (FIDA 2008).

The organization Keeping Alive Societies' Hope (KASH) recognized the impact that police violence had on sex workers, and in turn their vulnerability to HIV infection. In 2007, KASH approached police leaders in the Nyanza Province about launching a partnership to reduce police violence against sex workers. With the assistance of a lawyer, they piloted training workshops where police and sex workers together learned relevant human rights and Kenyan law pertaining to sex work and due process. These forums provided a non-adversarial forum for police to understand the concerns of sex workers, and for sex workers to build relationships with police. As of 2011, KASH has been invited to lead regular training courses at the Kisumu provincial police training centre. Through KASH's work, at least 600 police officers in the region have been trained on human rights and Kenyan law on sex work and due process, and KASH continues to reach another 120 regular police officers through the government-funded training (KASH 2011).

The result of KASH's work has been a reduction in police violence against sex workers. Through the human rights training workshops, for example, sex workers learn to ask for bond release to avoid lengthy detention that may make it difficult to find other employment. Sex workers also describe situations in which police who have participated in one of KASH's training workshops helped negotiate their release from illegal detention. For example, Wilson Lomali, a police peer educator with KASH who works as head of a provincial police training facility in Kisumu, has assisted sex workers in several circumstances. In one instance when a sex worker called him from the police station where she was being detained, Lomali asked her to pass the phone to the nearest officer and worked to secure her release (Thomas 2011). Lomali has also travelled to bars in the middle of the night to intervene when clients become violent, ready to mediate or make an arrest, based on the sex workers' needs. In one scenario in which a sex worker had been raped and stabbed, Lomali became involved when staff at a local health facility tried to charge the woman for the free form required to document sexual assaults. In another incident when several sex workers reported that a specific police officer was forcing them to have sex without a condom and stealing their money, Lomali and his colleagues worked to ensure that the man was fired (Thomas 2011).

Police likewise have benefited from the trainings in terms of improved community relations, reporting that patrolling areas where sex work is prevalent can feel less threatening when they see sex workers they have met through the trainings. In an illustration of support for the programme from high-ranking officers, consistent involvement with the training workshops is considered positively when weighing grounds for promotion. As the programme becomes recognized as a best practice for reducing violence and improving policing practices, police leaders are motivated to maintain and improve the initiative.

KASH engaged a lawyer, Joan, to assist in the development and implementation of the police training workshops. According to KASH, 'just by having Joan around our programme, we have noted fewer violations against sex workers. Joan's work with police officers and sharing on legal matters has greatly improved how police officers view our work' (KASH 2010: 5). In addition to offering substantive legal expertise in the development of the workshops, the lawyer contributes to other programmes that KASH offers to protect the human rights of sex workers. For example, she has trained a pool of sex workers as paralegals to receive and document complaints of human rights abuses through a mobile phone-based text services system known as Frontline SMS. If a sex worker is arrested, he or she is trained to immediately send a text message to a paralegal, who in turn responds or engages the lawyer to intervene immediately to attempt to stop the abuse. The information is then compiled to inform a legal and human rights advocacy strategy. KASH's lawyer also participates in a monthly advocacy planning session, which includes rotating members of police, sex workers, and other KASH programme staff, to continuously inform KASH's work on human rights and policy advocacy.

KASH's work attests not only to the importance of intervening at the pre-arrest stage, but also to the non-traditional role of the legal professional in contexts where due process and the rule of law are weak. To date, KASH's lawyer has not filed one case in court. Although her legal training and stature are likely critical to the success of KASH's efforts and to the police's willingness to participate in the training, her responsibilities are as much those of a trainer or programme officer as a practising lawyer. The services that she provides, while non-traditional for lawyers, are critical to sex workers obtaining justice and protecting their health.

'Legal first aid' in Indonesia: paralegals to keep people out of the system

If you can stop it, stop it. If you can't stop it, document it.

(Lembaga Bantuan Hukum Masyarakat [LBHM] 2011)

Indonesia is home to a concentrated HIV epidemic among people who inject drugs. The Indonesian government places the number of injecting drug users at 220,000 (Mathers *et al.* 2010), though harm-reduction NGOs have long noted that these are underestimates (Oppenheimer and Gunawan 2005). Almost half of Indonesia's injecting drug users are HIV positive (National AIDS Commission Republic of Indonesia 2009). Indonesian law allows for imposition of criminal penalties on those who fail to report illicit drug use voluntarily; though the law does provide for treatment alternatives to incarceration (Wardany 2009), judges rarely use this provision. This leaves drug users keenly aware of the potential dangers of going forward to trial: those caught with even small amounts of narcotics may serve a prison term of up to nine years, with pre-trial detention periods lasting months (Davis *et al.* 2009). More than 60 per cent of detainees in Indonesia's overcrowded detention centres are there on drug-related charges (LBHM 2011). Even before entry into the system, injecting drug users routinely experience beatings or torture, with a recent survey of more than 1,000 injecting drug users finding that 60 per cent had experienced abuses at the hands of police (Davis *et al.* 2009).

In a typical scenario encountered by a Jakarta-based NGO Lembaga Bantuan Hukum Masyarakat (LBHM), who provide paralegal services to people who use drugs, police break into a home with several suspected drug users and arrest two of them. The police accuse the arrestees of selling *putaw* (street-grade heroin) and search them, finding nothing. After an hour, three more police officers, including the head of the unit, arrive. They take the two suspects into a car, where they intimidate them through such things as beatings, a gun to the head, or pulling off their fingernails to force a confession. Later, they take them to police lock-up, where they are threatened with more beating and asked to pay money for their release.

To respond to this abuse, LBHM has trained drug users as paralegals to reduce detention and increase access to justice. In what is referred to by LBHM as 'legal first aid', those vulnerable to police harassment and detention, including drug users and fishermen deemed illegal residents in Jakarta, are trained as paralegals to educate their peers about due process and other legal issues (Global Campaign for Pretrial Justice 2011). Training is rigorous, with participants joining for a series of legal education groups and subsequently tested for accuracy of understanding. In the first cycle, approximately half of drug-using participants failed the examination. Those trained successfully visit at the initial stages of detention to take testimony from detainees, and where procedural violations have occurred, try to secure release. Other paralegals, notified when drug users are being beaten, have arrived at the scene and used their mobile phones to interview witnesses or otherwise document abuses. Paralegals consult frequently with lawyers working for the sponsoring organization, who represent drug users in court if necessary. The paralegals are also community educators, conducting trainings on specifics of Indonesian law at meetings convened by local AIDS organizations and drug user groups.

Paralegals thus serve a combined function of providing support, connecting the vulnerable to immediate legal assistance, and documenting human rights violations. In the context of a police raid such as the one described above, paralegals might follow the arresting officers' car to the police station, negotiate conditions of detention and release with police, and contact families when money is needed for bail. In some cases, paralegals perform functions many family members might be unable to do, such as delivering antiretroviral medications or taking testimony from those whose families may not know of their HIV infection or drug use. Drug users report that having peers as 'first responders' at the police station reduces the risk of extortion, since the arrival of a lawyer may signal that the detainee's family has money.

Working the system in Ukraine: lawyers securing pre-trial release

For drug users, 72 hours is too long to be held without drugs or treatment, but 144 hours is much longer – police take advantage of their state of withdrawal to get them to confess to anything.

(Kaminska 2011a)

Driven primarily by drug use, Eastern Europe's HIV epidemic is one of the fastest growing in the world. Weak investment in harm-reduction services combined with hyper-criminalization have resulted in a situation where people who use drugs are more likely to be detained by police than to be provided with community-based HIV prevention and treatment. Excessive detention is fuelled by rampant violations of due process. These have also exacerbated the health problems faced by people who use drugs, who – like all pre-trial detainees – are held in police interrogation units and in institutions, known as SIZOs, where they spend months or years in facilities that are rife with violence and lacking in basic medical care (Global Campaign for Pretrial Justice 2010; Tumanov and Telehov 2011). Pre-trial detainees are routinely denied diagnosis or treatment, with authorities citing the ostensibly temporary nature of the facilities as justification for inaction (Csete 2012; Global Campaign for Pretrial Justice 2010, 2011). With overcrowding common and infection control limited, tuberculosis infection is a particular danger – with some studies showing highest risk in the first weeks of detention (Global Campaign for Pretrial Justice 2010, 2011; Reyes 2003). Detainees have reported interruption of treatment, whether for HIV, diabetes, epilepsy, or multiple other life-threatening conditions (Barry 2011; Csete 2012; European Court of Human Rights 2007). Detention also exacerbates risk of blood-borne illnesses such as HIV and hepatitis C, since unprotected sex and drug injection are common, but condoms and clean needles are unavailable (Csete 2012; Global Campaign for Pretrial Justice 2011).

Ukraine, with an HIV epidemic concentrated among injecting drug users and the highest HIV prevalence in Europe (Ukraine Ministry of Health 2009), subjects pre-trial detainees to multiple health risks. Although laws limit the length of time during which criminal suspects can be held without appearance before a judge, officials routinely use procedural tricks to extend detention, often in hopes of coercing a bribe or confession (Kaminska 2011b). In an illustrative recent example, a client of the organization All Together in Lviv was detained on suspicion of distribution of drugs because a neighbour 'reported' him. The suspect was handcuffed and taken to the police station. A lawyer from All Together called by the detainee's parents the next day was refused a visit, after which she filed several complaints about violation of criminal and administrative procedures. On the third day of his detention, the client was released on the condition of admitting guilt. The lawyer later discovered that the police had registered a detention on administrative grounds, allowing them to hold the client for an initial 72 hours, and then filed a criminal detention order allowing for an additional 72 hours, that is a total of 144 hours of detention without any formal charge (Kaminska 2011c).

An extra 72 hours of detention carries particular risks for those dependent on opioids. Patients on medications such as methadone or buprenorphine, as well as drug-dependent individuals not on treatment, are routinely left to experience painful withdrawal symptoms, with police using the physical punishment of withdrawal as means of coercing confessions. 'This is how it works', the head of the Ukrainian association of substitution treatment patients explains. 'They have a needle with drugs in one hand, and a blank paper in the other. They tell you, "Sign the paper, and we'll give you the drugs"' (Belayeva 2008). A police notation that the detainee was using her apartment as a 'den' for sex work or drugs may result in an extended prison sentence, and in forfeiture of the property (Belayeva 2008).

Mariya Kaminska, the lawyer who leads the Ukrainian NGO All Together, and who intervened in the arrest described above, has developed an effective intervention of exploiting violations of internal procedure to get her clients, who are primarily people who use drugs, out of pre-trial detention. Kaminska recognized early on in her legal practice that respect for due process, much less a determination of guilt or innocence, is largely irrelevant to whether this population group remains detained. Even when evidence is absent to tie a drug user to a crime, the police will not hesitate to plant evidence, hire stand-in witnesses, or take other measures to pin an unsolved crime on an accused person (Schleifer 2006). Kaminska has consequently mastered procedures such as how to properly 'book' an arrestee as a negotiating tactic to persuade police to release a client rather than proceed with a trial that could easily result in a wrongful conviction (Kaminska 2011c). In the case described above, for example, Kaminska preemptively filed both criminal and administrative complaints against the police for their irregular booking procedures, undermining their claims of having legally obtained a confession and contributing to the criminal charges against her client to be dropped (Kaminska 2011c). In the climate of police acting '*bezpredel*' (without limits), it is mastery of these internal procedures, rather than due process claims or arguments made at trial, that constrain police action and result in release of detainees who might experience not only prolonged detention, but also exposure to or exacerbation of life-threatening illness.

Much of Kaminska's success has to do with the connections she has made between the basic principles of harm reduction, the provision of health services to drug users unable or unwilling to stop using drugs, and legal aid. Recognizing that establishing an alliance with her clients and 'meeting them where they are' is key to effectiveness, Kaminska is available to her clients 24 hours a day, and it is not unusual for her to receive text messages from those who are in the process of being detained or are en route to the police station. Her legal budget includes funds for sterile injection equipment, which she distributes on set dates in the areas of the city frequented by drug users. While on outreach, she also provides legal advice and distributes know-your-rights booklets, all of which list her contact information.

Restructuring risk: the role of the legal professional as health defender

Interventions that move risk reduction beyond the level of the individual, such as provision of sterile injection equipment and condoms, have been recognized as structural approaches that provide people who use drugs and sex workers with lifesaving commodities. In the HIV field generally, the provision of legal services has also been recognized as a structural intervention leading to decreased incarceration and improved health (Csete and Cohen 2010; UNAIDS *et al.* 2009). For legal services to be effective as a structural intervention, it is critical that they target the vast majority of injecting drug users and sex workers who are regularly detained by police, and for whom no court appearance or litigation occurs. Whether because of fear of painful withdrawal, police violence, public humiliation, or the need to get back to making money, these groups frequently submit to extortion or sexual abuse to 'plead out' of criminal justice systems they know to be too slow or inefficient to bring defendants to trial in a reasonable period. Reaching these individuals challenges our conventional understanding of legal services and, in turn, of structural interventions to prevent HIV. Non-traditional approaches to legal and paralegal services, and associated changes to police practices and patterns of detention, may ultimately be as critical to HIV prevention and other health protection as a clean needle or a condom.

Lawyers and paralegals seeking to bring their skills to bear on health protection of criminalized populations have redefined the role and locus of legal assistance. The legal and paralegal services provided to criminalized populations are not generally rendered in the court room, but rather in the training workshop, on the street, in the police van, or immediately at lock-up. These services may be less about defending someone in the criminal justice system than negotiating their way out of that system entirely. The provider of the services may be a lawyer, but it may equally be a paralegal drawn from the community who can triage services and make effective referrals. Shifting key tasks to paralegals may not only save money, but also build trust as people learn to provide legal advice and information to their own peers. The skills required of lawyers under this model also change. Strong trial skills are less essential then a mastery of procedures, relationships with the police, and perhaps most important, the capacity to listen to communities and officials and work with them to find innovative solutions to safeguard liberty.

In the context of HIV and AIDS, there is increasing recognition of the importance of shifting tasks traditionally performed by doctors towards community-based health workers who have the commitment, capacity, and community relationships to provide many needed health services. The legal profession is similarly recognizing the possibilities of 'task shifting' and the unique role played by community-based paralegals. The resulting blend of health and legal services is often expressed through physical as well as metaphoric integration: for example, providing food or clean needles as part of a legal or paralegal service gives lawyers and paralegals an opening to start a relationship and begin to build trust. In this regard, it is telling that the lawyer working in KASH, Joan, holds the title of programme officer, not unlike the sex workers KASH employs. In addition to her legal work, she assumes responsibilities such as developing programming and advocacy strategies, and recognizes that clients may need basic food or shelter before being able to discuss legal problems.

These kinds of legal and paralegal assistance also challenge police or public understanding of the social and legal position of sex workers and people who use drugs. Police actions against these populations, often conducted with attention to public display, play an important role in the formation of social attitudes about those undeserving of social support. Police in countries as varied as Macedonia and China have paraded 'prostitutes' in front of television cameras or jeering crowds in 'shame parades' (Doyle 2010; Watts 2006); China has also marked 26 June, the United Nations Day Against Illicit Drug Trafficking and Abuse, with public sentencing of alleged drug traffickers while crowds chant, 'Kill, kill!' (Wolfe 2007). In Thailand, Malaysia, Vietnam and Cambodia, government leaders have launched a variety of zero tolerance and 'strike hard' campaigns (Wolfe 2007), with Vietnam and Cambodia also devoting significant media attention to government plans to eliminate sex work (Human Rights Watch 2010). With detention so tied to social norms of good and evil, the appearance of a legal professional to help a drug user or sex worker signals that these individuals have social networks that extend beyond the criminal frame: those offering assistance outside the police van, station, or pre-trial facility affirm both the rights of those detained and their links to other social supports. In this sense, legal and paralegal assistance can be understood as stigma reduction, in a form that directly engages power relations in ways that many more generic approaches to stigma reduction campaigns may not (Parker and Aggleton 2003).

While the power of legal and paralegal services to secure liberty is lasting and deep, however, the interventions described in this chapter represent a stopgap solution to an unacceptable problem. Ultimately, it is the criminalization of populations at high risk of HIV combined with unaccountable police and weak rule of law that contributes to the abuses to which lawyers and paralegals must creatively respond. In the long term, the solution is to replace the *de jure* and de facto criminalization of sex workers and people who use drugs with a structural approach that minimizes or eliminates the intrusion of the criminal justice system into the arena of public health. Until such time as public health prevails over punishment, lawyers and paralegals will need to deploy all manner of tactics to protect the life, liberty, and health of some of society's most marginalized individuals, demonstrating a professional flexibility as 'without limits' as the abuse to which it must respond.

Acknowledgements

The authors thank Thomas Odhiambo at KASH (Kenya), Maria Kaminska of All Together (Ukraine), and Ricky Gunawan of LBHM (Indonesia) for their ongoing vision in use of legal and paralegal assistance to protect and improve health of criminalized groups. Rachel Thomas and David Scamell provided valuable insights and review, and Johna Hoey and Romina Kazandjian assisted ably with research and citations.

References

Alexander, P. (1998) 'Sex work and health: a question of safety in the workplace', *Journal of the American Medical Women's Association*, 53 (2): 77–82.

Barry, E. (2011) 'Poor care led to death of lawyer, Russia says', *New York Times*, 4 July. Online, available at: http://www.nytimes.com/2011/07/05/world/europe/05moscow.html (accessed 21 September 2011).

Barton, C. and Sovan, N. (2008) 'Poorhouse purgatory', *The Phnom Penh Post*, 29 June. Online, available at: http://ki-media.blogspot.com/2008/06/poorhouse-purgatory.html (accessed 21 September 2011).

Belayeva, O. (2008) 'Women, HIV and drug use in Ukraine', Open Society Institute Briefing on Women and Drug Use, Commission on Narcotic Drugs, Vienna, 7 March.

Beyrer, C., Jittiwutikarn, J., Teokul, W., Razak, M.H., Suriyanon, V., Srirak, N., Vongchuk, T., Tovanabutra, S., Sripaipan, T., and Celentano, D.D. (2003) 'Drug use, increasing incarceration rates, and prison-associated HIV risks in Thailand', *AIDS and Behavior*, 7 (2): 153–61.

Burris, S., Blankenship, K.M., Donoghoe, M., Sherman, S., Vernick, J.S., Case, P., Lazzarini, Z., and Koester, S. (2004) 'Addressing the "risk environment" for injection drug users: the mysterious case of the missing cop', *Milbank Quarterly*, 82 (1): 125–56.

Crago, A.L. (2009) *Arrest the Violence: Human Rights Abuses against Sex Workers in Central and Eastern Europe and Central Asia*, Budapest: Sex Workers' Rights Advocacy Network (SWAN).

Crago, A.L. and Arnott, J. (2009) *Rights Not Rescue: A Report on Female, Male, and Trans Sex Workers' Human Rights in Botswana, Namibia, and South Africa*, New York: Open Society Institute, Public Health Program.

Csete, J. (2012) *Pretrial Detention and Health: Unintended Consequences, Deadly Results*, New York: Open Society Institute Justice Initiative.

Csete, J. and Cohen, J. (2010) 'Health benefits of legal services for criminalized populations: the case of people who use drugs, sex workers and sexual and gender minorities', *Journal of Law, Medicine, and Ethics*, 38 (4): 816–31.

Daily Nation (2011) '37 held in raid on prostitution dens', 20 May, p. 6.

Davis, S.L., Triwahyuono, A., and Alexander, R. (2009) 'Survey of abuses against injecting drug users in Indonesia', *Harm Reduction Journal*, 6: 28.

Doyle, H. (2010) *You Must Know About Me: Sex Worker Voices in Macedonia*. Online, available at: http://blog.soros.org/2010/03/you-must-know-about-me-sex-worker-voices-in-macedonia/ (accessed 21 September 2011).

European Court of Human Rights (2007) *Khudobin v Russia*, no. 59696/00.

Federation of Women Lawyers Kenya (FIDA) (2008) *Documenting Human Rights Violations of Sex Workers in Kenya: A Report Based on Findings of a Study Conducted in Nairobi, Kisumu, Busia, Nanyuki, Mombasa and Malindi Towns in Kenya*, Nairobi: Federation of Women Lawyers Kenya.

Global Campaign for Pretrial Justice (2010) *Pretrial Detention and Public Health: Unintended Consequences, Deadly Results*, New York: Open Society Institute, Public Health Program.

Global Campaign for Pretrial Justice (2011) *Improving Health in Pretrial Detention: Pilot Interventions and the Need for Evaluation*, New York: Open Society Foundations.

Grover, A. (2010) United Nations General Assembly, Human Rights Council 14th Session. Promotion and Protection of all Human Rights, Civil, Political, Economic, Social and Cultural Rights, Including the Right to Development (A/HRC/14/20), 27 April 2010.

Hayashi, K., Milloy, M.-J., Fairbairn, N., Kaplan, K., Suwannawong, P., Lai, C., Wood, E., and Kerr, T. (2009) 'Incarceration experiences among a community – recruited sample of injection drug users in Bangkok, Thailand', *BioMed Central Public Health*, 9: 492.

Human Rights Watch (2010) *Off the Streets: Arbitrary Detention and Other Abuses against Sex Workers in Cambodia*, New York: Human Rights Watch.

Joint United Nations Programme on HIV/AIDS, International Development Law Organization, and United Nations Development Programme (UNAIDS, IDLO, UNDP) (2009) *Toolkit: Scaling Up HIV Related Legal Services*, Rome and Geneva: International Development Law Organization and Joint United Nations Programme on HIV/AIDS.

Jurgens, R., Ball, A., and Verster, M.A. (2009) 'Interventions to reduce HIV transmission related to injecting drug use in prison', *The Lancet Infectious Diseases*, 9 (1): 57–66.

Kaminska, M. (2011a) 'Re: Detention'. E-mail (19 September 2011).

Kaminska, M. (2011b) 'No subject'. E-mail (13 April 2011).

Kaminska, M. (2011c) 'No subject'. E-mail (12 April 2011).

Keeping Alive Societies' Hope (KASH) (2010) *Clarifications on Final Report to Open Society Institute – February 2010*. Kisumu: Keeping Alive Societies' Hope.

Keeping Alive Societies' Hope (KASH) (2011) Proposal to Open Society Foundations: *Intensifying the Focus on Sex Workers' and Men who Have Sex with Men's Human Rights amongst Judiciary, Civil/opinion Leaders and Law Enforcement Agents in Kisumu*, Kenya, Kisumu: Keeping Alive Societies' Hope.

Ki-Moon, B. (2009) United Nations General Assembly. *Progress made in the implementation of the Declaration of Commitment on HIV/AIDS and the Political Declaration on HIV/AIDS*. Document A/63/81. 7 May 2009.

Lembaga Bantuan Hukum Masyarakat (LBHM) (2011) *Empowering Drug Users: Strengthening Drug User Paralegals' Capacity in Documentation and Advocacy*, Jakarta: Lembaga Bantuan Hukum Masyarakat.

Mathers, B.M., Degenhardt, L., Ali, H., Wiessing, L., Hickman, M., Mattick, R.P., Myers, B., Ambekar, A., and Strathdee, S.A. (2010) 'HIV prevention, treatment, and care services for people who inject drugs: a systematic review of global, regional, and national coverage', *The Lancet*, 375 (9719): 1014–28.

Mbwambo, J.K. (2010) *Injection Drug Use and its Interventions in Africa: The Forgotten Continent – Some Examples from Tanzania*, Washington, D.C.: Center for Strategic and International Studies Africa Program.

Morison, L., Weiss, H.A., Buve, A., Carael, M., Abega, S.C., Kaona, F., Kanhonou, L., Chege, J., Hayes, R.J., and Study Group on Heterogeneity of HIV Epidemics in African Cities (2001) 'Commercial sex and the spread of HIV in four cities in sub-Saharan Africa', *AIDS*, 15: S61.

National AIDS Commission Republic of Indonesia (2009) *Republic of Indonesia Country Report on the Follow Up to the Declaration of Commitment on HIV/AIDS*, United Nations General Assembly Special Session on HIV/AIDS, Jakarta: National AIDS Commission Republic of Indonesia.

National AIDS Control Council (2010) *United Nations General Assembly Special Session on HIV and AIDS (UNGASS 2010) Country Report – Kenya*. Online, available at: http://www.unaids.org/en/dataanalysis/monitoringcountryprogress/2010progressreportssubmittedbycountries/kenya_2010_country_progress_report_en.pdf (accessed 21 September 2011).

Oppenheimer, E. and Gunawan, S. (2005) *A Review of Vulnerable Populations to HIV and AIDS in Indonesia*, Jakarta: Joint United Nations Programme on HIV/AIDS (UNAIDS) and National AIDS Commission.

Parker, R. and Aggleton, P. (2003) 'HIV and AIDS-related stigma and discrimination: a conceptual framework and implications for action', *Social Science & Medicine*, 57 (1): 13–24.

Pinkham, S. and Shapoval, A. (2010) *Making Harm Reduction Work for Women: The Ukrainian Experience*, New York: Open Society Institute, Public Health Program.

Ravi, A., Blankenship, K., and Altice, F.L. (2007) 'The association between history of violence and HIV risk: a cross-sectional study of HIV-negative incarcerated women in Connecticut', *Women's Health Issues*, 17 (4): 210–16.

Reyes, H. (2003) 'Pitfalls of TB management in prisons, revisited', *International Journal of Prisoner Health*, 3 (1): 43–67.

Richter, M. (2008) 'Sex work, reform initiatives and HIV/AIDS in inner-city Johannesburg', *African Journal of AIDS Research*, 7 (3): 323–33.

Sarang, A., Rhodes, T., Sheon, N., and Page, K. (2010) 'Policing drug users in Russia: risk, fear, and structural violence', *Substance Use and Misuse*, 45 (6): 813–64.

Schleifer, R. (2006) 'Rhetoric and risk: human rights abuses impeding Ukraine's fight against HIV/AIDS', *Human Rights Watch*, 18 (2): 1–88.

Shannon, K., Kerr, T., Strathdee, S.A., Shoveller, J., Montaner, J.S., and Tyndall, M.W. (2009) 'Prevalence and structural correlates of gender based violence among a prospective cohort of female sex workers', *British Medical Journal*, 339: b2939.

Shields, A. (2009) *The Effects of Drug User Registration Laws on People's Rights and Health: Key Findings from Russia, Georgia, and Ukraine*, New York: Open Society Institute, Public Health Program.

Sidibé, M. (2009) 'HIV and drugs: a total strategy', *The Bangkok Post*, 20 April. Online, available at: http://www.bangkokpost.com/opinion/opinion/15320/hiv-and-drugs-a-total-strategy (accessed 21 September 2011).

Singer, M. and Clair, S. (2003) 'Syndemics and public health: reconceptualizing disease in bio-social context', *Medical Anthropology Quarterly*, 17 (4): 423–41.

Strathdee, S.A., Hallett, T.B., Bobrova, N., Rhodes, T., Booth, R., Abdool, R., and Hankins, C.A. (2010) 'HIV and risk environment for injecting drug users: the past, present, and future', *The Lancet*, 376 (9737): 268–84.

Tais Plus (2008) *Shadow Report to the Third Periodic Report of Kyrgyzstan to the Committee on the Elimination of Discrimination against Women*, Bishkek: Tais Plus.

Thomas, R. (2011) *East Africa Trip Report: Law and Health Initiative and Sexual Health and Rights Project*, New York: Open Society Foundations, Public Health Program.

Tumanov, G. and Telehov, M. (2011) 'Detainees do not survive prison hospital', *Gazeta.ru*, 22 September. Online, available at: http://www.gazeta.ru/social/2011/08/10/3729165.shtml (accessed 1 July 2012).

Ukraine Ministry of Health (2009) *Ukraine: National Report on Monitoring Progress towards the UNGASS Declaration of Commitment on HIV/AIDS*, Kiev: Ukraine Ministry of Health.

Wardany, I. (2009) 'New drugs ruling not retroactive', *Jakarta Post*, 23 March. Online, available at: http://www.thejakartapost.com/news/2009/03/23/new-drugs-ruling-not-%E2%80%98retroactive%E2%80%99.html (accessed 7 July 2012).

Watts, J. (2006) 'Outrage at Chinese prostitutes' shame parade', *The Guardian*, 6 December. Online, available at: http://www.guardian.co.uk/world/2006/dec/06/china.jonathanwatts?INTCMP=SRCH (accessed 21 September 2011).

Wolfe, D. (2007) 'Paradoxes in antiretroviral treatment for injecting drug users: access, adherence and structural barriers in Asia and the former Soviet Union', *International Journal of Drug Policy*, 18 (4): 246–54.

Wolfe, D. and Cohen, J. (2010) 'Human rights and HIV prevention, treatment, and care for people who inject drugs: key principles and research needs', *Journal of Acquired Immune Deficiency Syndrome*, 55 (Suppl. 1): S56–62.

Wolffers, I. and van Beelen, N. (2003) 'Public health and the human rights of sex workers', *The Lancet*, 361 (9373): 1981.

12

STRUCTURED ENVIRONMENTS AND DIETARY-RELATED CHRONIC DISEASES

Deborah A. Cohen

> We prefer to take our chance with cholera and the rest than be bullied
> into health. There is nothing a man hates so much as being cleansed
> against his will, or having his floors swept, his walls whitewashed, his
> pet dung heaps cleared away, or his thatch forced to give way to slate, all
> at the command of a sort of sanitary bombaliff. It is a positive fact that
> many have died of a good washing.
>
> *The Times*, 1854 – Objecting to Sanitary Reform[1]

Before the sanitary revolution of the mid-nineteenth century, there were neither regulations nor standards that governed housing, sewage, trash and waste disposal, food sales, or pollution of the environment. When such regulations were proposed, they were not accepted blindly, but criticized as unreasonable, unfounded, and irrelevant to the promotion of public health. Yet, after standards were established, large declines in population mortality ensued. Ever since it was recognized that regulations and performance standards had a positive impact on health and well-being, the standards for housing, waste management, and food processing have become increasingly strict in developed countries. Furthermore, a large infrastructure has been created to enforce these regulations: inspectors daily check the construction of new buildings for safety concerns, assess and regulate the waste management practices of industry to protect air and water quality, and inspect farms, factories, and restaurants to reduce the likelihood of food contamination and infectious disease transmission. For the most part, a balance has been struck between regulators and industry, so that adherence to regulations does not spell bankruptcy and financial ruin for business.

Yet the gains made in the prevention of injury, toxic exposures, and infectious disease transmission have not been paralleled by gains in the prevention of chronic diseases. This may be due to the entirely different paradigm by which chronic diseases are conceptualized. While the former are generally considered to be due to exposures and conditions that individuals cannot easily avoid, chronic diseases associated with diet and physical activity are believed by many to be the result of conscious decisions and lifestyle choices freely chosen (US Department of Health and Human Services 2001). Thus, it has been argued, there is no need for regulation, since individuals have the right to determine the diets they consume and the amount of exercise they get.

Moreover, the relative risks of disease outcomes from dietary choices are quite modest compared to the risks that have been previously associated with exposures we now control, such as tobacco or asbestos. For example, compared to male non-smokers, the increased risk of lung cancer for males from smoking tobacco is about 22-fold for current smokers and 9.4 for former smokers (Fielding *et al.* 1998). In contrast, the relative risk of colon cancer attributable to eating red meat or processed meats frequently is 1.18 compared to a person consuming it only occasionally (Huxley *et al.* 2009). Obesity, however, may increase the overall risk of cancer twofold (Pischon *et al.* 2008). Table 12.1 lists the associations between dietary choices and chronic diseases. While the relative risks may appear modest, because such a large proportion of the population is at risk, these associations translate to millions of people who are adversely affected.

Overweight and obesity have become a global problem and in the United States, two of three adults and one of three children are affected. The influence of structural and contextual factors on energy balance behaviours has not been widely recognized nor accepted by elected officials and other policymakers, in light of the belief that individuals freely choose their consumption and behavioural patterns. Nevertheless, there is a great deal of evidence that lifestyle and behaviours are influenced more strongly by contextual factors than by individual preferences. This chapter will review how structural and contextual factors influence dietary behaviours,[2] and will discuss how a regulatory infrastructure could potentially protect people from the factors that lead to chronic diseases.

Table 12.1 The relationship between diet and chronic diseases

Disease	Toxin/nutrient/condition causing disease	Relative risk	Prevalence/incidence
Total mortality	Obesity (measured by waist-to-hip ratio)	2.0 men, 1.8 women[1]	2.4 million
	Excess refined grains	1.16[2]	
Coronary artery disease	Trans-fats	1.23[3]	12 million[13]
	Obesity	1.28[4]	
	Western-style diet	1.46 in women[5]	
	Dietary fibre	0.86[6]	
	Fruits and vegetables	0.85[7]	
Hypertension	Excess salt	62% of strokes	42 million[13]
	Lack of whole grains	49% of CHD[8]	
Cancers	Too much red meat	1.14–1.21[9]	12 million[13]
	Insufficient fibre	1.18[10]	141,405 with colon cancer
Diabetes	Sugar-sweetened beverages	1.83[11]	14.5 million[13]
	French fries	1.16[12]	

Sources: (1) Pischon *et al.* 2008; (2) Jacobs *et al.* 1999; (3) Sun *et al.* 2007; (4) Batty *et al.* 2007; (5) Fung *et al.* 2001; (6) Pereira *et al.* 2004; (7) Law and Morris 1998; (8) He and MacGregor 2009; (9) Huxley *et al.* 2009; (10) Park *et al.* 2005; (11) Schulze *et al.* 2004; (12) Halton *et al.* 2006; (13) Dall *et al.* 2009

Contextual influences on eating

Eyegaze is not fully consciously controllable; rather, our eyes reflexively look toward novel images in our environment. What we look at and pay attention to is dependent on what is located in our field of vision. Furthermore, as our eyes jump between different foci in a saccadic fashion, we only consciously perceive those images where our eyes dwell for at least 200 milliseconds (Berridge and Winkielman 2003). However, our eyes often move faster than that, and our brains can perceive images that we do not remember (Bargh 2005). We cannot ignore images in our visual fields, even if we do not focus on or consciously attend to them. Yet, even when we do not remember images, exposure to them can still influence our behaviours and decision-making (Chartrand 2005). This is particularly important when it comes to food and eating behaviours. Several studies have shown that just being exposed to images of food or advertisements that promote eating is associated with increases in the quantity of food subsequently consumed (Halford et al. 2004; Harris et al. 2009). Having no reference for comparison, individuals may not realize that they are eating larger quantities after such exposure.

Recent eye-tracking studies have documented that people preferentially orient their gaze to food where there are competing visual stimuli (Castellanos et al. 2009; Nijs et al. 2009). This means that food cues in our environment will be dominant over other kinds of visual stimuli and capture more of our attention. When people see what has been called 'palatable food' – foods that are high in sugar and fat – the human brain automatically secretes the neurohormone dopamine (Volkow et al. 2003). Dopamine causes the feeling of 'craving' and stimulates people to get into action to obtain the object (Volkow 2007). The neural pathways stimulated by palatable foods are believed to be the same ones involved in drugs of addiction (Volkow and Wise 2005). There is a distinct evolutionary advantage for having a heightened response to palatable foods, because they provide extra energy that may provide a survival advantage when food is scarce. However, in an era with excess available calories, this reflexive reaction may contribute to over-consumption of foods that increase the risk of chronic diseases (Polivy and Herman 2006).

In summary, people cannot avoid paying attention to food and food cues, and when we see palatable food, we automatically are stimulated to want to eat. Given its ubiquitous presence and availability, which likely plays a causal role in the obesity epidemic, societies suffering from diet-related chronic diseases must develop strategies to constrain its accessibility.

Limits on cognitive capacity

Unfortunately, people's abilities to counter natural impulses to eat when food is available are relatively limited. The capacity to control eating behaviours not only varies across individuals but also within individuals depending upon other tasks and demands to which the individual must concurrently respond. People typically can cognitively engage on only one task at a time (Dijksterhuis and Smith 2005). When people attempt to do more than one thing at a time, the tasks that require less attention occur automatically. Usually the automatic behaviours are related to motor activities, like walking or driving, but they also include activities that are generally thought of as requiring cognitive involvement, like decision-making. Decisions can be made without any thoughtful cognitive input and can be directed by heuristics – simple rules that guide automatic decision-making. Heuristics include factors, e.g. appearance, and superficial character-istics, e.g. size, price, and brand. Moreover, as information becomes overwhelming to people, or they are busy or distracted or stressed, they are more likely to resort to auto-matic heuristic processing, in which superficial characteristics govern decision-making, rather than using thorough cognitive and analytical processing (Dhar and Nowlis 1999; Dhar et al. 2000). For example, a busy or distracted person may choose products based upon the logo, price, or package appearance, rather than take the time to examine the product contents and fully appreciate its true value or contents (Vartanian et al. 2008).

Eating is a behaviour that is wired to occur automatically, and thus allows individuals to engage in other activities while they eat, such as paying attention to companions or scan-ning the environment for threats or opportunities (Cohen and Farley 2008). Eating can easily be accomplished without cognitive involvement or conscious direction. It is possible to drive, watch TV or listen to the radio and eat at the same time. As people multi-task and one of the tasks includes eating, they may be less able to control or limit their intake, because eating may be the activity least likely to require cognitive direction. Indeed, a variety of studies have shown that people eat more when they are distracted or if they try to control other factors, e.g. emotions, or other habitual behaviours, e.g. smoking (Bellisle and Dalix 2001; Brunstrom and Mitchell 2006; Hetherington et al. 2006).

People are hardwired to be automatically attracted to palatable foods, but refusing food is not automatic; it takes substantial cognitive effort. When people are cogni-tively depleted due to multiple demands or having had to exercise self-control, they are less able to refuse foods. This is one reason why people who are trying to change habitual behaviours tend to relapse under stress or at the end of a day (Baumeister and Schmeichel 2007; Muraven et al. 1998).

Modern retailing exploits hardwired attraction to food

The Green Revolution has made it possible for American society (and many others across the globe) to produce twice as many calories as are needed by all its residents (Putnam et al. 2002). The over-abundance of foods is a serious barrier to weight control, since these foods cannot easily be ignored or avoided and are very easy to obtain.

Agricultural policies in the United States have subsidized commodities that can be used to produce low-cost energy-dense food products. While the subsidy of commodi-ties has been considered a distal cause of the obesity epidemic, some scholars have argued that subsidies were the consequences of low prices, rather than the cause (Alston et al. 2007). Subsidies were intended to support farmers so they would not go out of business. Subsidies were not intended to make food cheap, but rather to keep farmers from producing too much, which would make food cheaper than it already is.

Nevertheless, most foods have become relatively much less expensive than they were in the past, in relationship to total income. Even most low-income individuals have the capacity to access more calories than they need. In the marketplace, there is continual encouragement to purchase and consume, to stimulate more sales and profits. There is no incentive for businesses to encourage individuals to restrain their consumption.

Marketers are constantly researching and developing new ways to encourage ever more consumption. The field of atmospherics was developed in the early 1970s when it was recognized that the design of buying environments enhanced purchasing prob-ability (Turley and Milliman 2000). Multiple marketing studies have identified how product presentation influences individuals to increase their purchases. The findings are continually being incorporated into marketing strategies. For example, pictures, symbols, logos, package appearance, and salient placement of goods influence what and how much people buy (Summers and Hebert 2001). People can be conditioned to be loyal to brands, and are frequently primed by a variety of cues that increase purchases (Fitzsimons *et al.* 2008). Placement near cash registers, in special displays, and on the ends of aisles are particularly influential. Now vendors pay retailers slotting fees to have their products placed in these salient locations (Sorenson 2009).

Marketers have also discovered the importance of impulse purchasing. Placing almost any item in a salient location increases its sale, but this may be especially effective for palatable foods (Sorenson 2009). Accordingly, impulse marketing of palatable foods has spread to a wide variety of retail businesses, and non-perishable products like candy, salty snacks, and sugar-sweetened beverages are sold in non-food outlets, like hardware stores, book stores, and car washes. This easy access to food and the concomitant cues stimulate the desire to eat. The strategy appears to be quite successful, given the increasing frequency of eating occasions over the past decade. Data from the National Health and Nutrition Examination Survey study indicate that between 1977 and 2006 the average American adult has added another eating occasion each day, increasing the percentage of calories consumed from snacks from 18 to 25 per cent (Piernas and Popkin 2009).

Another important change, which has been widely described, is the increase in portion sizes in retail food outlets (Young and Nestle 2002, 2003). The National Institutes of Health (NIH) even has a website called 'portion distortion' in which they document that over 20 years, increased portions have resulted in servings of burgers going from 333 to 590 calories, french fried potatoes from 210 to 610 calories, and sodas from 85 to 210 calories (National Heart Lung and Blood Institute 2003).

The availability of processed foods has grown geometrically. High fat foods are often difficult to prepare at home because they are labour intensive. But with the development of sophisticated manufacturing techniques and new technologies for packaging, delicate foods like chips that might otherwise crumble or become stale can be packaged and shipped around the world and remain intact, preserved for months and even years after the date of manufacture. Technology for food preservation coupled with lower costs compounds the easy availability of calories.

Structural cures

Given that excess calorie consumption is the consequence of either eating portions that are too large during meals and/or too many snacks between meals relative to what is expended, structural interventions should target the easy availability of large portions and high calorie snacks and beverages. However, introducing controls in a manner that is politically viable is the greatest challenge, especially because of the difficulty we face in attempting to convince the public that excess exposure to food should, in fact, be the primary intervention target, rather than individuals. Current approaches predominantly focus on giving people more information so they can make better decisions, such as the new regulations for calorie menu labelling. The current belief is that people are rational and will make choices in their best interest if information is available. However, the early evaluations of menu labelling are not very encouraging (Elbel *et al.* 2009; Finkelstein *et al.* 2011).

What is needed are policies that directly limit exposure to excess calories and environmental exposure to cues that cognitively stimulate the desire to eat. A few of these policies might include: (1) reducing access to low-nutrient foods: (2) portion control measures; and (3) taxes on foods most closely associated with chronic diseases. Policies that would indirectly influence consumption by reducing food cues include: (1) advertising regulations that counter cues that stimulate excess consumption; (2) policies that govern placement of items in locations that increase salience and exposure and thus impulse buying; and (3) warning labels on food items that increase the risk of obesity and chronic diseases (symbols or icons, rather than numbers).

Controlling accessibility of consumer products

There is a long history of using structural approaches to control the consumption of a variety of products, including those that have some harmful impact on individual and population health and for products that are in limited supply, but are vital to the functioning of society. The former products include alcohol, tobacco, and other drugs of addiction, items like poisons and guns, certain chemicals, and harmful materials. The latter include goods like gasoline, medications, and even food, in times of scarcity. Taxes have been particularly effective for tobacco control (Wakefield and Chaloupka 2000), and may be helpful for reducing consumption of low-nutrient foods. A relevant strategy that has worked to limit accessibility of a variety of products has been to license their sale and restrict the number of licences, as well as the location of licences, so they are not geographically concentrated. As applied to alcohol control, this strategy has been highly effective in reducing alcohol-related morbidity and mortality (Anderson et al. 2009). Licensure is currently required for the sale of food as well, but enforcement has been restricted to only those establishments that sell perishable, fresh foods. Certainly there is room to tighten the licensure requirements to reduce exposure to the foods most closely associated with obesity and dietary-related chronic diseases.

Consideration should be given to a density limit that would insure a limited minimum and maximum number of outlets that supply basic groceries to areas with specific population densities. The general specifications for the outlet sales can be part of the regulation. Where demand is high, licences can be more expensive; and where it is low, incentive or credits can be offered to attract outlets. Outlets that primarily supply foods whose consumption should be limited like candy stores, donut shops, and ice cream parlours, could face a limited availability of licences. Moreover, only outlets whose primary business is to sell food should be allowed to do so. Outlets that only sell non-perishable foods as a secondary part of their business, such as hardware stores or car washes, might be prohibited from selling any food items. This should protect individuals from being exposed to items that may stimulate feelings of hunger (like candy at the cash register) when they may have had no intention of eating.

Portion control and performance standards for away from home food

The Institute of Medicine (IOM) has established guidelines for school meal nutritional standards for breakfast and lunch to meet children's nutritional needs, foster healthy eating habits and safeguard their health (Stallings et al. 2009). While restaurants are not per se stewards of health or health care providers, there is a general expectation that the food available in commercial venues will not make people sick. Given that there is a consensus about what foods can increase or decrease the risk of chronic diseases, existing regulatory infrastructure could be expanded to cover the prevention of chronic diseases. The extent of regulation could include establishing standards for meals, certifying meals and menu items that meet standards, and clearly marking items that do not meet standards. Default portion sizes could be consistent with the Dietary Guidelines for Americans (DGA) or even the Food and Drug Administration sizes termed as reference amounts customarily consumed (RACC), which are based upon the amounts people ate in the 1980s. If all restaurants observed standard portion sizes, people would be able to gauge more easily what they consume, just as people can gauge their risks of becoming intoxicated by having alcoholic drinks come in standard sizes. Other standards may govern the nutritional content of meals. For example, a meal that could be certified as healthy might include 1 cup of fruit, 1 cup of vegetables, 2 ounces of meat or meat equivalent, and 2 ounces of whole grains. Based upon a daily maximum guideline of 1500 mg sodium per day, the sodium content might have to be <500 mg/meal and the saturated fat content <10 per cent (US Department of Agriculture 2010). The importance of requiring restaurants to at least have one or two options that are healthy is critical; no one should be forced to consume foods that will increase their risk for or exacerbate existing chronic diseases.

Limits on impulse marketing

Impulse marketing has grown geometrically over the past couple of decades as marketers have discovered the importance of placement and display characteristics. As mentioned, placement of products in specific locations such as end aisle displays, near cash registers, at eye-level, or in special displays is particularly effective in increasing the chance they will be sold. Research indicates that store factors are more important than individual factors in determining product sales (Curhan 1972). Indeed, placement is the strongest factor determining sales (Sorenson 2009). Moreover, nearly 60 per cent of all supermarket purchases are unplanned, and occur as a result of their placement and promotional strategies (Hausman 2000). Currently, the majority of large supermarket chains glean higher profits from vendors who pay slotting fees to buy display positions than they make from actual product sales to customers (Sorenson 2009). Shoppers often do not recognize and/or cannot resist these display marketing techniques. Regulations could limit the types of foods that can be displayed in salient locations, given that many are unable to defend themselves against this type of marketing. Currently regulations prohibit the display of certain materials where they are salient and easily accessed (e.g. pornography, tobacco, and alcohol). These types of restrictions could be reasonably extended to the foods most closely associated with chronic disease.

Advertising regulations to counter cues that stimulate excess consumption

Currently there is a great deal of effort and controversy regarding advertising of low-nutrient foods to children. Progress in achieving compliance with proposed standards to limit such advertising is quite slow; indeed, effective guidelines may be unattainable in a society that values free speech and capitalism. However, a strategy that has worked very well with tobacco control has been the use of counter-advertising. Messages can be developed that help people resist eating too much. A counter-advertising campaign could be implemented and funded the way the initial anti-tobacco campaign was funded, through the Fairness Doctrine (Warner 1977). This legislation had required broadcast media to match pro-tobacco advertising with anti-tobacco advertising. If people were equally likely to be exposed to messages that encourage eating as much as to resist eating too much, they may be in a better position to make healthier choices.

Discussion

While the obesity epidemic is broadly considered to be multi-factorial, the single most important and potentially malleable factor is food availability, particularly energy-dense, highly palatable foods and large portion sizes. As such, structural solutions hold significant promise in reversing the epidemic. However, to move forward, a variety of studies and demonstration projects will be necessary, given the vast amount of interest in preserving and indeed expanding the status quo. We need experimental restaurants and supermarkets where food cues are manipulated to determine which layouts, design and promotions result in healthier dietary choices. We need more communities that are willing to try policy-level regulations that fundamentally alter the availability of food.

Just as sanitary survey planning emerged as a useful practice, as it 'required the study of every street, lot, and building in a city to determine the precise location of any prevalent and all suspect environmental conditions' (Peterson 1979), similar measures are needed to identify the contextual factors that cause excess consumption without individual awareness and/or intention. Contextual factors need to be regulated to protect individuals from undue influences that exploit their hardwired, automatic responses to available food.

As a society we must embrace the reality that individual behaviours are guided or constrained by environmental factors that people cannot easily recognize or defend themselves against. Many exposures that lead to a poor diet and chronic diseases are essentially invisible to the majority of individuals, and they cannot easily gain insight into or learn how to resist these influences.

In the future, chronic disease control will need to adopt the same methods of infectious disease control in which performance standards exist for all outlets where food is served or procured, and compliance enforced. People should be able to obtain foods without too much difficulty, which will not increase the risk of chronic diseases. Future regulations should include portion control and limits on where low-nutrient foods can be displayed. Other regulations are also plausible, including taxes, permits governing outlet location, operations, and advertising standards. Although there is always a fear of intrusive government and an over-regulated society, the consequences of an absent government and a lack of regulations are untold misery, epidemics of chronic diseases, and premature mortality for hundreds of thousands of individuals.

Notes

1 Online, available at: http://www.bl.uk/learning/histcitizen/21cc/publichealth/sources/source17/economist.html (accessed 8 January 2012)
2 While structural factors also affect physical activity, which contributes to energy balance, I focus here on dietary behaviours, because there is strong evidence that diet is relatively more important in the onset of obesity. Increases in caloric consumption over time have been documented.

References

Alston, J.M., Sumner, D.A., and Sa, V. (2007) 'Farm subsidies and obesity in the United States', *Agricultural and Resource Economics Update*, 11 (2): 1–4.

Anderson, P., Chisholm, D., and Fuhr, D.C. (2009) 'Effectiveness and cost-effectiveness of policies and programmes to reduce the harm caused by alcohol', *The Lancet*, 373: 2234–46.

Bargh, J. (2005) 'Bypassing the will: toward demystifying the nonconscious control of social behavior', in R.R. Hassin and J.S. Uleman (eds) *The New Unconscious*, New York: Oxford University Press.

Batty, G.D., Kivimaki, M., Smith, G.D., Marmot, M.G., and Shipley, M.J. (2007) 'Obesity and overweight in relation to mortality in men with and without type 2 diabetes/impaired glucose tolerance: the original Whitehall Study', *Diabetes Care*, 30: 2388–91.

Baumeister, R.F. and Schmeichel, B. (2007) 'Self-regulation and the executive function: the self as controlling agent', in A.W. Kruglanski and E.T. Higgins (eds) *Social Psychology: Handbook of Basic Principles*, 2nd edition, New York: Guilford Press.

Bellisle, F. and Dalix, A.M. (2001) 'Cognitive restraint can be offset by distraction, leading to increased meal intake in women', *American Journal of Clinical Nutrition*, 74: 197–200.

Berridge, K.C. and Winkielman, P. (2003) 'What is an unconscious emotion? (The case for unconscious "liking")', *Cognition and Emotion*, 17: 181–211.

Brunstrom, J.M. and Mitchell, G.L. (2006) 'Effects of distraction on the development of satiety', *British Journal of Nutrition*, 96: 761–9.

Castellanos, E.H., Charboneau, E., Dietrich, M.S., Park, S., Bradley, B.P., Mogg, K., and Cowan, R.L. (2009) 'Obese adults have visual attention bias for food cue images: evidence for altered reward system function', *International Journal of Obesity*, 33: 1063–73.

Chartrand, T. (2005) 'The role of conscious awareness in consumer behavior', *Journal of Consumer Psychology*, 15: 203–10.

Cohen, D.A. and Farley, T.A. (2008) 'Eating as an automatic behavior', *Preventing Chronic Disease*, 5 (1). Online, available at: http://www.cdc.gov/pcd/issues/2008/jan/07_0046.htm (accessed 8 January 2012).

Curhan, R.C. (1972) 'The relationship between shelf space and unit sales in supermarkets', *Journal of Marketing Research*, 9: 406–12.

Dall, T.M., Fulgoni, V.L. 3rd, Zhang, Y., Reimers, K.J., Packard, P.T., and Astwood, J.D. (2009) 'Potential health benefits and medical cost savings from calorie, sodium, and saturated fat reductions in the American diet', *American Journal of Health Promotion*, 23: 412–22.

Dhar, R. and Nowlis, S.M. (1999) 'The effect of time pressure on consumer choice deferral', *Journal of Consumer Research*, 25: 369–84.

Dhar, R., Nowlis, S.M., and Sherman, S.J. (2000) 'Trying hard or hardly trying: an analysis of context effects in choice', *Journal of Consumer Psychology*, 9: 189–200.

Dijksterhuis, A. and Smith, P.K. (2005) 'What do we do unconsciously? And how?', *Journal of Consumer Psychology*, 15: 225–9.

Elbel, B., Kersh, R., Brescoll, V.L., and Dixon, L.B. (2009) 'Calorie labeling and food choices: a first look at the effects on low-income people in New York City', *Health Affairs*, 28: w1110–21.

Fielding, J.E., Husten, C.G., and Eriksen, M.P. (1998) 'Tobacco: health effects and control', in R.B.

Wallace, B.N. Doebbeling, and J.M. Last (eds) *Public Health and Preventive Medicine*, Stamford, CT: Appleton and Lange.

Finkelstein, E.A., Strombotne, K.L., Chan, N.L., and Krieger, J. (2011) 'Mandatory menu labeling in one fast-food chain in King County, Washington', *American Journal of Preventive Medicine*, 40: 122–7.

Fitzsimons, G.M., Chartrand, T.L., and Fitzsimons, G.J. (2008) 'Automatic effects of brand exposure on motivated behaviour: how Apple makes you "think different"', *Journal of Consumer Research*, 35: 21–35.

Fung, T.T., Willett, W.C., Stampfer, M.J., Manson, J.E., and Hu, F.B. (2001) 'Dietary patterns and the risk of coronary heart disease in women', *Archives of Internal Medicine*, 161: 1857–62.

Halford, J.C., Gillespie, J., Brown, V., Pontin, E.E., and Dovey, T.M. (2004) 'Effect of television advertisements for foods on food consumption in children', *Appetite*, 42: 221–5.

Halton, T.L., Willett, W.C., Liu, S., Manson, J.E., Stampfer, M.J., and Hu, F.B. (2006) 'Potato and french fry consumption and risk of type 2 diabetes in women', *The American Journal of Clinical Nutrition*, 83: 284–90.

Harris, J.L., Bargh, J.A., and Brownell, K.D. (2009) 'Priming effects of television food advertising on eating behavior', *Health Psychology*, 28 (4): 404–13.

Hausman, A. (2000) 'A multi-method investigation of consumer motivations in impulse buying behavior', *Journal of Consumer Marketing*, 17: 403–19.

He, F.J. and MacGregor, G.A. (2009) 'A comprehensive review on salt and health and current experience of worldwide salt reduction programmes', *Journal of Human Hypertension*, 23: 363–84.

Hetherington, M.M., Anderson, A.S., Norton, G.N., and Newson, L. (2006) 'Situational effects on meal intake: a comparison of eating alone and eating with others', *Physiology and Behavior*, 88: 498–505.

Huxley, R.R., Ansary-Moghaddam, A., Clifton, P., Czernichow, S., Parr, C.L., and Woodward, M. (2009) 'The impact of dietary and lifestyle risk factors on risk of colorectal cancer: a quantitative overview of the epidemiological evidence', *International Journal of Cancer*, 125: 171–80.

Jacobs, D.R. Jr., Meyer, K.A., Kushi, L.H., and Folsom, A.R. (1999) 'Is whole grain intake associated with reduced total and cause-specific death rates in older women? The Iowa Women's Health Study', *American Journal of Public Health*, 89: 322–9.

Law, M.R. and Morris, J.K. (1998) 'By how much does fruit and vegetable consumption reduce the risk of ischaemic heart disease?', *European Journal of Clinical Nutrition*, 52: 549–56.

Muraven, M., Tice, D.M., and Baumeister, R.F. (1998) 'Self-control as limited resource: regulatory depletion patterns', *Journal of Personality and Social Psychology*, 74: 774–89.

National Heart Lung and Blood Institute (NHLBI) (2003) *Portion Distortion!*, Bethesda: National Heart Lung and Blood Institute. Online, available at: http://hp2010.nhlbihin.net/portion/index.htm (accessed 20 September 2011).

Nijs, I.M.T., Muris, P., Euser, A.S., and Franken, I.H.A. (2009) 'Differences in attention to food and food intake between overweight/obese and normal-weight females under conditions of hunger and satiety', *Appetite*, 54: 243–54.

Park, Y., Hunter, D.J., Spiegelman, D., Bergkvist, L., Berrino, F., Van Den Brandt, P.A., Buring, J.E., Colditz, G.A., Freudenheim, J.L., Fuchs, C.S., Giovannucci, E., Goldbohm, R.A., Graham, S., Harnack, L., Hartman, A.M., Jacobs, D.R. Jr., Kato, I., Krogh, V., Leitzmann, M.F., Mccullough, M.L., Miller, A.B., Pietinen, P., Rohan, T.E., Schatzkin, A., Willett, W.C., Wolk, A., Zeleniuch-Jacquotte, A., Zhang, S.M. and Smith-Warner, S.A. (2005) 'Dietary fiber intake and risk of colorectal cancer: a pooled analysis of prospective cohort studies', *Journal of the American Medical Association*, 294: 2849–57.

Pereira, M.A., O'Reilly, E., Augustsson, K., Fraser, G.E., Goldbourt, U., Heitmann, B.L., Hallmans, G., Knekt, P., Liu, S., Pietinen, P., Spiegelman, D., Stevens, J., Virtamo, J., Willett, W.C. and Ascherio, A. (2004) 'Dietary fiber and risk of coronary heart disease: a pooled analysis of cohort studies', *Archives of Internal Medicine*, 164: 370–6.

Peterson, J.A. (1979) 'The impact of sanitary reform upon American urban planning, 1840–1890', *Journal of Social History*, 13 (1), 83–103.

Piernas, C. and Popkin, B.M. (2009) 'Snacking increased among U.S. adults between 1977 and 2006', *Journal of Nutrition*, 140: 325–32.

Pischon, T., Boeing, H., Hoffmann, K., Bergmann, M., Schulze, M.B., Overvad, K., Van Der Schouw, Y.T., Spencer, E., Moons, K.G.M., Tjã,Nneland, A., Halkjaer, J., Jensen, M.K., Stegger, J., Clavel-Chapelon, F., Boutron-Ruault, M.C., Chajes, V., Linseisen, J., Kaaks, R., Trichopoulou, A., Trichopoulos, D., Bamia, C., Sieri, S., Palli, D., Tumino, R., Vineis, P., Panico, S., Peeters, P.H.M., May, A.M., Bueno-de-Mesquita, H.B., Van Duijnhoven, F.J.B., Hallmans, G., Weinehall, L., Manjer, J., Hedblad, B., Lund, E., Agudo, A., Arriola, L., Barricarte, A., Navarro, C., Martinez, C., Quirãs, J.R., Key, T., Bingham, S., Khaw, K.T., Boffetta, P., Jenab, M., Ferrari, P. and Riboli, E. (2008) 'General and abdominal adiposity and risk of death in Europe', *New England Journal of Medicine*, 359: 2105–20.

Polivy, J. and Herman, C.P. (2006) 'An evolutionary perspective on dieting', *Appetite*, 47: 30–5.

Putnam, J., Allshouse, J., and Kantor, L.S. (2002) 'U.S. per capita food supply trends: more calories, refined carbohydrates, and fats', *Food Review*, 25 (3). Online, available at: http://www.ers.usda.gov/publications/FoodReview/DEC2002/frvol25i3a.pdf (accessed 8 January 2012).

Schulze, M.B., Manson, J.E., Ludwig, D.S., Colditz, G.A., Stampfer, M.J., Willett, W.C., and Hu, F.B. (2004) 'Sugar-sweetened beverages, weight gain, and incidence of type 2 diabetes in young and middle-aged women', *Journal of the American Medical Association*, 292: 927–34.

Sorenson, H. (2009) *Inside the Mind of the Shopper*, Upsaddle River, NJ: Pearson Education.

Stallings, V.A., Suitor, C.W., and Taylor, C.L. (eds) (2009) *School Meals: Building Blocks for Healthy Children*, Washington, D.C.: National Academies Press.

Summers, T.A. and Hebert, P.R. (2001) 'Shedding some light on store atmospherics: influence of illumination on consumer behavior', *Journal of Business Research*, 54: 145–50.

Sun, Q., Ma, J., Campos, H., Hankinson, S.E., Manson, J.E., Stampfer, M.J., Rexrode, K.M., Willett, W.C., and Hu, F.B. (2007) 'A prospective study of trans fatty acids in erythrocytes and risk of coronary heart disease', *Circulation*, 115: 1858–65.

Turley, L.W. and Milliman, R.E. (2000) 'Atmospheric effects on shopping behavior: A review of the experimental evidence', *Journal of Business Research Retail Atmospherics*, 49: 193–211.

United States Department of Agriculture (USDA) (2010) *Report of the Dietary Guidelines Advisory Committee on the Dietary Guidelines for Americans, 2010*, Washington, D.C.: US Department of Agriculture. Online, available at: http://www.cnpp.usda.gov/DGAs2010-DGACReport.htm (accessed 8 January 2012).

United States Department of Health and Human Services (DHHS) (2001) *Overweight and Obesity: The Surgeon General's Call to Action to Prevent and Decrease Overweight and Obesity*, Washington, D.C.: US Department of Health and Human Services.

Vartanian, L.R., Herman, C.P., and Wansink, B. (2008) 'Are we aware of the external factors that influence our food intake?', *Health Psychology*, 27: 533–8.

Volkow, N.D. (2007) 'This is your brain on food', Interview by Kristin Leutwyler-Ozelli, *Scientific American*, 297: 84–5.

Volkow, N.D., Wang, G.J., Maynard, L., Jayne, M., Fowler, J.S., Zhu, W., Logan, J., Gatley, S.J., Ding, Y.S., Wong, C. and Pappas, N. (2003) 'Brain dopamine is associated with eating behaviors in humans', *International Journal of Eating Disorders*, 33: 136–42.

Volkow, N.D. and Wise, R.A. (2005) 'How can drug addiction help us understand obesity?', *Nature Neuroscience*, 8: 555–60.

Wakefield, M. and Chaloupka, F. (2000) 'Effectiveness of comprehensive tobacco control programmes in reducing teenage smoking in the USA', *Tobacco Control*, 9: 177–86.

Warner, K.E. (1977) 'The effects of the anti-smoking campaign on cigarette consumption', *American Journal of Public Health*, 67: 645–50.

Young, L.R. and Nestle, M. (2002) 'The contribution of expanding portion sizes to the US obesity epidemic', *American Journal of Public Health*, 92: 246–9.

Young, L.R. and Nestle, M. (2003) 'Expanding portion sizes in the US marketplace: implications for nutrition counseling', *Journal of the American Dietetic Association*, 103: 231–4.

13

STRUCTURAL APPROACHES FOR UNINTENTIONAL INJURY PREVENTION

Adnan A. Hyder and Jeffrey C. Lunnen

Introduction

Unintentional injuries are responsible for a significant proportion of the global burden of disease; according to the World Health Organization (WHO), in 2004, unintentional injuries were estimated to have caused more than 3.9 million deaths worldwide. Road traffic injuries (RTIs), poisoning, falls, fire burns, drowning and other unintentional injuries leave tens of millions disabled each year and are thus responsible for over 138 million disability adjusted life years (DALYs), which present tremendous social and economic costs to societies across the globe. The consequences are greatest in low- and middle-income countries (LMICs), where over 90 per cent of injury-related deaths occur (WHO 2004).

Males are disproportionately affected by unintentional injuries, accounting for 65 per cent of all unintentional injury-related deaths (78 deaths and 2,686 DALYs per 100,000 males); in contrast, unintentional injuries cause 43 deaths per 100,000 females, corresponding to 1,611 DALYs per 100,000 (Table 13.1). If unexamined, it might appear that unintentional injuries are naturally occurring 'accidents' that strike down men and women in resource-poor settings by chance, but such a reading is far too simplistic (Norton *et al.* 2011). Unintentional injuries result from causes and risk factors that can be reduced, controlled, and prevented when properly identified and targeted appropriately.

However, effectively addressing unintentional injuries has remained a challenge because of the multifaceted nature of injury prevention and control, and the multi-sectoral nature of injuries. Unlike other health conditions, which mainly involve the health sector, injury prevention and control requires cooperation from a variety of sectors including transport, law, police, education, and others. Risk exposure is linked with myriad variables including a person's age, gender, and socio-economic status as well as the environments in which they interact (Peek-Asa and Hyder 2009). Research that identifies how effective interventions in high-income countries can be translated in LMICs is a priority, since injury prevention strategies need to be appropriate for local environments (Bishai and Hyder 2006).

This chapter thus seeks to address injury prevention and control in a multi-sectoral context, highlighting an evolution of approaches – from individual-level interventions to those that involve legislative, environmental, or structural changes. The chapter will introduce system-level interventions (i.e. structural interventions) for different types of injuries; discuss core components necessary for a successful intervention; and explore current knowledge on the effectiveness of these interventions. It hopes to broaden injury prevention discourse to include systematic changes in our social, physical, and legal environments and enhance global dialogue. The chapter will focus on LMICs with appropriate references to work in high-income countries (HICs).

Typology of injuries

Injury has been defined as physical damage of the human body that results from exposure to an excessive form of energy, either chemical, thermal, electrical, radioactive, or kinetic; or from a lack of essential life agents, such as oxygen or heat (Herbert *et al.* 2011; Krug *et al.* 2002; Norton *et al.* 2011). Injury is further classified according to the underlying intent – as intentional and unintentional. Unintentional injuries are those without evidence of pre-determined intent and include injuries sustained as a result of road traffic crashes, poisoning, falls, fire burns, and drowning. They also include occupational and sports injuries (Herbert *et al.* 2011; Krug *et al.* 2002; Norton *et al.* 2011). Intentional injuries (i.e. violence) are injuries where there is clear intent of harm and include homicide, assault, and suicide, among others. This chapter focuses solely on unintentional injuries.

The potential for energy transfer exists everywhere, but its ability to cause injury is limited to situations between an agent and a host. Only energy transmitted beyond a host's tolerance causes an injury. Injury prevention aims to either prevent the transfer of or reduce the amount of energy that is transferred from the environment to the host/ human. Prevention activities can thus focus on the host, the environment, vectors, or a combination of all these components (Peek-Asa and Hyder 2009).

Unintentional injuries

The WHO estimates over 3.9 million unintentional injury deaths occurred in 2004, accounting for 61 unintentional injuries per 100,000 population, or 6.6 per cent of the global mortality burden (WHO 2004). Of these injuries, nearly two-thirds affected men, or 78 unintentional injury-related deaths per 100,000 population among males, compared to 43 per 100,000 among females (Table 13.1). Unintentional injuries were responsible for more than 138 million DALYs in 2004 or 2,153 DALYs per 100,000 population. DALY rates are also higher among males than females.

Over 90 per cent of unintentional injury-related deaths occurred in LMICs; compare 3.6 million deaths in LMICs with 340,497 in HICs (WHO 2004) (Table 13.1). In 2004, RTIs represented the largest proportion of unintentional injury deaths (33 per cent). Falls, drowning, poisoning, and fire burns represent small but similar proportions (Figure 13.1).

Unintentional injury-related deaths per 100,000 population increase by age (Figure 13.2). Differences among the sexes are obvious with male mortality rates much higher

Table 13.1 Global burden of unintentional injuries by sex (per 100,000 population), 2004

	Deaths per 100,000			DALYs per 100,000		
	Males	*Females*	*All*	*Males*	*Females*	*All*
All unintentional injuries	78	43	61	2,686	1,611	2,153
Road traffic injuries	29	10	20	901	375	640
Falls	8	5	7	322	210	267
Drowning	8	4	6	945	629	788
Poisoning	7	4	5	151	80	116
Fire burns	4	6	5	140	211	175
Other unintentional injuries	22	14	18	945	629	788

Source: World Health Organization 2004

Note: DALYs = disability adjusted life years

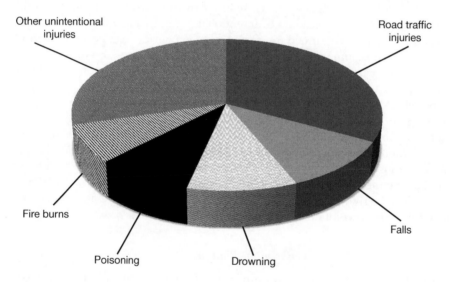

Figure 13.1 Proportion of global unintentional injury deaths by cause, 2004 (n = 3.9 million)
Source: World Health Organization 2004

than females. Rates peak at approximately 296 deaths per 100,000 population among persons aged 80 years or more (350 per 100,000 males, 265 per 100,000 females).

The burden of disease from unintentional injuries was responsible for more than 138 million DALYs in 2004; 94 per cent occurred in LMICs (WHO 2004). RTIs contribute to high DALYs in HICs and LMICs (Table 13.2). The DALY rate is three times as high in LMICs (2,398 per 100,000) as compared to HICs (775 per 100,000) (Table 13.2). Five key types of unintentional injuries (Figure 13.1) are described below using global data from the WHO.

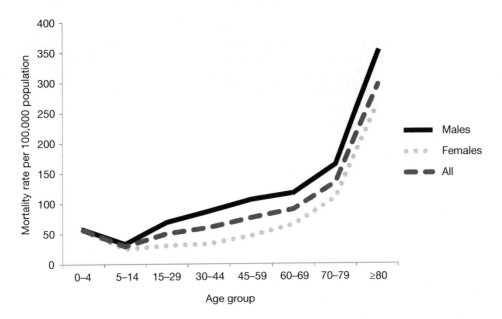

Figure 13.2 Global unintentional injury-related mortality rates by age groups and sex per 100,000 population, 2004

Source: World Health Organization 2004

Table 13.2 Global unintentional injury death rates by cause and income level (per 100,000 population), 2004

	Deaths per 100,000			DALYs per 100,000		
	High Income	Low and middle income	All	High income	Low and middle income	All
All unintentional injuries	35	65	61	775	2,398	2,153
Road traffic injuries	12	21	20	319	698	640
Falls	8	6	7	133	290	267
Drowning	2	7	6	31	191	167
Poisoning	3	6	5	70	124	116
Fire burns	1	6	5	19	203	175
Other unintentional injuries	10	20	18	202	893	788

Source: World Health Organization 2004

Note: DALYs = disability adjusted life years

Road traffic injuries

A road traffic crash is defined as a collision occurring on a public road involving at least one moving vehicle. A road traffic injury (RTI) is defined as a fatal or non-fatal injury that results from a road traffic crash (WHO 2008). RTIs are the ninth leading cause of death worldwide, and were responsible for over 1.2 million deaths in 2004 or 2.2 per cent of global mortality. The WHO predicts RTIs will become the fifth leading cause of death by 2030 without immediate action (WHO 2009). RTIs are estimated to have caused 29 deaths and contribute to 901 DALYs per 100,000 in males, much higher than the ten deaths and 375 DALYs per 100,000 for females (Table 13.1). The burden of RTI mortality is disproportionately high in LMICs; in 2004 more than 1 million RTI deaths occurred in LMICs, corresponding to 20 deaths per 100,000 population (WHO 2004).

Falls

A fall is an event that results in a person coming to rest inadvertently on the ground, floor, or other lower level (WHO 2008). Falls caused more than 424,000 deaths in 2004 with a reported mortality rate of seven and a loss of 267 DALYs per 100,000 population. Falls are one of the leading complaints for visits to hospitals and emergency departments and comprise the third highest proportion of all unintentional injury-related deaths (11 per cent; Figure 13.1). Approximately 82 per cent of falls and 92 per cent of DALYs from falls occurred in LMICs (Table 13.2). The mortality rate due to falls was higher among males than among females: compare 8 per 100,000 males to 5 per 100,000 females (Table 13.1).

Drowning

Drowning refers to an event in which a person's airway is submerged in liquid leading to breathing impairment. The outcome can be fatal or non-fatal, the latter often leading to significant neurological damage (WHO 2008). In 2004, an estimated 388,000 people drowned, making drowning the third leading cause of unintentional death globally (Table 13.2). These estimates exclude drowning deaths that result from floods, boating, water transport, and intentional injury (Norton et al. 2011; Herbert et al. 2011). Approximately 97 per cent of all drowning deaths occur in LMICs (Peden and McGee 2003), and drowning accounts for nearly 11 million DALYs (Table 13.2). Fatal drowning rates are twice as high in males as females (Table 13.1) (WHO 2004).

Poisoning

Poisoning refers to acute cellular injury or death caused by inhalation, ingestion, injection, or absorption of a toxic substance or 'poison'. Key factors that predict the severity and outcome of poisoning are the nature, dose, formulation, and route of exposure of the poison; co-exposure to other poisons; state of nutrition; age; and pre-existing health conditions (WHO 2008). The WHO estimates 346,000 deaths were caused by poisoning in 2004 (five deaths per 100,000) with rates of seven per 100,000 for males and four per 100,000 for females (Table 13.1). While over 90 per cent of poison-related deaths occurred in LMICs, poisoning is also the fourth leading cause of death and DALYs in HICs (Herbert *et al.* 2011). Poisoning contributes nearly 7.5 million DALYs lost, corresponding to 116 DALYs per 100,000 population (Table 13.2).

Fire burns

A burn is defined as an injury to the skin or other body tissue caused by heat. It occurs when some, or all, of the cells in the skin or other tissue are destroyed by hot liquids (scalds), hot solids (contact burns), or flames (flame burns). Injuries to the skin or other body tissue as a result of radiation, radioactivity, electricity, friction, or contact with chemicals are also considered burns (WHO 2008). Unfortunately, WHO data includes only fire burns, labelled 'fires', and not scalds or contact burns (Herbert *et al.* 2011). Fire burns were responsible for over 310,000 deaths in 2004, resulting in more than 175 DALYs per 100,000 population (Table 13.2). Approximately 97 per cent of fatal fire-related burns occurred in LMICs corresponding to more than 200 DALYS per 100,000 population (Table 13.2). The mortality rate due to fire burns and corresponding DALYs are higher among females than males, reflecting the higher risks to women and girls especially due to cooking with faulty cook stoves or unsafe fuels; compare six deaths and 211 DALYs per 100,000 females with four deaths and 140 DALYs per 100,000 males (Table 13.1).

'Other' unintentional injuries

Injuries that result from insect and animal bites, or those which are otherwise unspecified were grouped together in WHO data. 'Other' unintentional injuries represent approximately 30 per cent of the proportion of unintentional injury-related deaths, which suggests a greater specificity of data is necessary. The mortality rate due to 'other' unintentional injuries is twice as high in LMICs as HICs (Table 13.2).

Defining structural approaches

The matrix developed by William Haddon, Jr in 1970 is the most common framework used in injury prevention. It is useful for identifying the components of injury and for describing injury-causing events in terms of time along the pre-event, event and post-event phases (Haddon 1972). The matrix helps locate interventions by host, vector and environmental factors (Table 13.3). Interventions are also often framed in terms of the *three E's*: education, enforcement, and engineering.

A successful injury intervention often affects multiple people and targets the physical or sociocultural environments where people live; such interventions are, therefore, focusing on 'systems' of governance, livelihood, care, and community that surround people. This approach to injury prevention is synonymous with a 'structural' approach. Structural approaches to injury prevention focus on systemic risk factors and can include developing appropriate national strategies, establishing agencies to promote action, improving existing legislation to ensure safety, investing in evidence-based programmes, and supporting research to modify interventions in local contexts. These structural approaches can be applied to specific risk factors for different types of injuries (described below). This chapter will provide a number of effective structural approaches

Table 13.3 Example of Haddon's Matrix applied to drowning

	Host	*Vector*	*Environment*

Pre-event	• Information
	• Education
	• Supervision
	• Knowledge
	  of swimming
	  instruction
		• Access to water blocked	• Ensuring safe water systems, i.e.
			  drainage, piped water systems,
			  flood control embankments
			• Covering wells, open cisterns, or
			  buckets
			• Mandating four-sided pool fences
			  in HICs and barriers in LMICs
			• Requiring lifeguards at swimming
			  areas

Event	• Access to personal
	  flotation device
	• Access to swimming
	  instruction
		• Use of personal flotation
		  device
		• Use of swimming
		  instruction skills
			• Requiring lifeguards at swimming
			  areas

Post-event	• Access to first
	  responders
		• Ease of access to drowning
		  victim
		• Promptness of first
		  responders
		• First responders' knowledge
		  of cardiopulmonary
		  resuscitation
			• Rescue and rehabilitative care
			  facilities

Source: World Health Organization 2008

that have been used, or are recommended, to address the problem of specific unintentional injuries.

Examples of structural risks and interventions for unintentional injuries

Structural risk factors that influence road traffic crash involvement include economic development, social inequality, demographic factors, land use planning, the ratio of motorized traffic to vulnerable road users, and poor road design (Peden *et al.* 2004). Risk is exacerbated by speeding, alcohol use, and fatigue, not to mention young inexperienced drivers, while the risk of severe injury is higher with lack of safety restraints or helmets and insufficient vehicle crash protection. Risk factors that affect post-crash outcomes include access to appropriate pre-hospital and hospital care (Herbert *et al.* 2011; Peden *et al.* 2004). Effective structural interventions in road safety therefore must address risk factors associated with all three phases – crash involvement, crash severity, and post-crash outcomes.

Risk factors for falls in the elderly are categorized into four dimensions – biological, behavioural, environmental, and socio-economic – the latter two being more structural (WHO 2007). Environmental risk factors include individuals' physical living conditions, such as hazards in the home; and socio-economic factors include low income and education levels, inadequate housing, and limited access to health care (WHO 2007). Among children, risk factors for falls include developmental stage, gender (boys), poverty, underlying disabilities, and unsafe physical environment, such as playground equipment. The incidence and severity of fall injuries are influenced by structural factors such as the height of the fall, type of surface involved, and mechanism (WHO 2008). The literature suggests that in HICs, children fall from playground equipment whereas children in LMICs fall at home (De Sousa Petersburgo *et al.* 2010; Sherker *et al.* 2009; Wakes and Beukes 2011). Structural interventions to prevent falls among children emphasize redesigning children's furniture, legislating for window guards, and the provision of safer playground equipment (Table 13.4) (Herbert *et al.* 2011; WHO 2008).

Drowning in HICs is often associated with recreational swimming, while drowning in LMICs often occurs with everyday activities near bodies of water (Hyder *et al.* 2008). Evidence regarding the effectiveness of drowning prevention interventions in both HICs and LMICs is relatively sparse. Data from case-controlled studies, for example, suggest fencing around domestic swimming pools reduces the risk of drowning in HICs (see Table 13.4, and Thompson and Rivara 2000). Interventions to prevent water-related transport drowning include providing well-maintained and functional flotation devices; however, evidence regarding the effectiveness of these interventions is currently not available (Callaghan *et al.* 2010; Peden and McGee 2003).

In HICs, product accessibility, such as safe packaging and storage, is a key risk factor for poisoning (Wilkerson *et al.* 2005). Storage and availability of poisons are also risk factors in LMICs, as several studies show paraffin (kerosene) and pesticides are commonly ingested by children from unlocked kitchen cabinets and old cola bottles (Koueta *et al.* 2009; Manzar *et al.* 2010; Oguche *et al.* 2007; Pillai *et al.* 2004). Structural interventions to reduce exposure to poisoning include appropriate storage of poisons in terms of position and vessels, warning labels, and first aid education (Nixon *et al.* 2004; WHO 2008).

Structural risk factors for burn injuries differ according to geographic regions, but generally include use of open fires for space heating, use of ground-level stoves for cooking, high-set water heater temperatures, and sub-standard electrical wiring (Mock *et al.* 2008). Burn research in LMICs identified childhood risk factors that include use of kerosene, cooking in open spaces, overcrowding, and lack of parental supervision (Dissanaike and Rahimi, 2009; Herbert *et al.* 2011; Mashreky *et al.* 2010; Petrass *et al.* 2009; Van Niekerk *et al.* 2010). Interventions that have been proposed, but have yet to be shown to be effective, include separating the cooking area from the living area, reducing the amount of flammable substances available in the household, and enhancing child supervision (Table 13.4) (Atiyeh *et al.* 2009; Turner *et al.* 2004; WHO 2008; Ytterstad and Sogaard 1995).

The next section will provide examples of five interventions as a part of a structural approach to prevent five unintentional injuries. The section will highlight their successes as well as the associated challenges, and the examples focus on LMICs to the extent possible.

Structural approaches to unintentional injury prevention

Strong governance: the importance of a lead agency

RTIs affect young adults, particularly males, reflected in the very high mortality rates in the 15 to 29 (32 per 100,000) and 30 to 44 (38 per 100,000) age groups (WHO 2004). Since these age groups correspond to one of the most economically productive segments of any population, RTIs have serious implications for national economies (Norton *et al.* 2011). At the same time, the number of vehicles on the world's roadways has doubled since 1986 from 500 million to over 1 billion at present (Sousanis 2011). Accordingly, a structural approach to RTI prevention and control is necessary

Table 13.4 Examples of interventions for unintentional injuries recommended by the World Health Organization

Road traffic injuries	Falls	Drowning	Poisoning	Fire burns
Introducing (and enforcing) minimum drinking-age limits	Implementing multifaceted community programmes	Removing or covering water hazards	Removing the toxic agent	Setting (and enforcing) laws on smoke alarms
Setting (and enforcing) lower blood-alcohol level for novice drivers and zero tolerance for offenders	Redesigning nursery furniture and other products	Requiring isolation fencing (4-sided) around swimming pools	Legislating for (and enforcing) child-resistant packaging of medicines and poisons	Developing a standard for child-resistant lighters
Utilizing appropriate child restraints and seat belts	Establishing playground standards for the depth of appropriate surface material, height of equipment, and maintenance	Wearing personal flotation devices	Packaging drugs in non-lethal quantities	Setting (and enforcing) laws on hot tap water temperature and educating the public
Wearing motorcycle and bicycle helmets	Legislating for window guards	Ensuring immediate resuscitation	Establishing poison control centres	Treating patients at dedicated burn centres
Forcing a reduction of speed around schools, residential areas, play areas		Ensuring the presence of lifeguards at swimming areas		
Separating different types of road users		Conducting targeted awareness-raising on drowning		
Introducing daytime running lights for motorcycles				
Introducing graduated driver licensing systems				

Source: World Health Organization 2008

that promotes institutionalization of road safety. Such an approach requires increased governance to mandate and enforce safe behaviours, ensure proper standards for the construction of roads and production of vehicles, and promote the use of road safety equipment in a country (Peden *et al.* 2004).

In 2009, 178 countries participated in the WHO *Global Status Report on Road Safety*; 58 per cent reported having a national road safety strategy, although 16 per cent were not formally endorsed by their respective governments (WHO 2009). In addition, 86 per cent of countries reported having a 'lead agency', and 79 per cent of these received funds from their national budgets. A lead agency at country level not only has the mandate for road safety, but also the authority to make decisions, and the finances to implement them. This lead agency might be a national road safety council, committee, authority, or a new dictate for an existing ministry. Such an institution can spearhead the implementation of effective road safety interventions with good governance, appropriate financial resources, and continued monitoring and technical support (Table 13.5).

Infrastructure safety: playground injuries

In HICs, falls from playground equipment present unnecessary, costly, and painful injuries, some of which are fatal. Consequently, governments require that playground equipment be redesigned to limit or reduce the levels of injury from falls (Wakes and Beukes 2011). The risk of fall-related injury is significantly reduced when the height of equipment is below 1.5 metres, so it is important to build or resize climbing equipment below that height (Wakes and Beukes 2011). Redesigning existing playgrounds, especially in schools, in LMICs in accordance with these recommendations should also reduce the risk and severity of fall injuries.

However, experience in HICs shows that fall-related injury hospitalization rates may not decrease even with height restrictions on equipment unless the playground surface depth recommendations are followed (Sherker *et al.* 2009). These structural changes ensure that the impacts of a fall are minimized with shock-absorbing surfaces several inches thick. Local councils and schools tasked with ensuring the safety of playgrounds in Western countries cited a lack of resources as a reason for non-compliance (Sherker *et al.* 2009). Thus, appropriate financial investments and subsidies would need to be explored in LMIC settings, especially because playgrounds are less common (Table 13.5). Empowering community members to keep playgrounds safe may also be an option where resources are deficient.

Home protection: barriers for drowning

In Bangladesh, drowning is one of the most common causes of death in children aged 1 to 4 years (Borse *et al.* 2011). What is more the critical risk factor – water – abounds; a single district alone might have 50,000 or more ditches and ponds (Hyder *et al.* 2008). A useful structural approach for rural Bangladesh has been piloted in the form of barrier-based interventions for drowning prevention in children less than 5 years old. Door barriers and playpens may work, especially for Bangladeshi children aged 1 to 3 years who are at high risk of drowning during the morning times when their mother is performing household tasks (Borse *et al.* 2011). Blocking children's access to waterways with barriers, or blocking their unsupervised exit from a dwelling, might be effective ways to ease the burden on mothers (Table 13.5). Producing such barriers in the community or making them available at little or no cost to low-income families in LMICs is an important agenda for future research.

Safe production: child resistant containers

Paraffin or kerosene poisoning is one of the most common forms of childhood poisoning in most LMICs, linked to its dominance as a household fuel (Ahuja *et al.* 2011; De Wet *et al.* 1994). Poisoning occurs in children who mistake paraffin for a beverage and ingest the fuel often directly from the source, or from old cola and juice bottles used for storage (De Wet *et al.* 1994; Krug *et al.* 1994; Schwebel and Swart 2009). Containers with skull and crossbones attract young children although they were meant to warn them of the dangers (De Wet *et al.* 1994). Child-resistant containers (CRCs) are an intervention strategy to combat paraffin poisoning in the same way they were utilized in HICs to combat poisoning from prescription drugs (Ozanne-Smith *et al.* 2001; US Consumer Product Safety Commission 2005).

At approximately 20 million paraffin users per day, South Africa has one the of world's largest paraffin-using populations (Schwebel and Swart 2009). An earlier study by Krug *et al.* (1994) identified paraffin ingestion as the most common cause of poisoning among black South African children and distributed CRCs in an intervention site reducing the incidence of paraffin ingestion by 47 per cent (Krug *et al.* 1994). A cost-effectiveness analysis by Bishai and Hyder (2006) reveals that an investment of US $16,000 could save 490 life years or US $61 per DALY, making CRCs one of the most cost-effective health interventions (Bishai and Hyder 2006).

All paraffin should be sold in CRCs and changes to the environments in which paraffin is manufactured, stored, and used are needed (Schwebel and Swart 2009). The most effective way to reduce poisoning from paraffin lies in producing CRCs for all paraffin storage (Table 13.5). This requires buy-in from the government and private sector to develop and market safer products (De Wet *et al.* 1994). A structural approach of safe production is both appropriate and cost-effective in this instance.

Equipment safety: new cook stoves

Cook stove burns from equipment explosion have been reported as a leading cause of severe house burns in women and children in Asia and Africa (Godwin *et al.* 1996; Mabrouk *et al.* 2000; Peck *et al.* 2008). In a prospective study of flame stove patients' admissions in a Cape Town, South Africa hospital, 25 per cent of those patients were injured in stove-related incidents, of which the majority (60 per cent) were due to stove explosions (Peck *et al.* 2008; Steenkamp *et al.* 2002). Poor manufacturing standards, low quality control, and lack of safety features define the cook stoves in LMICs. Cook stoves which utilize paraffin may burst into flame, especially when the paraffin is contaminated.

Malfunctioning cooking appliances are an important risk factor for fire burn injury. Many LMICs do not have infrastructures in place to regulate fuel integrity, specifically whether the fuel has been contaminated with another type of fuel (Peck *et al.* 2008). The Global Alliance for Clean Cook Stoves, led by the United Nations Foundation, seeks to encourage 100 million homes in LMICs to adopt clean cook stoves and fuels by 2020 as well as support a clean and innovative cook stove industry (Global Alliance

2011). Efficient cook stoves that are affordable in the context of LMICs can dramatically reduce fuel consumption, exposure to harmful emissions and smoke, and reduce the risk of fire burns (Table 13.5).

Challenges to structural approaches for injury prevention

In order to implement comprehensive structural strategies for injury prevention, countries, states, and local communities need to develop the infrastructure and indigenous capacity to conduct the essential activities needed for an effective programme. Infrastructure includes the identification of lead agencies to oversee injury control policies and their implementation. Capacity includes the availability of appropriate human, financial, and technical resources (Peek-Asa and Hyder 2009). Many governments, especially in LMICs, still lack dedicated injury prevention units in their health departments, often leaving injuries to be managed as a part of non-communicable disease programmes. This creates a situation where good intentions or a policy alone do not provide the conditions necessary for effective action. In fact, unless there is institutional support for injury prevention, even investments in training and development of individual capacity are at risk of being lost to other fields. Trained injury professionals or practitioners may apply their skills in other areas where there are better institutional incentives and career pathways. Therefore, the success of injury prevention efforts will be contingent not only on human resources, but also on the strength of the institutions that engage these individuals. As the science and evidence base for injury prevention evolves, so too must these institutional arrangements (Tran and Hyder 2008).

Despite evidence of effective structural approaches that prevent unintentional injuries in HICs, many policies and interventions are not directly transferable in LMIC contexts. Structural approaches to injury prevention that include developing national policies, building agencies to promote action, improving older legislation to ensure safety, investing in evidence-based programmes, and supporting relevant research all need to be modified to suit local and national contexts in LMIC. The use of public health sciences to help identify the local causes of injuries and support their solutions in LMICs is essential; and these actions must be multi-sectoral so that all relevant groups are engaged in the solution.

Table 13.5 Examples of structural approaches and effective interventions for unintentional injuries

Structural approach	Strong governance	Infrastructure safety	Home protection	Safe production	Equipment safety
Example of an intervention	Lead agency or national organization with mandate and funding for road safety	Height constrained and shock absorbing playground design	Barriers separating children (host) from hazard (ponds, bodies of water)	Containers with child-resistant tops	Safer and environmentally friendly cook stoves
Injury targeted	Road traffic injuries	Falls	Drowning	Poisoning	Fire burns

Source: Global Alliance 2011

Conclusion

Structural approaches must be prioritized as part of injury prevention work. Professionals from public health, medicine, engineering, social services, urban planning, and law enforcement, among others, can all help create safer environments and programmes. The public health community must play a leadership role in galvanizing a multi-sectoral, structural response to unintentional injuries; advocate for investments at local, national, and international levels; and encourage information-sharing around the world. The growing impact of injury on global health makes it imperative that the international community invest in injury research and prevention, and actively work towards reducing this unacceptable burden.

References

Ahuja, R.B., Dash, J.K., and Shrivastrava, P. (2011) 'A comparative analysis of liquefied petroleum gas (LPG) and kerosene related burns', *Burns*, 37 (8): 1403–10.

Atiyeh, B.S., Costagiola, M., and Hayek, S.N. (2009) 'Burn prevention mechanisms and outcomes: pitfalls, failures and successes', *Burns*, 35 (2): 181–93.

Bishai, D.M. and Hyder, A.A. (2006) 'Modeling the cost effectiveness of injury interventions in lower and middle income countries: opportunities and challenges', *Cost Effectiveness and Resource Allocation*, 4: 2.

Borse, N.N., Hyder, A.A., Streatfield, P.K., Arifeen, S.E., and Bishai, D. (2011) 'Childhood drowning and traditional rescue measures: case study from Matlab, Bangladesh', *Archives of Disease in Childhood*, 96: 675–80.

Callaghan, J.A., Hyder, A.A., Khan, R., Blum, L.S., Arifeen, S., and Baqui, A.H. (2010) 'Child supervision practices for drowning prevention in rural Bangladesh: a pilot study of supervision tools', *Journal of Epidemiology and Community Health*, 64: 645–7.

De Sousa Petersburgo, D., Keyes, C.E., Wright, D.W., Click, L.A., Macleod, J.B., and Sasser, S.M. (2010) 'The epidemiology of childhood injury in Maputo, Mozambique', *International Journal of Emergency Medicine*, 3 (3): 157–63.

De Wet, B., Van Schalkwyk, D., Van der Spuy, J., Du Plessis, J., Du Toit, N., and Burns, D. (1994) 'Paraffin (kerosene) poisoning in childhood – is prevention affordable in South Africa?', *South African Medical Journal*, 84 (11): 735–8.

Dissanaike, S., and Rahimi, M. (2009) 'Epidemiology of burn injuries: highlighting cultural and socio-demographic aspects', *International Review of Psychiatry*, 21 (6): 505–11.

Global Alliance for Clean Cookstoves (2011) *Overview: The Solution*, New York: The United Nations Foundation. Online, available at: http://cleancookstoves.org/overview/solution/ (accessed 7 September 2011).

Godwin, Y., Hudson, D.A., and Bloch, C.E. (1996) 'Shack fires: a consequence of urban migration', *Burns*, 23: 151–3.

Haddon, W. (1972) 'A logical framework for categorizing highway safety phenomena and activity', *Journal of Trauma*, 12 (3): 193–207.

Herbert, H.K., Hyder, A.A., Butchart, A., and Norton, R. (2011) 'Global health: injuries and violence', *Infectious Disease Clinics of North America*, 25: 653–68.

Hyder, A.A., Borse, N.N., Blum, L., Khan, R., Arifeen, S.E., and Baqui, A.H. (2008) 'Childhood drowning in low- and middle-income countries: urgent need for intervention trials', *Journal of Paediatrics and Child Health*, 44: 221–7.

Koueta, F., Dao, L., Ye, D., Fayama, Z., and Sawadogo, A. (2009) 'Acute accidental poisoning in children: aspects of their epidemiology, aetiology, and outcome at the Charles de Gaulle paediatric hospital in Ouagadougou (Burkina Faso)', *Sante*, 19 (2): 55–9.

Krug, A., Ellis, J.B., Hay, I.T., Mokgabudi, N.F., and Robertson, J. (1994) 'The impact of resistant containers on the incidence of paraffin (kerosene) ingestion in children', *South African Medical Journal*, 84 (11): 730–4.

Krug, E.G., Dahlberg, L.L., Mercy, J.A., Zwi, A.B., and Lozano, R. (2002) *The World Report on Violence and Health*, Geneva: World Health Organization.

Mabrouk, A., El Badawy, A., and Sherif, M. (2000) 'Kerosene stove as a cause of burns admitted to the Ain Shams burn unit', *Burns*, 26 (5): 474–7.

Manzar, N., Saad, S.M., Manzar, B., and Fatima, S.S. (2010) 'The study of etiological and demographic characteristics of acute household accidental poisoning in children – a consecutive case series study from Pakistan', *BMC Pediatrics*, 10: 28.

Mashreky, S.R., Rahman, A., Khan, T.F., Svanström, L., and Rahman, F. (2010) 'Determinants of childhood burns in rural Bangladesh: a nested case-control study', *Health Policy*, 96 (3): 226–30.

Mock, C., Peck, M., Peden, M., and Krug, E. (eds) (2008) *A WHO Plan for Burn Prevention and Care*, Geneva: World Health Organization.

Nixon, J., Spinks, A., Turner, C., and McClure, R. (2004) 'Community based programs to prevent poisoning in children 0–15 years', *Injury Prevention*, 10 (1): 43–6.

Norton, R., Hyder A.A., and Butchart, A. (2011) 'Unintentional injuries and violence', in M.H. Merson, R. Black and A.J. Mills (eds) *Global Health: Diseases, Programs, Systems and Policies*, 3rd edition, Burlington, MA: Jones & Bartlett Learning.

Oguche, S., Bukbuk, D.N., and Watila, I.M. (2007) 'Pattern of hospital admissions of children with poisoning in the Sudano-Sahelian North Eastern Nigeria', *Nigerian Journal of Clinical Practice*, 10 (2): 111–15.

Ozanne-Smith, J., Day, L., Parsons, B., Tibbals, J., and Dobbin, M. (2001) 'Childhood poisoning: access and prevention', *Journal of Paediatric Child Health*, 37: 262–5.

Peck, M.D., Kruger, G.E., Van der Merwe, A.E., Godkaumbura, W., and Ahuja, R.B. (2008) 'Burns and fires from non-electric domestic appliances in low and middle income countries Part I. The scope of the problem', *Burns*, 34 (3): 303–11.

Peden, M. and McGee, K. (2003) 'The epidemiology of drowning worldwide', *Injury Control and Safety Promotion*, 10 (4): 195–9.

Peden, M., Scurfield, R., Sleet, D., Mohan, D., Hyder, A.A., Jarawan, E., and Mathers, C. (2004) *World Report on Road Traffic Injury Prevention*, Geneva: World Health Organization.

Peek-Asa, C. and Hyder, A.A. (2009) 'Injury prevention and control: the public health approach', in R. Detels, R. Beaglehole, M.A. Lansang, and M. Guilliford (eds) *Oxford Textbook of Public Health*, 5th edition, Oxford: Oxford University Press.

Petrass, L.A., Finch, C.F., and Blitvich, J.D. (2009) 'Methodological approaches used to assess the relationship between parental supervision and child injury risk', *Injury Prevention*, (15) 2: 132–8.

Pillai, G.K., Boland, K., Jagdeo, S., and Persad, K. (2004) 'Acute poisoning in children. Cases hospitalized during a three-year period in Trinidad', *West Indian Medical Journal*, 53 (1): 50–4.

Schwebel, D.C. and Swart, D. (2009) 'Preventing paraffin-related injury', *Journal of Injury and Violence Research*, 1 (1): 3–5.

Sherker, S., Ritchie, J., Eager, D., and Dennis, R. (2009) 'Soft landings: encouraging compliance with safety standards in Local Government Authority playgrounds', *Health Promotion Journal of Australia*, 20 (1): 31–6.

Sousanis, J. (2011) *World Vehicle Population Tops 1 Billion Units*. Online, available at: http://wardsauto.com/ar/world_vehicle_population_110815/ (accessed 7 September 2011).

Steenkamp, W.C., Van der Merwe, A.E., and De Lang, R. (2002) 'The prevention of burn injuries: problems with paraffin stove burns', *South African Medical Journal*, 92: 445.

Thompson, D.C. and Rivara, F.P. (2000) 'Pool fencing for preventing drowning in children', *Cochrane Database of Systematic Reviews*, 2: CD001047.

Tran, N.T. and Hyder, A.A. (2008) 'Securing the future of injury prevention: people and institutions', *Injury Prevention*, 14 (4): 277.

Turner, C., Spinks, A., McClure, R., and Nixon, J. (2004) 'Community-based interventions for the prevention of burns and scalds in children', *Cochrane Database of Systematic Reviews*, 3: 1–19.

United States Consumer Product Safety Commission (2005) *Poison Prevention Packaging: A Guide for Healthcare Professionals*, Washington, D.C.: United States Consumer Product Safety Commission.

Van Niekerk, A., Menckel, E., and Laflamme, L. (2010) 'Barriers and enablers to the use of measures to prevent pediatric scalding in Cape Town, South Africa,' *Public Health Nursing*, 27 (3): 203–20.

Wakes, S. and Beukes, A. (2011) 'Height, fun and safety in the design of children's playground equipment', *International Journal of Injury Control and Safety Promotion*, 1: 1–8.

World Health Organization (WHO) (2004) *Global Burden of Disease: 2004 Update*, Geneva: World Health Organization.

World Health Organization (WHO) (2007) *WHO Global Report on Falls Prevention in Older Age*, Geneva: World Health Organization.

World Health Organization (WHO) (2008) *World Report on Child Injury Prevention: Summary*, Geneva: World Health Organization.

World Health Organization (WHO) (2009) *Global Status Report on Road Safety: Time for Action*, Geneva: World Health Organization.

Wilkerson, R., Northington, L., and Fisher, W. (2005) 'Ingestion of toxic substances by infants and children: what we don't know can hurt', *Critical Care Nurse*, 25 (4): 35–44.

Ytterstad, B. and Sogaard, A.J. (1995) 'The Harstad injury prevention study: prevention of burns in small children by a community-based intervention', *Burns*, 21 (4): 259–66.

Part 3

EVALUATING STRUCTURAL INTERVENTIONS

14

EVALUATING STRUCTURAL INTERVENTIONS IN PUBLIC HEALTH

Challenges, options and global best practice

Paul Pronyk, Jennifer Schaefer, Marie-Andrée Somers, and Lori Heise

Introduction

Structural interventions in public health pose a host of challenges to evaluation. They operate through indirect pathways and are often complex and cross-sectoral. Programmes may require extended time horizons for health effects to be observed, and their delivery at the level of communities, institutions, or populations carries major implications for sampling. Finally, issues of ethics, logistics, and/or political feasibility may limit opportunities for random assignment and the use of experimental designs.

Nonetheless, evaluation is vital – both for strengthening the link between good science and sound policy, as well as ensuring public confidence in how limited resources are deployed. This chapter will explore the range of potential options and considerations when evaluating structural interventions in public health. We will draw upon global experience to explore the merits and limitations of adequacy assessments, plausibility evaluations, and randomized experiments, including stepped-wedge designs. We will discuss the challenges of choosing an appropriate comparison group, the importance of impact pathway assessment, and the use of time-series monitoring. Finally, we will highlight the value of mixed-methods approaches, both to assess impact and to document the implementation principles that carry wider application to public health policy and programme development.

Here we define structural interventions in public health as interventions that attempt to engage the complex social, economic, and political determinants of health as a way of influencing more downstream outcomes (Blankenship *et al.* 2000). Such interventions operate at the level of groups or populations and generally attempt to shape an individual's risk of disease through indirect mechanisms. In his seminal work, Rose argued that disease in populations is more a reflection of the mean level of risk in that society, rather than simply a product of cumulative, independent, individual choices (Rose 1985). Structural interventions seek to influence this mean level of risk by engaging upstream dynamics and conditions, with the aim of shaping norms, behaviours, and health outcomes in the population as a whole.

Why evaluate?

There is an ever increasing demand for accountability and evidence-based decision-making in public health. Unfortunately, in the past, many structural interventions have been poorly evaluated, evaluated only in retrospect, or not at all (Savedoff *et al.* 2006). The paucity of evaluation literature, particularly for complex interventions, means that policymakers can be forced to make decisions in a vacuum, risking the repetition of mistakes from the past and failing to benefit from the lessons of successful interventions (Campbell *et al.* 2000).

There is a clear need to improve the evidence base for structural interventions in public health. This chapter underscores the many challenges encountered when evaluating structural interventions, highlighting implications for evaluation design. Drawing from a diverse range of disciplinary perspectives, we then profile a range of tools and methods that can be employed to conduct appropriate and rigorous programme evaluations.

What makes structural interventions difficult to evaluate?

Policymakers and programme managers in public health are accustomed to weighing, synthesizing, and applying new evidence in relatively standardized ways that are heavily influenced by evaluations of discrete, downstream, technical interventions. Evidence from randomized controlled trials, systematic reviews, and cost-effectiveness studies has played an important role in shaping policy and informing practice. However, for numerous reasons, weighing evidence from structural interventions may be different – with such 'gold-standard' evaluations often unavailable or inappropriate (Bonell *et al.* 2006a; McKee *et al.* 1999; Shepperd *et al.* 2009; Victora *et al.* 2004). We outline a number of the reasons for this below.

Context

Structural interventions are by nature contextual. Strategies to address economic barriers, engage legal systems, or shift cultural norms and power relationships will differ from place to place. Contextual factors influence implementation, affect uptake and utilization, and carry implications for reproducibility and external validity of evidence generated from programme evaluations (Campbell *et al.* 2000). Evaluation designs should, therefore, employ an appropriate mix of methods to describe and document context, noting the ways this might affect the interpretation of programme results.

Understanding contextual factors often requires qualitative research, which can be conducted during or prior to an intervention. For example, a pre-intervention observational study assessing the feasibility of introducing school-based sexual health programmes in Tanzania identified many potential barriers, including low attendance rates, lack of trust between students and teachers, and limited teacher training (Plummer *et al.* 2007b). This knowledge allows such barriers to be considered in the subsequent process and impact evaluations (Plummer *et al.* 2007a; Ross *et al.* 2007).

Multi-sector focus

The design and evaluation of interventions to address structural determinants of health often require input from multiple sectors. Despite this, cross-disciplinary work happens too infrequently – with funding mechanisms, the design of academic institutions, and the organization of government departments creating many barriers to such partnerships. New insights and novel innovations have the potential to be important by-products of working between sectors. In an interdependent world with many complex and interrelated challenges, cross-sectoral perspectives are necessary now more than ever.

Complexity

Complex interventions have multiple interacting components, with the behaviour of implementers and the response of programme recipients influencing intervention delivery and results (UK Medical Research Council 2006). Progression from one programme phase to another may be non-linear, iterative, and adaptive, making strict adherence to an implementation protocol potentially inappropriate (Campbell *et al.* 2000). This poses obvious challenges to conventional evaluation methods, where standardized exposures, discrete hypothesis testing, and pre-stated effect measurement are generally the norm.

Examples of complex interventions include health systems strengthening programmes – such as the Integrated Management of Childhood Illness (IMCI – see Case Study 1), which simultaneously addressed improvements in case management, health systems, and family and community practices to improve child survival (Arifeen *et al.* 2009; Bryce *et al.* 2004) – and multi-layered interventions with legal, policy, and media components, such as the Avahan programme, which aimed to reduce violence and HIV risk among sex workers in India (Beattie *et al.* 2010) (see Case Study 2; also, see Chapter 10, Swendeman and Jana, in this volume).

Timeframes

Because structural interventions act indirectly, longer time horizons may be required to detect measurable effects on downstream outcomes. It has also been suggested that gains achieved through addressing the structural roots of problems, rather than targeting more immediate risk behaviours, may be better sustained over time. Both issues have implications for the duration of programme evaluations. Furthermore, governments and donors are often themselves bound by short-term time horizons, creating pressure for more immediate results.

While longer-term evaluations are required to measure some downstream outcomes and assess sustainability, there is also ample evidence suggesting that structural interventions have the potential to exert effects over relatively short time horizons. A comprehensive structural intervention to address undernutrition across nine rural sites in sub-Saharan Africa reduced rates of childhood stunting by over 40 per cent in just three years (Remans *et al.* 2011) (see Case Study 3). The Intervention with Microfinance for AIDS and Gender Equity (IMAGE Study) demonstrated major reductions in rates of intimate partner violence and HIV-related risk behaviour after just two years of exposure to an integrated microfinance and training programme (Pronyk *et al.* 2006; Pronyk *et al.* 2008b) (see Case Study 4). Thus, while longer time horizons are advocated for evaluations of structural interventions, shorter-term interim follow-up should also be included in the timing of assessment rounds.

Sampling

As structural interventions are often delivered at the level of institutions or communities, these become the primary unit of assessment. Detecting statistical differences between exposed and unexposed groups is generally more strongly influenced by the total number of units sampled rather than the number of individuals within each unit (Hayes and Bennett 1999; Hayes *et al.* 2000). This has serious time and resource implications for programme evaluations as interventions must be delivered to sufficient numbers of units with adequate intensity of exposure achieved in each, and sufficient follow-up time to discern measurable effects.

Random allocation

Random assignment of structural interventions is often difficult. It may not be appropriate (such as in the case of a national policy shift or media campaign), ethical (such as a poverty reduction programme that cannot be politically withheld from some groups over others), or politically feasible (where governments feel political imperatives are critical in determining who is exposed or unexposed) (Bonell *et al.* 2006a). Non-random choices of intervention groups have the potential to introduce selection bias – where exposed and unexposed groups may differ or not be sufficiently representative. In addition, because it is difficult to conduct blinded assessments or offer placebos for structural interventions, issues of response bias are important to consider. A more detailed discussion of whether and when to randomize is presented below.

Secular change

Secular change includes the background mix of local and national policies and programmes, and other dynamic factors affecting the health outcomes of intervention participants and the wider community, including any comparison group. Secular change can pose major challenges to the evaluation of structural interventions. Factors such as unanticipated policy and programme shifts, forces in the media, and/or economic changes all carry the potential to shape social attitudes, behaviours, and health outcomes. Unlike a clinical trial, where control groups are generally unexposed to an intervention, evaluations of structural interventions are often confounded by secular change. For example, major long-term evaluations of community-level programmes to address cardiovascular disease have yielded disappointing results partially as a result of the rapid pace of social change around healthier diets, greater levels of exercise, and reductions in smoking (Susser 1995). Similar challenges are faced for evaluations of programmes to scale up proven interventions in programme-rich environments, where many similar interventions are being implemented by governments or NGOs. In such contexts, reference groups may be exposed to a host of similar interventions to those being assessed, carrying the potential to understate intervention effects (Victora *et al.* 2010).

Intervention diffusion also has the potential to complicate effects. As opposed to secular change, which affects the population as a whole, diffusion happens when some individuals in the comparison or reference group are exposed to the specific intervention through migration or spillover of the intervention services between groups. Such effects are also called 'spillover effects' and 'externalities' in other disciplines. Spillover can be accounted for in the analysis, but it is better addressed in the design phase, ensuring proper site selection and sufficient distance between groups at the outset.

Synergies

As structural interventions often have multiple moving parts, the 'active ingredient' or 'mechanism of action' can be difficult to pin down. In addition, questions of potential synergies may also be important – where the effects of the whole (combined package) may be greater than the sum of the component parts.

There are a number of steps evaluators can take to address these challenges. They include the use of detailed impact pathway monitoring, time-series data, or qualitative implementation research and the assessment of the degree to which observed effects of combined programmes compare to those predicted from evaluations of single interventions. These will be described in more detail in the following section.

Evaluation options for structural interventions

Robust evaluations of structural interventions generally require a mix of methods to respond to the challenges highlighted above (Bamberger et al. 2010; Leeuw and Vaessen 2009). Decisions about *what* and *how* to evaluate must be made through careful consideration of *why* an evaluation is being done – with methods reflecting those most appropriate for the questions being posed (Habicht et al. 1999; Victora et al. 2004). In this section, we review a range of complementary methods in the menu of options for evaluating structural interventions, including impact assessment, implementation research, and economic analysis.

Impact assessment

Impact assessments answer questions about whether project goals were achieved and whether these effects were caused by the intervention. There are three main designs that may be suitable for evaluating structural interventions – adequacy, plausibility, and probability (Victora et al. 1999).

Adequacy

An *adequacy* assessment compares the performance of the intervention package against a fixed set of goals or targets. The purpose is to demonstrate that the intervention is adequate to meet the designated objectives. The types of targets can be performance indicators such as whether clinics were opened or how many teachers have been trained in a school, or outcome-related indicators such as levels of intervention coverage and disease-specific endpoints. Adequacy assessments may also measure change over time but without any attempt to account for secular change.

Adequacy assessments generally lack a control group, and thus the main limitation is the inability to make statements regarding causality or attribution. For structural interventions, each point in the causal chain is important, and in the absence of adequate programme performance, it is unrealistic to expect changes in health outcomes.

Plausibility

A *plausibility* assessment compares observed changes against a non-randomly selected reference group, as a way of accounting for the effects of secular change and confounding. This reference group may be a historical control group (a before and after assessment); or an external control group. The allocation of groups to receive an intervention in a plausibility assessment is generally non-random; therefore, factors such as selection bias and confounding cannot be completely excluded.

Strategies to enhance plausibility

There are a number of strategies that can improve the case for attribution – whether exposure to an intervention has caused the observed changes. *Impact pathway mapping* involves applying a pre-defined and theoretically grounded impact pathway that systematically maps proposed mechanisms through which an intervention is expected to lead to changes in outcomes. In a complex and multi-component structural intervention, it is important to track indicators at each point in a causal chain. The size and consistency of changes across a range of activities and outcomes also helps enhance the plausibility that observed effects were a result of an intervention, while helping to distinguish between interventions that are inherently faulty (failure of intervention concept or theory), those that were simply poorly delivered (implementation failure), or those that were truly ineffective (an intervention that was well-conceived, well-implemented, but ultimately not effective) (Rychetnik *et al.* 2002).

Supporting evidence can also be derived from assessing a *dose–response relationship*, which correlates the magnitude of exposure with the level of response. If better outcomes are associated with individuals or groups exposed to a greater intensity of the intervention, this supports the case for attribution. Instrumental variables analysis may be a useful analytical tool in this regard (Greenland 2000). In this approach, the association between intervention dose (such as number of visits to a health clinic) and health outcomes is adjusted for by using an independent predictor of dosage (such as distance to a health clinic).

Changes observed can also be compared to *national or sub-national trends*. This provides a weaker reference point than a designated comparison group as external data may not be available on the exact outcomes of interest; national surveys may be conducted at different time points; and, they may be subject to uncertain and inconsistent enumerator and respondent bias. However, if intervention participants are outpacing both the designated comparison group as well as regional trends, this provides further support of intervention effectiveness.

Finally, if time-series data are available on outcomes of interest – with multiple time points both before and after the start of an intervention – then an *interrupted time-series design* can be employed. An 'inflection point' in the time-series trend at the start of the intervention provides supportive evidence for the existence of a causal effect (Shadish *et al.* 2002).

Probability

A *probability* assessment employs randomization. For structural interventions, similar units are designated for participation in an evaluation, with the final selection of exposed and unexposed groups taking place using a random selection process. If a sufficient number similar of units are studied, this design minimizes the effect of *selection bias* (McKee *et al.* 1999).

When to employ a randomized design

One of the major challenges faced by evaluators of structural interventions is whether to opt for a randomized design. This choice is an important one. Evidence from randomized studies can be summarized in systematic reviews and used to accumulate a body of evidence for a particular intervention. Such information can shape global consensus, inform policy decisions, and influence resource allocation.

However, the random allocation of structural interventions may be difficult for a number of reasons. As described above, randomization may be perceived to be unethical or politically unfeasible. For example, a recent evaluation of a cash transfer programme noted the intervention could not be withheld from poor control groups for extended periods as originally planned (IFPRI 2002). Alternatively, intervention funding may have been pre-designated to particular groups based on non-random criteria. Second, for an intervention delivered to very large units (e.g. a media campaign in a city), random selection may be logistically complex, and having sufficient numbers of exposed and unexposed groups may not be possible (Mensah *et al.* 2010). Third, the time required for expected outcomes may be longer than is practical for informing decision-making (Bonell *et al.* 2006a). Fourth, randomization may not be necessary – such as where an intervention is expected to have a large and immediate effect that is unlikely to be explained by secular changes (UK Medical Research Council 2006). Fifth, some structural interventions may be so complex, adaptive, or context-specific that the type of impact questions best answered by randomized experiments may be less relevant. Here, the most relevant question might not be 'did it work?', but 'why and how did the various elements of an intervention influence the outcome, and are they likely to work in a similar way in another context?' Finally, randomized studies may not be appropriate in settings where secular change is pronounced or in programme-rich environments in which relatively untouched control groups are not possible.

In summary, these challenges should be carefully weighed when making choices regarding evaluation design. Randomized evaluations should be strongly considered for structural interventions under the following circumstances (Victora *et al.* 2010; Bonell *et al.* 2006a):

- When the aim is to assess the efficacy of unproven interventions;
- Where interventions can be delivered in a consistent manner across treatment areas;
- Where an intervention is reasonably 'discrete' and operates through pre-specified impact pathways;
- Where a relatively large number of units can be randomized;
- Where relatively unexposed control groups can be maintained throughout the assessment period.

Alternative approaches: stepped-wedge design and regression discontinuity

A variant of the randomized experiment is the *stepped-wedge design*. This design may be used to overcome practical or ethical objections to experimental evaluations, especially for potentially effective interventions that cannot be made available to entire populations simultaneously (Brown and Liliford 2006). This approach involves the advanced random selection of intervention clusters, with implementation sequenced according to this random allocation. All clusters are assessed at project inception and at each point when a new group is enrolled, with late adopters serving as comparison groups for early initiators. Eventually, the whole population receives the intervention. The stepped-wedge design has been used in diverse settings, including assessment of the effect of cash transfer programmes on health and nutrition outcomes in Mexico (IFPRI 2002); examination of how housing improvements affect respiratory ailments in England (Somerville *et al.* 2002); and evaluation of the effects of water treatment on community health in South Africa (Bailey and Archer 2004).

It is also worth noting that in non-health sectors, *regression discontinuity designs* have been employed as an equally rigorous option for evaluating programme impact (Bloom 2009; Imbens and Lemieux 2008). In this type of design, assignment to the intervention is based on a cut-off for some external criterion such as income; those above or below the cut-off receive the treatment, while others do not. In public health, for example, services could be offered to the poorest third of the families in a community. Though exposure to the programme is not randomized, it is based on a measured criterion that can be modelled in the analysis. Under reasonable assumptions, the causality of this design is as strong as a randomized experiment. The appeal of this design is that unlike random assignment, the neediest individuals or communities receive the intervention. The limitation of this approach, however, is that it requires two to five times the sample size of a randomized experiment.

Implementation research

Implementation research, also known as process evaluation, is an essential component in the evaluation of structural interventions. While impact assessments respond to questions of whether an intervention works, implementation research is more exploratory in nature, asking *how* an intervention exerts its effects (Wight and Obasi 2003). This is particularly important for structural interventions given their multifaceted nature and dependence on social context (Oakley *et al.* 2006). Such assessments are increasingly recommended for evaluations of complex interventions (Guba and Lincoln 1989; Oakley *et al.* 2004), including randomized trials and interventions that are introduced at the level of populations or clusters (Bamberger *et al.* 2010; Campbell *et al.* 2000; Hawe *et al.* 2004; Hayes and Bennett 1999; Leeuw and Vaessen 2009).

The primary aim of implementation research is to examine how the process of implementation affects project outcomes (Koepsell *et al.* 1992; Rychetnik *et al.* 2002; Shiell *et al.* 2008; Wight and Obasi 2003). This has implications for internal and external validity, addresses issues of equity and acceptability, and also reveals unintended consequences, both negative and positive. Despite the importance of process evaluation, especially of complex interventions, the creative use of qualitative methods alongside impact evaluation remains rare (Lewin *et al.* 2009).

Qualitative research

While the specific methods of implementation research are by nature contextual, a set of best practice guidelines are emerging to guide implementation science. *Qualitative research* examines the perspectives of participants in the intervention – implementers, project partners, and beneficiaries. This may involve key informant interviews with implementers to discuss the theory and programme design, community engagement, local adaptation, and barriers and facilitators to implementation. Interviews with government and other stakeholders document the alignment of the intervention within national policies and programmes, and wider implications for integration and scale-up. Focus groups with project beneficiaries help unpack the accessibility and acceptability of an intervention and generate insight about key ingredients of an intervention's failure or success – which are critical in complex adaptive systems, where seemingly small inputs or omissions can have disproportionate effects on uptake or impact (WHO 2009).

To be most useful, qualitative investigations should be closely linked to implementation and quantitative assessments, with process evaluation investigators also being involved in the interpretation of the study findings. Too often qualitative research accompanying trials and other impact studies ends up being largely a parallel effort with little influence on study outcomes (Lewin *et al.* 2009). When reference groups are used, it is also important to use qualitative research to understand and document 'business as usual' or secular change, and the presence of other (similar or different) interventions in these comparison groups.

Performance monitoring

Performance monitoring examines programme activities, outputs, and outcomes along a range of thematic areas. The emphasis is on systematically documenting the timing, sequence, and uptake of various intervention components in the participating sites. Data are often generated from routinely collected source documents such as health facility forms, attendance or participation registers, or programme management reports.

If performance data are collected on a regular basis, this yields time-series data that can be used to help understand when 'tipping or inflection points' took place – whether the introduction of specific investments or activities led to changes in levels of coverage or outcomes. This strategy is often used to enhance plausibility in observational data. Examples include the decline in hospital admissions due to childhood pneumonia that coincided with the introduction of pneumococcal vaccination to the routine immunization schedule in the United States (Grijalva *et al.* 2007), or reductions in child mortality that took place in Tanzania alongside increased government spending on efforts to expand coverage of child health interventions (Masanja *et al.* 2008).

Context mapping

Investigating *contextual factors* that might influence the delivery, uptake, or effects of structural interventions is another important dimension of a comprehensive evaluation. A deeper understanding of contextual drivers may help interpret the presence or absence of programme effects. Factors such as policy change, shifting norms, or major financial investments may drive wider secular changes and accelerate outcomes, while economic and political shocks may attenuate intervention effects. In addition, better understanding contextual issues may enhance the generalizability of findings (Bonell *et al.* 2006b; Hawe *et al.* 2004). For example, key cultural messages and a multi-component media campaign were felt to play a major role in stimulating policy change on domestic violence in South Africa (Usdin *et al.* 2005). While the content of the intervention may not have external validity beyond the immediate region, there may be processes and lessons around simultaneously engaging stakeholders at multiple levels to evoke policy shifts that are generalizable across a range of settings.

Methods for tracking contextual factors may be difficult to standardize, and may require detailed understandings of a range of secular forces that might influence intervention effects. A diverse set of methods can be employed to facilitate this process and include – but are not limited to – qualitative interviews with key stakeholders, monitoring media reports, tracking budgets and financial flows, satellite imagery, and remote sensing. Tools that assess shifting norms, attitudes, levels of service delivery, and the presence of external partnerships in comparison sites are also important. Systems for monitoring context are best initiated prospectively, and should document the timing, nature, and scope of potential influences, in both intervention and control groups.

Economic evaluation

A final component to the evaluation of structural interventions is assessing economic returns on investment, which can be challenging for a number of reasons. First, valuing the inputs for complex, multi-component structural interventions is often more difficult than for more discrete interventions. Second and more importantly, structural interventions may generate a wide range of health and non-health benefits or outputs, which may extend well beyond the timeframe of the intervention, and may be poorly captured using conventional health economics methods such as cost-effectiveness analyses (Jamison *et al.* 2006).

Cost-effectiveness analyses (CEA) are used in health economics to compare 'usual practice' with an intervention under consideration. These outcomes use standard measures such as cases prevented, lives saved or life years saved, as well as composite measures such as disability adjusted life years (DALYs) or quality adjusted life years (QALYs). CEAs work best when one can specify a health intervention in some detail – such as the dose, frequency and duration of vitamin A, who will be delivering it, and the level at which it will be delivered – as all have associated costs. These costs must then be paired against measurable health endpoints, such as reductions in disease rates or mortality. CEA works less well for interventions that have a range of benefits that may be difficult to quantify in terms of health endpoints.

An alternative approach is cost–benefit analysis (CBA), which involves appraising a programme in terms of costs and benefits to society, with benefits measured in monetary units (Mishan 1971). This approach may be more appropriate for interventions with multiple effects and provides a basis for valuing non-health benefits as well as 'spill-overs' – where benefits extend beyond programme participants (Mooney 1994; Ryan 1995). This is particularly true in relation to changes in the social environment – including improvements in social and economic well-being – which are not captured as immediate health benefits but may nevertheless be important (McKinlay 1993).

Within the health economics literature there is growing interest in assessing the value of more diffuse outcomes, with the community rather than the individual as the unit of interest (Jan 1998; Shiell and Hawe 1996). One of the methodological tools used is a *willingness-to-pay (WTP) assessment* (Mishan 1971), which is based on the assumption that a consumer is the best judge of the value of the goods and services they consume. There are some concerns about using WTP in the health sector, particularly because willingness-to-pay tends to be directly related to ability to pay and thus this approach gives lower values to goods and services consumed by people of lower income. Although there are examples in the literature where a WTP approach has been successfully applied in low-income settings (Bhatia and Fox-Rushby 2002; Onwujekwe *et al.* 1998, 2000), its validity among very poor communities, particularly those which rely heavily on bartering or subsistence farming, has yet to be firmly established. Further methodological innovation in valuing the costs and returns of structural interventions remains a major priority.

Conclusions

While there are a number of challenges to evaluating structural interventions, high-quality evaluation is vital. Too often, structural interventions have been under-developed and under-researched as their rigorous evaluation seems beyond the scope of established tools and methods. While discrete technical interventions may seem more easily engaged scientifically, addressing complex public health challenges will likely require broader approaches that extend the useful limits of conventional evaluation models.

This chapter has presented a range of complementary methods to assist the design of evaluations for structural interventions in public health. We have described approaches to impact assessment, implementation research, and economic evaluation. Many challenges can be overcome through adequate planning, setting realistic evaluation objectives, optimizing evaluation design, defining clear impact pathways, using an appropriate mix of methods, careful monitoring of secular trends, and drawing upon perspectives and expertise from partners outside the health sector. Taken together, these approaches may foster new insights and a deeper understanding the role of structural drivers in shaping health outcomes.

1 Multi-Country Evaluation of Integrated Management of Childhood Illness (MCE-IMCI)

Intervention overview

In the mid-1990s, the World Health Organization (WHO) and the United Nations Children's Fund (UNICEF) launched the IMCI strategy to improve health and development of under-five-year-old children by targeting diarrhoeal disease, pneumonia, malaria, and malnutrition, which together accounted for approximately 70 per cent of global under-five deaths. The IMCI strategy includes a combination of structural interventions addressing improvements in case management, health systems, and family and community practices (Arifeen *et al.* 2009; Bryce *et al.* 2004).

Evaluation design

Impact assessment: While the individual IMCI interventions had proven efficacy in controlled settings, there was a need to evaluate programme effectiveness in 'real-world' settings. The multi-country evaluation (MCE) ran for seven years and included feasibility studies in 12 countries and in-depth evaluations in five countries. The impact assessment combined adequacy and plausibility evaluations using non-randomized comparison groups in Tanzania, Peru, Brazil, and Uganda, and a probability evaluation using a cluster-randomized design in Bangladesh (Bryce *et al.* 2004). The intervention operated in a programme-rich environment, with many IMCI components already being scaled nation-wide, making overall interpretation of the results difficult.

Implementation research: Demonstrating the adequacy of the provision, utilization, and coverage indicators was deemed essential for interpreting impact results. The evaluators conducted detailed impact pathway mapping, employing a range of implementation research tools. Although no effect on mortality was seen within the timeframe of the Bangladesh study, positive changes were seen in all input, output, and outcome indicators (Arifeen *et al.* 2009). Conversely, in Peru, no associations between IMCI and outpatient utilization, vaccine coverage, mortality, or malnutrition were demonstrated and implementation research showed inadequate health systems support for IMCI and low uptake of IMCI training by health workers (Huicho *et al.* 2005).

Economic costing: All five in-depth evaluations also included cost-effectiveness studies (Bishai *et al.* 2008; Armstrong Schellenberg *et al.* 2004). For a more detailed discussion on the methodological lessons learned through design and implementation of the evaluation, see Bryce *et al.* 2004, and Bryce and Victora 2005.

2 Avahan – the India AIDS Initiative

Intervention overview

Avahan, the India AIDS Initiative, is a ten-year intervention that commenced in 2003 with the goal of preventing the expansion of the HIV epidemic in India. The intervention operated in the six states with the majority of HIV cases and focused on high-risk groups such as female sex workers and their clients, men who have sex with men, and injecting drug users (Bill and Melinda Gates Foundation). The initiative addressed downstream risk factors such as sexually transmitted infections (STIs) and condom use, while simultaneously addressing more upstream risk factors including stigma, violence, legal, environmental, and health infrastructure factors. The initiative was a complex, multi-layered structural intervention that was adapted to suit local needs, involving peer-support activities alongside work with the police, journalists, and government officials.

Evaluation design

Impact assessment: To monitor intervention effects on violence (Beattie *et al.* 2010), condom use (Lowndes *et al.* 2010; Ramesh *et al.* 2010), and HIV and STI prevalence

(Ramesh *et al.* 2010), evaluators employed primarily an adequacy assessment – conducting cross-sectional surveys among female sex workers (a pre–post design using historical controls). In addition, several strategies were used to enhance plausibility:

- Using temporal data linking observed changes to the timing of programme activities (Lowndes *et al.* 2010)
- Associating the duration of exposure to shifts in key outcomes (Ramesh *et al.* 2010)
- Documenting the adequacy (whether goals were achieved) of each step along the impact pathway (Chandrasekaran *et al.* 2008).

Because Avahan focused on high-risk individuals in high-prevalence districts, and because of the potential for diffusion and overlap with existing interventions, it was deemed impractical or unethical to employ randomization or matched comparison groups (Chandrasekaran *et al.* 2008). Rapid scale-up was considered essential to containing the spread of the epidemic, so a stepped-wedge design was also not possible.

Implementation research: The evaluation framework addressed each step along the impact pathway. Routine programme monitoring indicators were collected to assess provision, utilization, coverage, and quality of services before considering questions of impact. Daily tracking of news articles was used to assess levels of stigma and effects of the community component of the intervention. The use of data-driven management tools to modify and improve the programme is considered one of the reasons why successful rapid scale-up has been achievable (Bertozzi *et al.* 2010).

3 The Millennium Villages Project

Intervention overview

The Millennium Villages (MV) project is a ten-year initiative that delivers a package of scientifically proven interventions with the central aim of achieving the Millennium Development Goals (MDGs) across diverse sub-Saharan African field sites (Sanchez *et al.* 2007; Earth Institute and Millennium Promise 2010). The project operates in rural areas of the continent where MDG-related progress has been insufficient. Activities are coordinated across multiple sectors (including health, agriculture, environment, business development, education, and infrastructure) and adapted to local needs, systems challenges, and disease profiles. Inputs are cost-limited, with a modest annual ceiling of US $120 per capita across all sectors sustained over a ten-year period.

Evaluation design

Impact assessment: To maximize external validity, rural clusters of approximately 40,000 people with high rates of poverty and undernutrition were purposively selected from ten countries to represent over 90 per cent of the agro-ecological zones in sub-Saharan Africa. Assessment rounds are conducted at two-year intervals to measure the adequacy of the intervention in relation to effects on MDG-related outcomes. To account for secular change and enhance the plausibility that observed changes were the result of intervention exposure, a controlled design with comparison clusters selected at random from among matched candidates was chosen. Finally, national and sub-national MDG outcomes provide an additional reference group. Initial results highlight positive synergies on critical health- and nutrition-related outcomes (Remans *et al.* 2011).

Implementation research: Performance metrics across all sectors are collected on a monthly to quarterly basis using health facility and school registers, infrastructure mapping, and other available sources of information. Qualitative research includes focus groups and key informant interviews with intervention recipients, programme managers, and key partners on the ground. Detailed intervention timelines are constructed for activities across all sectors. Context mapping takes place in parallel to survey rounds using purpose-built inventories of community-level characteristics such as shocks, changes in service delivery, policy changes, and so forth.

Economic costing: An economic assessment examines year-on-year MDG-related spending by sector and by stakeholder. These data will be used to estimate returns on investment and cost-effectiveness in relation to impacts observed.

4 The Intervention with Microfinance for AIDS and Gender Equity (IMAGE Study)

Intervention overview

IMAGE was a structural intervention for the prevention of HIV and intimate partner violence (IPV). The initiative brought together two components: a poverty-focused microfinance programme and a gender and HIV training curriculum. A major focus of the training programme was community mobilization and collective action, which was by nature fluid and adapted to local needs and priorities (Pronyk *et al.* 2006; Pronyk *et al.* 2008b).

Evaluation design

Impact assessment: A cluster-randomized trial was undertaken using a matched-pair design to examine village-level effects. As the total number of clusters was low (n=8), the evaluators considered this a plausibility assessment. Detailed impact pathways examined effects on a range of pathway variables, including dimensions such as economic well-being, empowerment, and social capital, where the size and consistency of changes were profiled in the reporting of results (Kim *et al.* 2007; Pronyk *et al.* 2008a). In an attempt to assess the relative effects of the two intervention components, a separate sub-study was conducted among women who received microfinance alone (Kim *et al.* 2009).

Implementation research: Routine records of microfinance loan performance and attendance at training sessions examined feasibility and exposure to the intervention. Gender trainers employed diaries and 'key events timelines' to document the narratives of individual loan centres and systematically document community mobilization efforts. Qualitative interviews with programme managers, participants, local partners, and policymakers examined barriers and facilitators to implementation, as well as opportunities for replication and scale-up (Hargreaves *et al.* 2010).

Economic costing: A full cost-effectiveness study was done to examine the costs relative to intervention effects on DALY saved from observed reductions in levels of IPV (Jan et al. 2010).

References

Arifeen, S.E., Hoque, D.M.E., Akter, T., Rahman, M., Hoque, M.E., Begum, K., Chowdhury, E.K., Khan, R., Blum, L.S., Ahmed, S., Hossain, M.A., Siddik, A., Begum, N., Rahman, Q.S.U., Haque, T.M., Billah, S.M., Islam, M., Rumi, R.A., Law, E., Al-Helal, Z.A.M., Baqui, A.H., Schellenberg, J., Adam, T., Moulton, L.H., Habicht, J.P., Scherpbier, R.W., Victora, C.G., Bryce, J., and Black, R.E. (2009) 'Effect of the Integrated Management of Childhood Illness strategy on childhood mortality and nutrition in a rural area in Bangladesh: a cluster randomised trial', *The Lancet*, 374: 393–403.

Armstrong Schellenberg, J.R.M., Adam, T., Mshinda, H., Masanja, H., Kabadi, G., Mukasa, O., John, T.J., Charles, S., Nathan, R., Wilczynska, K., Mgalula, L., Mbuya, C., Mswia, R., Manzi, F., De Savigny, D., Schellenberg, D., and Victora, C.G. (2004) 'Effectiveness and cost of facility-based Integrated Management of Childhood Illness (IMCI) in Tanzania', *The Lancet*, 364: 1583–94.

Bailey, I.W. and Archer, L. (2004) 'The impact of the introduction of treated water on aspects of community health in a rural community in Kwazulu-Natal, South Africa', *Water Science and Technology*, 50: 105–10.

Bamberger, M., Rao, V., and Woolcock, M. (2010) *Using Mixed Methods in Monitoring and Evaluation: Experiences from International Development*, Policy Research Working Paper No 5245, Washington, D.C.: The World Bank.

Beattie, T.S., Bhattacharjee, P., Ramesh, B.M., Gurnani, V., Anthony, J., Isac, S., Mohan, H.L., Ramakrishnan, A., Wheeler, T., Bradley, J., Blanchard, J.F., and Moses, S. (2010) 'Violence against female sex workers in Karnataka state, south India: impact on health, and reductions in violence following an intervention program', *BMC Public Health*, 10: 476.

Bertozzi, S.M., Padian, N., and Martz, T.E. (2010) 'Evaluation of HIV prevention programmes: the case of Avahan', *Sexually Transmitted Infections*, 86: I4–5.

Bhatia, M. and Fox-Rushby, J. (2002) 'Willingness to pay for treated mosquito nets in Surat, India: the design and descriptive analysis of a household survey', *Health Policy and Planning*, 17: 402–11.

Bill and Melinda Gates Foundation (2008) 'Avahan – the India AIDS initiative: the business of HIV prevention at scale', New Delhi: Bill and Melinda Gates Foundation.

Bishai, D., Mirchandani, G., Pariyo, G., Burnham, G., and Black, R. (2008) 'The cost of quality improvements due to integrated management of childhood illness (IMCI) in Uganda', *Health Economics*, 17: 5–19.

Blankenship, K.M., Bray, S.J., and Merson, M.H. (2000) 'Structural interventions in public health', *AIDS*, 14: S11–21.

Bloom, H. (2009) *Modern Regression Discontinuity Analysis*. MDRC Working Papers on Research Methodology, New York: MDRC.

Bonell, C., Hargreaves, J., Strange, V., Pronyk, P., and Porter, J. (2006a) 'Should structural interventions be evaluated using RCTs? The case of HIV prevention', *Social Science & Medicine*, 63: 1135–42.

Bonell, C., Oakley, A., Hargreaves, J., Strange, V., and Rees, R. (2006b) 'Assessment of generalisability in trials of health interventions: suggested framework and systematic review', *British Medical Journal*, 333: 346–9.

Brown, C.A. and Liliford, R.J. (2006) 'The stepped wedge trial design: a systematic review', *BMC Medical Research Methodology*, 6: 54.

Bryce, J., Victora, C.G., Habicht, J.P., Vaughan, J.P., and Black, R.E. (2004) 'The multi-country evaluation of the integrated management of childhood illness strategy: lessons for the evaluation of public health interventions', *American Journal of Public Health*, 94: 406–15.

Bryce, J. and Victora, C.G. (2005) 'Ten methodological lessons from the multi-country evaluation of integrated management of childhood illness', *Health Policy and Planning*, 20 (Supplement 1): i94–105.

Campbell, M., Fitzpatrick, R., Haines, A., Kinmonth, A.L., Sandercock, P., Spiegelhalter, D., and Tyrer, P. (2000) 'Framework for design and evaluation of complex interventions to improve health', *British Medical Journal*, 321: 694–6.

Chandrasekaran, P., Dallabetta, G., Loo, V., Mills, S., Saidel, T., Adhikary, R., Alary, M., Lowndes, C.M., Boily, M.C., Moore, J., and Avahan Evaluation Partners (2008) 'Evaluation design for large-scale HIV prevention programmes: the case of Avahan, the India AIDS initiative', *AIDS*, 22: S1–15.

Earth Institute and Millennium Promise (2010) *Harvests of Development in Rural Africa: The Millennium Villages after Three Years*, New York: Earth Institute, Columbia University.

Greenland, S. (2000) 'An introduction to instrumental variables for epidemiologists', *International Journal of Epidemiology*, 29: 722–9.

Grijalva, C.G., Nuorti, J.P., Arbogast, P.G., Martin, S.W., Edwards, K.M., and Griffin, M.R. (2007) 'Decline in pneumonia admissions after routine childhood immunisation with pneumococcal conjugate vaccine in the USA: a time-series analysis', *The Lancet*, 369: 1179–86.

Guba, E.G. and Lincoln, Y.S. (1989) *Fourth Generation Evaluation*, Newbury Park, CA: Sage.

Habicht, J., Victora, C., and Vaughan, J. (1999) 'Evaluation designs for adequacy, plausibility and probability of public health programme performance and impact', *International Journal of Epidemiology*, 28: 10–18.

Hargreaves, J.R., Hatcher, A., Strange, V., Phetla, G., Busza, J., Kim, J.C., Watts, C., Morison, L.A., Porter, J.D.H., Pronyk, P.M., and Bonnel, C. (2010) 'Process evaluation of the Intervention with Microfinance for AIDS and Gender Equity (IMAGE) in rural South Africa', *Health Education Research*, 25: 27–40.

Hawe, P., Shiell, A., and Riley, T. (2004) 'Complex interventions: how "out of control" can a randomised controlled trial be', *British Medical Journal*, 328: 1561–3.

Hayes, R.D., Alexander, N.D.E., Bennett, S., and Cousens, S.N. (2000) 'Design and analysis issues in cluster-randomized trials of interventions against infectious diseases', *Statistical Methods in Medical Research*, 9: 95–116.

Hayes, R.J. and Bennett, S. (1999) 'Simple sample size calculation for cluster randomised trials', *International Journal of Epidemiology*, 28: 319–26.

Huicho, L., Davila, M., Gonzales, F., Drasbek, C., Bryce, J., and Victora, C.G. (2005) 'Implementation of the integrated management of childhood illness strategy in Peru and its association with health indicators: an ecological analysis', *Health Policy and Planning*, 20 Suppl. 1: i32–41.

International Food Policy Research Institute (IFPRI) (2002) *PROGRESA: Breaking the Cycle of Poverty*, Washington, D.C.: International Food Policy Research Institute.

Imbens, G. and Lemieux, T. (2008) 'Regression discontinuity designs: a guide to practice', *Journal of Econometrics*, 142: 615–35.

Jamison, D.T., Breman, J.G., Measham, A.R., Alleyne, G., Claeson, M., Evans, D.B., Jha, P., Mills, A., and Musgrove, P. (2006) *Priorities in Health: Disease Control Priorities Project*, Washington, D.C.: World Bank.

Jan, S. (1998) 'A holistic approach to the economic evaluation of health programs using institutionalist methodology', *Social Science & Medicine*, 47: 1565–72.

Jan, S., Ferrari, G., Watts, C.H., Hargreaves, J.R., Kim, J.C., Morison, L.A., Phetla, G., Porter, J.D.H., and Pronyk, P.M. (2010) 'Economic evaluation of a combined microfinance and gender training intervention for the prevention of intimate partner violence in rural South Africa', *Health Policy and Planning*, 26 (5): 366–72.

Kim, J.C., Watts, C.H., Hargreaves, J.R., Morison, L.A., Porter, J.D.H., Phetla, G., Buzsa, J., Ndhlovu, L., and Pronyk, P.M. (2007) 'Understanding the impact of a microfinance-based intervention on women's empowerment and the reduction of intimate partner violence in the IMAGE Study, South Africa', *American Journal of Public Health*, 97: 1794–802.

Kim, J.C., Ferrari, G., Abramsky, T., Watts, C.H., Hargreaves, J.R., Morison, L.A., Phetla, G., Porter, J.D.H., and Pronyk, P.M. (2009) 'Assessing the incremental benefits of combining health and economic interventions: experience from the IMAGE Study in rural South Africa', *Bulletin of the World Health Organization*, 87: 824–32.

Koepsell, T.D., Wagner, E.H., Cheadle, A.C., Patrick, D.L., Martin, D.C., Diehr, P.H., Perrin, E.B., Kristal, A.R., Allan-Andrilla, C.H., and Dey, L.J. (1992) 'Selected methodological issues in evaluating community-based health promotion and disease prevention programs', *Annual Review of Public Health*, 13: 31–57.

Leeuw, F. and Vaessen, J. (2009) *Impact Evaluations and Development: NONIE Guidance in Impact Evaluation*, Washington, D.C.: Network of Networks for Impact Evaluation.

Lewin, S., Glenton, C., and Oxman, A.D. (2009) 'Use of qualitative methods alongside randomised controlled trials of complex healthcare interventions: methodological study', *British Medical Journal*, 339: b3496.

Lowndes, C.M., Alary, M., Verma, S., Demers, E., Bradley, J., Jayachandran, A.A., Ramesh, B.M., Moses, S., Adhikary, R., and Mainkar, M.K. (2010) 'Assessment of intervention outcome in the absence of baseline data: "reconstruction" of condom use time trends using retrospective analysis of survey data', *Sexually Transmitted Infections*, 86: 149–55.

Masanja, H., De Savigny, P., Schellenberg, J., John, T., Mbuya, C., Upunda, G., Boerma, T., Victora, C.G., Smith, T., and Mshinda, H. (2008) 'Child survival gains in Tanzania: analysis of data from demographic and health surveys', *The Lancet*, 371: 1276–83.

McKee, M., Britton, A., Black, N., McPherson, K., Sanderson, C., and Bain, C. (1999) 'Interpreting the evidence: choosing between randomised and non-randomised studies', *British Medical Journal*, 319: 312–15.

McKinlay, J.B. (1993) 'The promotion of health through planned sociopolitical chance', *Social Science & Medicine*, 36: 109–17.

Mensah, J., Oppong, J.R., and Schmidt, C.M. (2010) 'Ghana's national health insurance scheme in the context of the health MDGs: an empirical evaluation using propensity score matching', *Health Economics*, 19: 95–106.

Mishan, E.J. (1971) 'Evaluation of life and limb: a theoretical approach', *Journal of Political Economy*, 79: 687–706.

Mooney, G. (1994) 'What else do we want from our health services?', *Social Science & Medicine*, 39: 151–4.

Oakley, A., Strange, V., Stephenson, J. M., Forrest, S., and Monteiro, H. (2004) 'Evaluating processes: an example from a randomised controlled trial of sex education: rationale and methods', *Evaluation*, 10 (4): 440–62.

Oakley, A., Strange, V., Bonell, C., Allen, E., and Stephenson, J. (2006) 'Process evaluation in randomised controlled trials of complex interventions', *British Medical Journal*, 332: 413–16.

Onwujekwe, O.E., Shu, E.N., Nwagbo, D., Akpala, C.O., and Okonkwo, P.O. (1998) 'Willingness to pay for community-based ivermectin distribution: a study of three onchocerciasis-endemic communities in Nigeria', *Tropical Medicine and International Health*, 3: 802–8.

Onwujekwe, O.E., Shu, E., Chima, R., Onyido, A., and Okonkwo, P.O. (2000) 'Willingness to pay for the retreatment of mosquito nets with insecticide in four communities of south-eastern Nigeria', *Tropical Medicine and International Health*, 5: 370–6.

Plummer, M.L., Wight, D., Obasi, A.I.N., Wamoyi, J., Mshana, G., Todd, J., Mazige, B.C., Makokha, A., Hayes, R.J., and Ross, D.A. (2007a) 'A process evaluation of a school-based adolescent sexual health intervention in rural Tanzania: the MEMA kwa vijana programme', *Health Education Research*, 22: 500–12.

Plummer, M.L., Wight, D., Wamoyi, J., Nyalali, K., Ingal, T., Mshana, G., Shigong, Z.S., Obasi, A.I.N., and Ross, D.A. (2007b) 'Are schools a good setting for adolescent sexual health promotion in rural Africa? A qualitative assessment from Tanzania', *Health Education Research*, 22: 483–99.

Pronyk, P.M., Hargreaves, J.R., Kim, J.C., Morison, L.A., Phetla, G., Watts, C., Busza, J.A., and Porter, J.D.H. (2006) 'Effect of a structural intervention for the prevention of intimate partner violence and HIV in rural South Africa: a cluster randomized trial', *The Lancet*, 368: 1973–83.

Pronyk, P.M., Harpham, T., Busza, J., Phetla, G., Morison, L.A., Hargreaves, J.R., Kim, J.C., Watts, C.H., and Porter, J.D.H. (2008a) 'Can social capital be intentionally generated? A randomized trial from rural South Africa', *Social Science & Medicine*, 67 (10): 1559–70.

Pronyk, P.M., Kim, J.C., Abramsky, T., Phetla, G., Hargreaves, J.R., Morison, L.A., Watts, C.H., Busza, J., and Porter, J.D.H. (2008b) 'A combined microfinance and training intervention can reduce HIV risk behaviour among young female participants', *AIDS*, 22: 1659–65.

Ramesh, B.M., Beattie, T.S., Shajy, I., Washington, R., Jagannathan, L., Reza-Paul, S., Blanchard, J.F., and Moses, S. (2010) 'Changes in risk behaviours and prevalence of sexually transmitted infections following HIV preventive interventions among female sex workers in five districts in Karnataka state, south India', *Sexually Transmited Infections*, 86 Suppl. 1: i17–24.

Remans, R., Pronyk, P.M., Fanzo, J., Chen, J., Palm, C.A., Nemser, B., Muniz, M., Radunsky, A., Abay, A.H., Coulibaly, M., Mensah-Homiah, J., Wagah, M., An, X., Mwaura, C., Quintana, E., Somers, M., Sanchez, P.A., McArthur, J.W., Sachs, S.E., and Sachs, J.D. (2011) 'A multi-sector intervention to accelerate reductions in child stunting: an observational study from nine sub-Saharan African countries', *American Journal of Clinical Nutrition*, 94 (6): 1632–42.

Rose, G. (1985) 'Sick individuals and sick populations', *International Journal of Epidemiology*, 14: 32–8.

Ross, D.A., Changalucha, J., Obasi, A.I.N., Todd, J., Plummer, M.L., Cleophas-Mazige, B., Anemona, A., Everett, D., Weiss, H.A., Mabey, D.C., Grosskurth, H., Hayes, R.J., Balira, R., Wight, D., Gavyole, A., Makokha, M.J., Mosha, F., Terris-Prestholt, F., and Parry, J.V. (2007) 'Biological and behavioural impact of an adolescent sexual health intervention in Tanzania: a community-randomized trial', *AIDS*, 21: 1943–55.

Ryan, M. (1995) *Economics and the Patient's Utility Function: An Application to Assisted Reproductive Techniques*, Ph.D. thesis, University of Aberdeen.

Rychetnik, L., Frommer, M., Hawe, P., and Shiell, A. (2002) 'Criteria for evaluating evidence on public health interventions', *Journal of Epidemiology and Community Health*, 56: 119–27.

Sanchez, P., Palm, C., Sachs, J., Denning, G., Flor, R., Harawa, R., Jama, B., Kiflemariam, T., Konecky, B., Kozar, R., Lelerai, E., Malik, A., Modi, V., Mutuo, P., Niang, A., Okoth, H., Place, F., Sachs, S.E., Said, A., Siriri, D., Teklehaimanot, A., Wang, K., Wangila, J., and Zamba, C. (2007) 'The African Millennium Villages', *Proceedings of the National Academy of Sciences*, 104: 16775–80.

Savedoff, W., Levine, R., and Birdsall, N. (2006) *When Will We Ever Learn? Improving Lives through Impact Evaluation*. Report of the Evaluation Gap Working Group. Washington, D.C.: Center for Global Development.

Shadish, W.R., Cook, T.D., and Campbell, D.T. (2002) *Experimental and Quasi-experimental Designs for Generalized Causal Inference*, Boston: Houghton Mifflin.

Shepperd, S., Lewin, S., Straus, S., Clarke, M., Eccles, M.P., Fitzpatrick, R., Wong, G., and Sheikh, A. (2009) 'Can we systematically review studies that evaluate complex interventions?', *Public Library of Science Medicine*, 6 (8): e1000086.

Shiell, A. and Hawe, P. (1996) 'Health promotion, community development and the tyranny of individualism', *Health Economics*, 5: 241–7.

Shiell, A., Hawe, P., and Gold, L. (2008) 'Complex interventions or complex systems? Implications for health economic evaluation', *British Medical Journal*, 336: 1281–3.

Somerville, M., Basham, M., Foy, C., Ballinger, G., Gay, T., Shute, P., and Barton, A.G. (2002) 'From local concern to randomised trial: the Watcombe Housing Project', *Health Expectations*, 5: 127–35.

Susser, M. (1995) 'The tribulations of trials – intervention in communities', *American Journal of Public Health*, 85: 156–9.

United Kingdon Medical Research Council (2006) *Developing and Evaluating Complex Interventions: New Guidance*, London: United Kingdom Medical Research Council.

Usdin, S., Scheepers, E., Goldstein, S., and Japhet, G. (2005) 'Achieving social change on gender-based violence: a report on the impact evaluation of Soul City's fourth series', *Social Science & Medicine*, 61: 2434–45.

Victora, C.G., Habicht, J.P., and Vaughan, J.P. (1999) 'Evaluation designs for adequacy, plausibility and probability of public health programme performance and impact', *International Journal of Epidemiology*, 28: 10–18.

Victora, C.G., Habicht, J.P., and Bryce, J. (2004) 'Evidence-based public health: moving beyond randomized trials', *American Journal of Public Health*, 94: 400–5.

Victora, C.G., Black, R.E., Boerma, J.T., and Bryce, J. (2010) 'Measuring impact in the millennium development goal era and beyond: a new approach to large-scale effectiveness evaluations', *The Lancet*, 377 (9759): 85–95.

World Health Organization (WHO) (2009) *Systems Thinking for Health Systems Strengthening*, Geneva: Alliance for Health Policy and Systems Research, World Health Organization.

Wight, D. and Obasi, A. (2003) 'Unpacking the "black box": the importance of process data to explain outcomes', in J. Stephenson, J. Imrie, and C. Bonell (eds) *Effective Sexual Health Interventions: Issues in Experimental Evaluation*, Oxford: Oxford University Press.

15

DEVELOPING AND EVALUATING STRUCTURAL-ENVIRONMENTAL INTERVENTIONS TO REDUCE HIV RISK AMONG FEMALE SEX WORKERS AND THEIR SEXUAL PARTNERS IN THE DOMINICAN REPUBLIC

Deanna Kerrigan, Clare Barrington, and Luis Moreno

Introduction

The purpose of this chapter is to outline the collaborative process of developing and evaluating structural-environmental interventions to reduce the risk of HIV acquisition among female sex workers (FSWs) and their sexual partners in the Dominican Republic (DR). We will first describe the formative, qualitative research methods utilized to define feasible and culturally appropriate intervention models. The models included a community solidarity or 'collective commitment' intervention component, as well as governmental policy to promote and enable HIV prevention among establishment-based FSWs. We will then discuss the research design and methods utilized to evaluate the intervention models, including the development of methods and indicators to assess the influence of individual and structural-environmental factors and the use of methodological triangulation, including self-reported and observed data, to provide a more robust understanding of intervention processes and outcomes. We will present key findings and lessons learned from both the process and impact evaluations and consider their implications for future structural-environmental HIV prevention interventions and evaluations.

Intervention and measure development

Intervention development

Following the results of Thailand's 100% Condom Use Programme in the early 1990s, including significant increases in consistent condom use and reductions in sexually transmitted infections (STIs) among establishment-based FSWs (Rojanapithayakorn and Hanenberg 1996) (see Chapter 9, Rojanapithayakorn and Steen, in this volume), the Dominican non-governmental organization (NGO) Centro de Orientación e Investigación Integral (COIN) became interested in adapting this programme model to the female sex work industry in the DR (Kerrigan *et al.* 2001). Since 1989, COIN had trained a cadre of FSW peer educators who conduct outreach to provide health education and social support around a holistic set of topics, including self-esteem, gender and sexuality, occupational rights, HIV prevention, and reproductive health. COIN also supported the development of Movimiento de Mujeres Unidas (MODEMU), a union of FSWs that works to protect and promote sex workers' legal rights, health, and economic development through individual and political advocacy efforts (Moreno and Kerrigan 2000). Results of behavioural surveys conducted since the late 1980s to evaluate COIN's FSW peer education efforts indicated significant gains, particularly in terms of reported consistent condom use with new clients, which reached over 90 per cent by the mid-1990s (Kerrigan *et al.* 2003). However, reported consistent condom use by FSWs with their regular paying and non-paying partners remained significantly lower than rates with new clients, suggesting ongoing risk for HIV acquisition (Murray *et al.* 2007).

The Thai model was one of the earliest examples of a structural approach to HIV prevention in the context of sex work. This governmental initiative included policies and regulations to promote access to condoms, condom use in all brothel-based sexual activity, and sex worker attendance at regular STI screenings. Rather than holding sex workers responsible to comply with these policies, an innovative aspect of this model was that sex establishment owners/managers were held accountable for creating an environment where these policies could be upheld, and local authorities could impose sanctions on establishments for non-compliance (Rojanapithayakorn and Hanenberg 1996). It is important to note that despite the success of the Thai 100% Condom Use Programme, many sex worker advocates have remained concerned about its top-down strategy and have argued that empowerment and rights-based approaches are critical to a sustainable response to HIV prevention among sex workers (Kendall and Razali 2010).

As noted above, peer-led, community-driven approaches to HIV prevention among FSWs had been used in the DR and in turn, it was critical that any new intervention models built upon this pre-existing grassroots base. An additional structural intervention model studied during this formative period was the Sonagachi community mobilization model in Kolkata, India, which was highly successful in increasing condom use and reducing STIs (Jana and Singh 1995) (see Chapter 10, Swendeman and Jana, in this volume). Sonagachi's bottom-up approach to preventing HIV among sex workers was squarely in line with the types of HIV prevention interventions conducted and valued in the DR. Ultimately, the formative research phase of the project inquired into the strengths and applicability of using both community mobilization and governmental approaches to HIV prevention among sex workers in the DR, and examined how specific elements of these differing paradigms might be adapted and integrated in a feasible, effective, and culturally appropriate manner.

From 1996 to 1998, formative research using both qualitative and quantitative methods was conducted by an interdisciplinary team composed of investigators and key stakeholders from COIN and the Johns Hopkins Bloomberg School of Public Health (Kerrigan *et al.* 1997, 2001, 2003). During the initial phase from June to September 1996, a purposive sample of 62 participants was recruited from five sex work establishments in Santo Domingo, including 25 FSWs, 22 male paying clients, eight male non-paying steady partners and seven establishment owners/managers. In addition, key informant interviews were conducted with individuals from 14 government and non-governmental agencies. A socio-demographic survey and in-depth interviews were administered to all study participants recruited at sex establishments. Each participant was interviewed approximately three times to facilitate an iterative analysis process and obtain greater depth of data. The use of multiple interviews with participants was crucial, as it allowed participants to reflect on previous discussions and topics and share those reflections in subsequent interviews. The interviews examined ongoing, organic means of building social solidarity and establishing and enforcing internal policies and regulations within the sex establishments to prevent HIV among sex workers and their partners. A hypothetical 100% condom use programme was also described to participants as a law or policy that would be enforced by the Ministry of Health, whereby sex establishment owners and managers would be responsible for ensuring that condoms were used in all sexual activity between sex workers and their clients. Participants were asked to comment on the advantages, disadvantages and potential barriers to implementing such a programme in the Dominican Republic (Kerrigan et al. 2001).

Among participants, there was general consensus that a 100% condom use programme would be appropriate in the DR context and most believed that the norms and policies of such a programme would be health promoting rather than repressive. Sex workers found the hypothetical programme helpful because it would help to protect their health and the health of their children, and also because it would save time and energy spent on trying to convince clients to use condoms. Sex workers also mentioned improved solidarity and a sense of group protection as potential advantages of a 100% condom use programme. Owners and managers believed the policies would create the perception that their establishments were 'clean' and 'STD-free', which would improve prestige and profits. For the most part, clients were supportive of such policies as they worried about their health and the health of their families. Steady and non-paying partners supported the concept of the programme because they believed it would assist sex workers in using condoms more consistently with their paying clients (Kerrigan et al. 2001).

While there was overall support for the 100% condom use programme, some participants did raise concerns about the government's ability to implement and/or enforce such a programme, arguing that condom use cannot be controlled solely by policy or regulation, and must also be addressed by consciousness raising and what participants termed a *compromiso colectivo*, or collective commitment, to preventing HIV. Stakeholders also felt strongly that policy alone, without a community mobilization base, was not appropriate in the DR, given the importance placed on grassroots organizing and community-led interventions. Based on these findings and the historical commitment to community-led, participatory health promotion among NGOs and sex workers in the DR, the intervention models developed for this project included locally appropriate versions of condom promotion policies and mechanisms for enforcement. The models also incorporated continued community mobilization efforts to sustain a collective commitment to condom use and HIV prevention among sex workers, similar to the strategies utilized in the Sonagachi Project (Basu et al. 2004). The resulting intervention models were among the first attempts to integrate the strengths of two structural-environmental-level HIV prevention paradigms and strategies – government policy and community mobilization – to prevent HIV infection in the context of female sex work.

Model refinement and measure development

Building on findings from the first phase of the formative research, which indicated that implementing a structural-environmental intervention to reduce HIV risk among sex workers in the DR was feasible and acceptable, the second phase sought to identify specific intervention components that should be included in such a model by assessing the quantitative association between structural-environmental factors and consistent condom use in the context of female sex work. This second phase of formative research also served as an opportunity to develop new measures to use in the subsequent process and impact evaluations.

From March to June 1998, a cross-sectional survey was conducted in Santo Domingo with 288 establishment-based FSWs and 296 of their male, regular paying partners. Findings from formative research with FSWs showed lower reported levels of consistent condom use with regular paying partners, higher vulnerability to HIV with these partners, and the need for innovative HIV prevention strategies. Thus, this study focused on partner dynamics between FSWs and their regular paying partners. Participants were recruited from approximately 40 direct and indirect sex establishments in Santo Domingo, where clients are charged a fee to go out with FSWs employed there (Kerrigan et al. 2003; Murray et al. 2007).

The survey instrument was informed by findings from the previous formative research, review of the existing literature, and input from NGO staff and sex worker peer educators and included items on individual, relational, and structural-environmental factors. Multivariate analysis was conducted to determine which of these factors were significantly associated with consistent condom use between sex workers and their regular, paying partners. Structural-environmental variables were generated largely from the first phase of formative research conducted with sex workers and their clients. Nine individual items were included in the final aggregate measure of structural-environmental support for condom use and HIV prevention including those at physical, social and policy levels. This measure included both individual perceptions of the environment and observed establishment-level variables. Reported items included participan''s perceived levels of condom access and quality in the establishment; communication from establishment employees at the beginning of employment about the importance of condom use; notification from the owner of a clear policy that condoms are to be used during all sexual activity with clients; ongoing reminders from employees regarding condom use; encouragement from the owner to attend monthly STI check-ups required by the government; and establishment-based monitoring checks performed by government health inspectors regarding condom supplies and STI clinic attendance. In addition, study interviewers physically observed whether condoms were available at each establishment and whether the establishment had an updated government health certificate posted at the time of the survey (Kerrigan et al. 2003).

The main finding from the analysis of survey data was that multiple levels of factors are at play in the process of HIV-related sexual decision-making in the context of female sex work in the DR. In the case of FSWs, for example, significant associations between consistent condom use and individual, relational, and structural-environmental factors were documented. Consistent condom use with regular partners was significantly higher among sex workers who on average charged more than US $22 per date with clients (OR 1.99; CI 1.10–3.59); had a strong sense of self-efficacy in the context of commercial sex negotiations (OR 2.80; CI 1.31–5.97); perceived low levels of relationship intimacy with that partner (OR 7.20; CI 3.49–14.83); and worked in establishments with high levels of structural-environmental support for condom use and HIV/STI prevention (OR 2.16; CI 1.18–3.97). These findings confirmed the need to integrate factors at all three levels into the conceptual framework, intervention strategies, evaluation methods, and measures of a structural-environmental HIV prevention model to facilitate and reinforce protective behaviour and reduce HIV-related vulnerability (Kerrigan *et al.* 2003; Murray *et al.* 2007).

In summary, mixed-method formative research was critical for the effective cultural adaptation of existing structural models of HIV prevention in the context of female sex work to the local environment in the DR. The participatory approach used to obtain opinions and perspectives from multiple key stakeholders and potential target populations provided a comprehensive understanding of what a structural-environmental model should look like in the DR. Through this process, we also developed aggregate measures for capturing the multiple levels of influence on condom use that were critical for a comprehensive evaluation of the intervention.

Process and impact evaluation: design, methods, and key findings

Intervention implementation

A comparative pre–post study design was utilized to examine the relative effects of the two structural-environmental HIV prevention intervention models in the DR. Final intervention elements were determined based on findings from the formative qualitative and quantitative research described above, as well as extensive consultation with local NGO staff members, MODEMU members, and national, regional, and local Dominican governmental health officials. The models were implemented in two cities in the DR: Santo Domingo, the country's capital, and Puerto Plata, a tourist town in the north-eastern region of the country, as indicated in Figure 15.1.

In each city, 34 sex establishments located in areas with a high number of entertainment venues were chosen to participate. Both cities implemented community-based solidarity promotion and mobilization activities related to HIV prevention, while Puerto Plata additionally enacted government policies and regulations. As discussed earlier, key stakeholders felt strongly that testing the effects of a policy component alone, without a community empowerment and mobilization base, was not appropriate in the DR. Additionally, given the population-level impact of policy interventions, it was impossible to randomize participants or communities into intervention and control conditions (Issel 2009). Both cities selected for study participation had NGOs with a long history of facilitating peer-led FSW interventions. Puerto Plata was purposively selected to receive the additional policy intervention component, as the former director of a local NGO, Centro de Promoción y Solidaridad Humana (CEPROSH), was then the provincial health director and able to facilitate the creation of an enabling policy environment for HIV prevention in the context of female sex work (Kerrigan *et al.* 2004, 2006).

During the intervention period, participating sex establishments from both cities received workshops to foster solidarity and collective commitment, as well as monthly follow-up visits to reinforce these principles. These workshops were conducted with

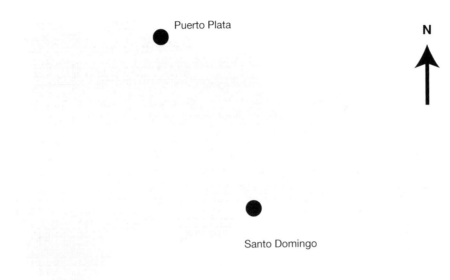

Figure 15.1 Map of and location of study sites within the Dominican Republic

Source: Adapted with permission from Kerrigan *et al.* (2004: 1) 'Horizons research summary'

both FSWs and establishment owner/managers and other employees. Workshops with sex workers also explored the dynamics of regular, paying and non-paying partners and the influence of trust and intimacy on condom use given formative research findings on the importance of these issues. Environmental cues were implemented in the sex work establishment, such as condom promotion posters, visibly displayed condoms, deejay messages, and HIV prevention information booths for clients at the entrance of sex establishments. Clinical services were improved in each city to make them more accessible and sex worker-friendly. Sensitization training was provided to clinicians and health inspectors involved in clinical care and STI screening and management. Sex worker peer educators were placed inside government clinics to counsel their peers – the first time peer education was allowed within Dominican government clinics. Monitoring and support for intervention adherence also occurred across both sites. However, in Puerto Plata, all participating sex establishment owners were informed that a regional policy requiring condom use between sex workers and their clients had been established and would be monitored by government health inspectors and NGO workers (Kerrigan *et al.* 2004, 2006).

Process evaluation

To examine intervention implementation, including exposure and adherence to the intervention, process indicators were measured at both the individual and environmental levels. Using the measures developed from formative research, the level of structural-environmental support for HIV prevention in each city was assessed through the pre- and post-test cross-sectional surveys and utilized as a marker of individual-level exposure to the intervention. Additionally, local government health inspectors and NGO workers jointly collected observational data from participating sex establishments on a monthly basis for the following five environmental benchmarks: (1) presence of condom promotion posters; (2) visibly placed condoms; (3) stocks of at least 100 condoms; (4) sex worker attendance at monthly STI checks; and (5) number of STI diagnoses among sex workers. NGO workers collaborated with government health inspectors to provide monthly feedback to owners and managers regarding the establishment's degree of adherence to these key elements of intervention implementation. In the case of Puerto Plata, where the policy and regulatory component of the intervention was implemented, establishments that did not adhere to the intervention were exposed to a gradual sanction system, including notifications, fines, and temporary closing. Figure 15.2 presents changes in compliance with the intervention across the two cities during the one-year study period. While individual-level exposure to the intervention increased significantly in both cities, adherence to the five environmental intervention elements described above increased significantly only in Puerto Plata.

Impact evaluation

To evaluate the impact of the two structural-environmental intervention models, pre- and post-test socio-behavioural surveys were conducted with cross-sections of approximately 200 FSWs from participating sex establishments in each of the two cities. Primary

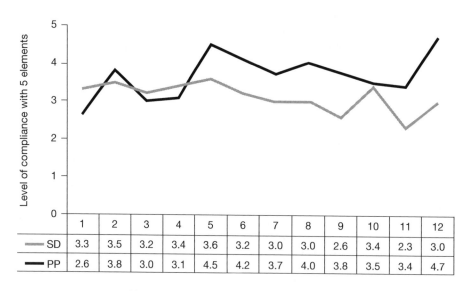

	1	2	3	4	5	6	7	8	9	10	11	12
SD	3.3	3.5	3.2	3.4	3.6	3.2	3.0	3.0	2.6	3.4	2.3	3.0
PP	2.6	3.8	3.0	3.1	4.5	4.2	3.7	4.0	3.8	3.5	3.4	4.7

Months (0–12) during intervention evaluation period

Figure 15.2 Compliance with structural-environmental HIV prevention intervention elements during the course of programme implementation in Santo Domingo and Puerto Plata

Source: Adapted with permission from Kerrigan *et al.* (2004: 21) 'Horizons final report'

behavioural outcomes included consistent condom use with new clients, as well as with regular paying and non-paying partners. All women participating in these surveys were screened for common STIs including gonorrhoea, chlamydia, and trichomoniasis.

Positive findings in terms of both behavioural and STI-related changes from pre- to post-intervention were documented in both cities; however, the combined intervention model in Puerto Plata demonstrated a statistically significant impact on STI prevalence and a range of other process and impact indicators, beyond what was achieved in Santo Domingo. For example, consistent condom use with regular partners increased significantly from 13 to 29 per cent, which was a major accomplishment given the historical difficulty of achieving this behavioural change in the DR. As seen in Figure 15.3, STI prevalence was reduced by approximately 40 per cent in both cities, going from 29 to 16 per cent in Puerto Plata and 26 to 16 percent in Santo Domingo. However, statistically significant changes in STI prevalence (p <0.01) were only achieved in Puerto Plata. At the environmental level, the percentage of establishments achieving the goal of zero STIs on a monthly basis increased significantly and dramatically from 25 to 65 per cent over the one-year period in Puerto Plata, as did adherence to the intervention from pre- to post-intervention. Adherence to the five key establishment-level intervention elements was the only aggregate variable found to be significantly associated with STI prevalence among participating FSWs in multivariate analyses (Kerrigan *et al.* 2004, 2006).

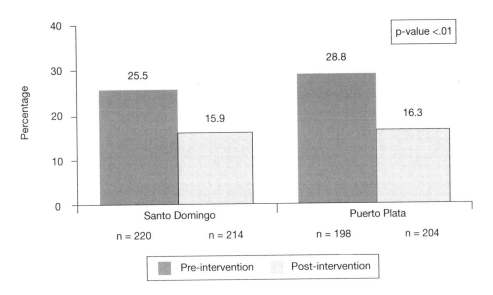

Figure 15.3 Prevalence of STIs among female sex workers in Santo Domingo and Puerto Plata, pre- to post-intervention

Source: Adapted with permission from Kerrigan *et al.* (2004: 3) 'Horizons research summary'

Cost-effectiveness analysis

The cost-effectiveness of each intervention model was also assessed by collecting detailed financial data from the budgets of both implementing NGOs. While the costs of implementing the two models were found to be comparable, the combined community solidarity and government policy model was found to be significantly more cost-effective than community solidarity alone. The cost per HIV infection averted in Puerto Plata, for example, was US $10,856, substantially less than that of Santo Domingo, which was US $28,208. When converted, the average cost per disability adjusted life year (DALY) saved was US $457 (ranging from US $153–1,317) in Puerto Plata, compared to US $1,186 (ranging from US $291–6,841) in Santo Domingo (Sweat *et al.* 2006). While there are no strict guidelines for comparing the cost-effectiveness of health interventions across countries, the World Health Organization (WHO) recommends that an intervention can be considered 'highly cost-effective' if the cost per DALY saved is less than the gross domestic product (GDP). At the time this analysis was conducted, the GDP in the DR was US $7,000, making both the Santo Domingo and Puerto Plata models highly cost-effective approaches to HIV prevention (Goldie *et al.* 2006; Sweat *et al.* 2006; WHO 2011).

Implications for future structural–environmental HIV prevention interventions and evaluations

The importance of mixed-method approaches

From the initial phase of intervention development through the implementation and evaluation of its structural-environmental components, we integrated both qualitative and quantitative methods and multiple categories of participants to obtain a wide range of perceptions, suggestions, and markers – both behavioural and biological – of the model's potential, and actual processes and impact. During the formative phase, we were able to assess what potential target populations and stakeholders thought about structural-environmental approaches and what would be acceptable and feasible to implement in the DR. The integration of qualitative and quantitative methods provided a richer and more robust understanding of what the model should look like, how it should be implemented, and later during the process evaluation, how well it was working, than we would have obtained by using only one type of research method or approach.

In our evaluation we utilized pre–post, cross-sectional surveys as the main source of data regarding changes in HIV risk behaviours and the influence of exposure to structural-environmental interventions on those changes. Our approach reflects the technical and logistical challenges to evaluating structural-environmental interventions with vulnerable populations. First, while randomizing individuals or communities to intervention versus control groups is considered the most rigorous way to test a new intervention model, there was no way to meaningfully randomize in this context. We only implemented the policy component in one city, Puerto Plata. This was facilitated by the fact that our local NGO partner's director became the provincial health leader during this time period. We would not have been able to control for the effects of that policy within Puerto Plata through randomization and would not have had enough participants to effectively test the model. A second alternative to our design would have been to follow a cohort of intervention participants over time, which would have allowed us to conduct a more controlled assessment of the intervention intensity and effects. Due to limited resources and high mobility of sex workers, this approach was also considered logistically and financially infeasible. However, with sufficient resources, a longitudinal design could provide a strong alternative to a randomized controlled trial (Lippman *et al.* 2010).

Multiple outcomes provide greater understanding of effects

The incorporation of both behavioural and biological markers in our pre- and post-intervention surveys allowed us to triangulate findings and address the limitations of self-reports of condom use and other sexual risk behaviours in the context of HIV prevention interventions. Our measures of structural-environmental support for condom use also provided a comprehensive assessment of how factors beyond individual knowledge and attitudes influenced changes in the political, social, and physical environments during the intervention, which has been identified as a key priority for the effective evaluation of structural interventions (Blankenship *et al.* 2006). Additionally, qualitative interviews conducted with FSWs with positive STI tests at the conclusion of the intervention provided critical insight regarding the limitations of the model and identified future directions for HIV prevention efforts, including the need for further work with their male, regular partners (Barrington *et al.* 2009; Kerrigan *et al.* 2006). These interviews also aided immensely in the interpretation of pre- to post-intervention changes in behaviour and improved understanding of the ways in which structural-environmental factors operated, and were influenced by power dynamics within and beyond the sex establishment, such as with owner/managers and government health officials.

Structural factors require dynamic evaluation processes

While environmental and policy-level interventions are often lauded for their ease of implementation and potential for sustainability, in reality these contextual factors are complex and require dynamic and long-term evaluation processes in order to effectively capture both short- and long-term impacts (Blankenship *et al.* 2006). By addressing factors beyond individual knowledge and attitudes, these models may also be influenced by structural shifts beyond those directly targeted by the intervention. In our experience, the policy implemented in Puerto Plata was relatively stable during the course of the intervention. However, the provincial health leader who was so critical to approving the policy did not continue indefinitely in that role and the policy was not sustained, reflecting how political positions generally shift every few years in this and many other settings. Sustaining the policy and intensity of the structural-environmental intervention components beyond the context of the intervention has been a significant challenge.

Since this initial evaluation, there has been no formal assessment of the continuity and sustainability of the policy and other structural-environmental elements of the intervention. While ongoing HIV surveillance efforts do suggest stabilization and even slow decline of HIV prevalence in areas of the DR where the intervention was implemented, these data do not permit determination of causal relationships (Kerrigan *et al.*

2008). In addition, despite the positive findings of the model in Puerto Plata, it has been extremely challenging to find sufficient support, both financial and political, to scale up the model to other areas of the country. While COIN and CEPROSH have continued to implement peer education and some level of community mobilization, engaging with sex workers, establishment staff and owner/managers and, to an increasing degree, clients and regular partners, they have not been able to sustain and build on the governmental policy and regulatory elements of the structural-environmental intervention that were found to be highly effective in Puerto Plata.

Despite these challenges, informal observations and discussions with COIN and CEPROSH leadership and staff suggest that while they have not been able to find support to sustain and scale up the structural-environmental intervention models, they have been able to maintain activities beyond individual-level health education targeting only FSWs, which reflects how the experience of adapting and implementing the models did have a lasting impact on their work. Examples of this expansion include continued engagement with sex establishment owners in COIN and CEPROSH's efforts to maintain a collective commitment to HIV prevention at the level of the sex establishment, even if the policy component of the intervention model has not been scaled up. Additionally, pilot efforts to reach more male clients through male peer educators and community-based HIV testing activities reflect a key lesson learned from the trial of the need for greater male involvement in HIV prevention efforts in the female sex industry.

Finally, in collaboration with MODEMU, FSW peer educators continue to fight for the rights of FSWs, recognizing that the human rights and labour violations experienced by women working in the DR's sex industry are as influential on their HIV-related risk and protective behaviours as individual knowledge and attitudes about condoms.

References

Barrington, C., Latkin, C., Sweat, M.D., Moreno, L., Ellen, J., and Kerrigan, D. (2009) 'Talking the talk, walking the walk: social network norms, communication patterns, and condom use among the male partners of female sex workers in La Romana, Dominican Republic', *Social Science & Medicine*, 68: 2037–44.

Basu, I., Jana, S., Rotheram-Borus, M.J., Swendeman, D., Lee, S.J., Newman, P., and Weiss, R. (2004) 'HIV prevention among sex workers in India', *Journal of Acquired Immune Deficiency Syndromes*, 36: 845–52.

Blankenship, K.M., Friedman, S.R., Dworkin, S., and Mantell, J.E. (2006) 'Structural interventions: concepts, challenges and opportunities for research', *Journal of Urban Health*, 83: 59–72.

Goldie, S.J., Yazdanpanah, Y., Losina, E., Weinstein, M.C., Anglaret, X., Walensky, R.P., Hsu, H.E., Kimmel, A., Holmes, C., Kaplan, J.E., and Freedberg, K.A. (2006) 'Cost-effectiveness of HIV treatment in resource-poor settings – the case of Côte d'Ivoire', *New England Journal of Medicine*, 355: 1141–53.

Issel, L.M. (2009) *Health Program Planning and Evaluation: A Practical, Systematic Approach for Community Health*, Sudbury, MA: Jones and Bartlett.

Jana, S. and Singh, S. (1995) 'Beyond medical model of STD intervention – lessons from Sonagachi', *Indian Journal of Public Health*, 39: 125–31.

Kendall, M. and Razali, K. (2010) *HIV and Sex Work in Thailand*, Bangkok: HIV/AIDS Data Hub. Online, available at: http://www.nswp.org/sites/nswp.org/files/sex_work_hiv_thailand.pdf (accessed 17 December 2011).

Kerrigan, D., Moreno, L., Rosario, S., Butler, M., De Moya, E., and Sweat, M.D. (1997) *Formative Research for a 100% Condom Program in the Dominican Republic*, Arlington, VA: AIDS Control and Prevention Project/Family Health International/United States Agency for International Development.

Kerrigan, D., Moreno, L., Rosario, S., and Sweat, M. (2001) 'Adapting the Thai 100% condom programme: developing a culturally appropriate model for the Dominican Republic', *Culture, Health & Sexuality*, 3: 221–40.

Kerrigan, D., Ellen, J.M., Moreno, L., Rosario, S., Katz, J., Celentano, D.D., and Sweat, M. (2003) 'Environmental-structural factors significantly associated with consistent condom use among female sex workers in the Dominican Republic', *AIDS*, 17: 415–23.

Kerrigan, D., Moreno, L., Rosario, S., Gomez, B., Jerez, H., Weiss, E., Van Dam, J., Roca, E., and Sweat, M. (2004) *Combining Community Approaches and Government Policy to Prevent HIV Infection in the Dominican Republic*, Washington, D.C.: Horizons/Population Council/United States Agency for International Development.

Kerrigan, D., Moreno, L., Rosario, S., Gomez, B., Jerez, H., Barrington, C., Weiss, E., and Sweat, M. (2006) 'Environmental-structural interventions to reduce HIV/STI risk among female sex workers in the Dominican Republic', *American Journal of Public Health*, 96: 120–5.

Kerrigan, D., Barrington, C., and Moreno, L. (2008) 'The state of HIV/AIDS in the Dominican Republic: guarded optimism amidst sustainability concerns', in D.D. Celentano and C. Beyrer (eds) *Pubic Health Aspects of HIV/AIDS in Low and Middle Income Countries: Epidemiology, Prevention and Care*, New York: Springer.

Lippman, S.A., Shade, S.B., and Hubbard, A.E. (2010) 'Inverse probability weighting in sexually transmitted infection/human immunodeficiency virus prevention research: methods for evaluating social and community interventions', *Sexually Transmitted Diseases*, 37: 512–18.

Moreno, L. and Kerrigan, D. (2000) 'The evolution of HIV prevention strategies among female sex workers in the Dominican Republic', *Research for Sex Work*, 3: 8–10.

Murray, L., Moreno, L., Rosario, S., Ellen, J., Sweat, M., and Kerrigan, D. (2007) 'The role of relationship intimacy in consistent condom use among female sex workers and their regular paying partners in the Dominican Republic', *AIDS and Behavior*, 11: 463–70.

Rojanapithayakorn, W. and Hanenberg, R. (1996) 'The 100% Condom Program in Thailand', *AIDS*, 10: 1–7.

Sweat, M., Kerrigan, D., Moreno, L., Rosario, S., Gomez, B., Jerez, H., Weiss, E., and Barrington, C. (2006) 'Cost-effectiveness of environmental-structural communication interventions for HIV prevention in the female sex industry in the Dominican Republic', *Journal of Health Communication*, 11 (Suppl. 2): 123–42.

World Health Organization (WHO) (2011) 'Choosing interventions that are cost-effective'. Online, available at: http://www.who.int/choice/costs/CER_thresholds/en/index.html (accessed 17 December 2011).

16

HELMET DAY! STRUCTURAL INTERVENTION AND STRATEGIC LEARNING IN VIETNAM

Mary Byrne McDonnell and Alyson Metzger

Vietnam's swift economic transition picked up speed in the mid-1990s, ushering in a rapid and dramatic shift for ordinary Vietnamese from bicycle to motorcycle use. The chaotic street scene intensified as the growing numbers of wealthy Vietnamese imported cars and the booming economy packed roads and highways with heavily laden trucks. The corresponding increase in the risk and reality of motorcycle-related head injuries and deaths indicated a need for structural intervention to make helmet use a matter of course for motorcycle riders and passengers of all ages. While the economically vulnerable were the most exposed to the dangers of traffic accidents – both on the seats of their motorcycles and in their limited transportation options – the entire country was paying the price, with road accidents estimated to cost Vietnam at least US $900 million each year, equal to 2.7 per cent of gross domestic product (GDP) (ADB/ASEAN 2003).

On 15 December 2007, motorcycle helmets became mandatory in Vietnam, with almost immediate universal compliance, as this chapter will describe. This achievement was years in the making and depended on two enabling factors coming together in full measure: (1) the political will to identify, create, and implement needed regulation; and (2) the coalescing of funding, passion, vision, and leadership to both promote and support necessary action. The story of Helmet Day provides a lens on this process of creating achievable policy and behavioural change, and offers a set of lessons learned that in whole or in part may be applicable to interventions for other public health issues and in different national settings where changing individual behaviour and culturally accepted norms of behaviour is a goal.

Helmet Day also tells a story about evaluation and how evaluation can assist learning. Ideally, process evaluation should be fully integrated into structural interventions to allow for continuous assessment and improvement as the work itself is being accomplished. The incorporation of a learning agenda into a programmatic agenda aimed at improving population health through behaviour change enables real-time adjustments that can improve the efficiency and effectiveness of the programme process, reducing the time required to achieve the goal and limiting missteps along the way. While the evaluation of the helmet intervention in Vietnam described here began 'after the fact' and, therefore, could not contribute to incremental learning in the course of pre-2007 programming, it was an opportunity to look back at a successful intervention to determine what worked, why it worked, and what lessons might be applicable to future interventions. The resulting report helped the players involved identify and understand their accomplishments and determine what still needs to be done.

Evaluating structural intervention in Vietnam

In 2006, the Atlantic Philanthropies (Atlantic) asked the Social Science Research Council (SSRC) to develop and undertake a strategic learning and assessment project to evaluate their Population Health Programme in Vietnam. Atlantic sees evaluation as a critical part of its grant-making strategies, and evaluation components are built in to its Vietnam grants. Each grantee is required to assess whether funded activities have been carried out properly and the extent of project impact, but these evaluation criteria rarely capture the entire process of a structural intervention, particularly when multiple players are involved.

Atlantic sought a partner who would step back from the day-to-day work of each grantee and carry out a continuous assessment of its multifaceted Vietnam programme against its overall programmatic goals, with an eye toward providing a comprehensive understanding of what was and was not working, determining what further interventions should be added to programming, and developing a strong feedback loop for strategic learning for both programme officers and grantees that could continue independently after the programme's funding expired. Atlantic would use the evaluation as a basis for both the design of sustainability strategies for its own work and the communication of lessons learned that were relevant to the broader philanthropic enterprise.

Atlantic had been working in Vietnam, and specifically in injury prevention, since 1997 and saw another decade of work ahead. Thus, the evaluation project needed to be both retrospective and prospective. When the project began in 2006, there was no way of knowing that the culmination of the helmet intervention – the launch of a universal helmet law – planned for the following year would be so successful. As part of the SSRC's ongoing evaluation, a team set out to investigate what made Helmet Day possible.[1]

The work was interdisciplinary and involved anthropological, historical, and oral history research. The team reviewed grant-related documents, programme records, and intervention materials, as well as contextual factors, such as relevant laws, policies, attitudes, and economic actualities. All stakeholders who could be identified were interviewed and re-interviewed. As information was collected, analyzed, and interpreted, the team began to integrate ideas about the meaning of individual pieces of evidence into a larger theory of what happened and why. Trends, patterns, and transitional moments were identified, and the critical roles of key institutions and external forces became apparent. Gradually, over many months, the story of the helmet intervention in Vietnam began to unfold.

The story of Helmet Day

When the people of Ha Noi stepped outside on Saturday, 15 December 2007, they faced a beautiful, colourful sea of helmets on the heads of the adults and children riding by. Bui Huynh Long, secretary of the National Traffic Safety Committee (NTSC) and Vietnam's helmet use champion, was there to document the occasion:

On the morning of 15 December, other dignitaries and I planted ourselves at the Daewoo Hotel intersection with TV crews and other journalists. We wanted to find four or five people who were not wearing helmets, who could be filmed getting fined by police. There was no job for the police to do and nothing for TV to film. ... There was 100 per cent compliance.

(Long 2008)

On 14 December, no one in all of Vietnam would have predicted this enormous success. There was no stampede to buy helmets. Certainly, almost no one had them on their heads. As the workweek drew to a close, it was mostly business as usual and traffic chaos as on any other Friday evening. There was a sense of anticipation among people working with helmet use projects, but no one was betting on anything. Nothing on the streets signalled that the next morning would display such a radical change.

The journey to Helmet Day was not simple or easy. Multiple players, from government ministries and global non-governmental organizations (NGOs) to local police and international movie stars, contributed in a variety of ways over many stages across decades. During each particular time period, different factors enabled – or set up obstacles to – each step taken and contributed to the intervention's overall momentum.[2]

1990–1996: Understanding connections

In Vietnam's initial wave of motorization, there was very little movement toward helmet imperatives. The government saw the emerging chaos on the roads as a problem but had not recognized the significance of motorcycle accidents or injuries and did not draw a connection between accidents, serious head injuries, and helmets. The magnitude of the problem had yet to be realized internally, and external pressure had not yet come to bear.

Political will and government action: a local false start and a national champion

This early period did see a brief local attempt at requiring helmet use. In 1993, Ho Chi Minh City – already facing a dramatic rise in motorcycle accident injuries and deaths that the rest of Vietnam would experience later – mandated helmet use within the city. A year later, city authorities halted implementation and repealed the law. One explanation given for this about-face was that the city exceeded its regulatory authority when there was no national helmet mandate. It was also reported that there were not enough helmets available amid public complaints about helmet cost and necessity.

Bui Huynh Long, working in the legal department of the Ministry of Transport on the first national set of rules for traffic order and safety, recognized the legal obstacle and included a helmet-wearing clause in the rules but was unable to promote it. However, Mr Long emerged as a champion of the helmet cause and would become a strong partner for international players as their involvement and influence grew around the helmet issue.

Funding, passion, vision, and leadership: a gradual realization

The first stirrings of international interest in helmet use came in 1991 with the establishment of the World Health Organization (WHO) and FIA Foundation Helmet Initiative to promote the use of motorcycle and bicycle helmets worldwide. Awareness was spreading that needlessly large numbers of people were being killed or permanently disabled as a result of head injuries received from motorcycle falls or crashes that could have been prevented, or less severe, through the use of a simple and inexpensive helmet.

At this time, the only significant funding available for injury prevention work in Vietnam was bilateral aid through the Swedish International Development Authority (SIDA – now the Swedish International Development Cooperation Agency). In 1994, Vietnam and Sweden entered into a five-year health cooperation agreement to develop a legal framework for the health sector, in general, and to address accidents and injuries as urgent health problems. A Safe Community model was piloted by the Ministry of Health, with the guidance of the model's originator, Swedish professor of social medicine Leif Svanström. Although a few pilot projects were carried out, universal, mandatory helmet use had not yet been identified as an urgently needed solution.

A tipping point: 1997

1997 was a year destined to change the direction of injury prevention work in Vietnam. Two actors appeared on the scene who would stress that it was time to stop the carnage on roads and highways and time to put helmets on everyone's heads. First, when the first post-war US ambassador, Pete Peterson, arrived in Vietnam in 1997, he began to raise the profile of road traffic safety and helmet use. Having lost a son in a traffic accident, he was a man with a personal passion for injury prevention work. He also believed that accidents were a great waste of Vietnam's resources and therefore a drag on development. But most of all, he wanted to save lives. Ambassador Peterson saw injury prevention as a non-controversial area for US participation and wanted to find a way to build capacity inside existing systems. Also in 1997, the government of Vietnam created the National Traffic Safety Committee (NTSC) to advise the prime minister on strategic and policy directions for ensuring traffic order and safety, coordinate public information and education outreach efforts, and report on the activities of ministries, sectors, and localities ensuring traffic order and safety. A purely Vietnamese initiative, the NTSC would become a major partner to many international groups that would come to work on the helmet issue.

1997–2001: Sudden awakening and some momentum

This interim period saw major changes in attitudes toward helmet use. There was much energy, enthusiasm, commitment, and leadership shown by various individuals and international groups and their Vietnamese partners working on injury prevention and helmet-related programming. This increase in interest and the growing number of players – both inside and outside the government – began to produce forward momentum. Nonetheless, as we shall see, for every step forward there was often a setback.

Political will and government action: more drive but disjointed action

Although there began to be a significant increase in political will and government action around the helmet issue, with more political actors joining the movement, legislative efforts became disjointed. The result was a pattern of legislation and implementation attempts that lacked clarity and appropriate sanction.

The National Assembly gave the government legal authority to mandate and sanction helmet use in the 2001 Law on Road Traffic. However, the law's helmet provisions covered only a few highways and imposed only a minor fine, and there were not enough police for enforcement. The responsibility for controlling traffic accidents was still seen as the sole purview of the Ministry of Transport and the traffic police, making it hard to forge the needed cooperation between relevant ministries.

Still, the combined efforts began to pay off as the different parties learned how to cooperate and coordinate. A major breakthrough came at the end of 2001 with the adoption of the National Policy on Accident and Injury Prevention and Control for 2002–2010. At the same time, a multi-sector National Steering Committee on Injury Prevention and Control formed, chaired by the Ministry of Health and including the Ministry of Transport.

Funding, passion, vision, and leadership: joining forces

Alongside the growing domestic political will, a vibrant international community was developing around injury prevention work, in particular helmet use programming. It was an unusual time, rich with people who were highly motivated and completely committed to success. Many more international groups became involved, pushed and prodded initially by US Ambassador Peterson and Mike Linnan, the US embassy health attaché for the Centers for Disease Control and Prevention (CDC). In 1999, Pete Peterson and Mike Linnan, in collaboration with the Ministry of Health and Morten Giersing, the United Nations Children's Fund (UNICEF) country representative, started The Safe Viet Nam Initiative, a network including the NTSC, the Ministry of Health, other ministries and agencies, and a range of international organizations, such as the Asia Injury Prevention Foundation (AIPF), UNICEF, SIDA, and the US and Australian embassies.

American funding became an important factor, and here too Ambassador Peterson served as a catalyst. After tapping the CDC and USAID for help, he and Mike Linnan convinced Chuck Feeney, the founder of the Atlantic Philanthropies, to invest in injury prevention work and put him in touch with AIPF and UNICEF Vietnam. In 2000, Atlantic gave its first injury prevention grants to the US Fund for UNICEF (for UNICEF Vietnam) and AIPF, deeming AIPF's project feasible largely based on the grounding provided by The Safe Viet Nam Initiative. As a condition of its grant-making, Atlantic's funding was matched by resources from the corporate sector, foundations, and others.

In 2001, as Vietnam was growing more receptive to a public health approach to reducing accidents and injuries, the prime minister issued a decree establishing the Hanoi School of Public Health (HSPH) as a new agent of change. The first sound research on which to base injury-related policy and public education and advocacy was accomplished that same year – the 2001 Vietnam Multi-Center Injury Survey, which determined that 'a national helmet use policy is urgently needed' (Linnan *et al.* 2003: 56). Funded by UNICEF and carried out by the HSPH in collaboration with the Ministry of Health, this was Vietnam's first national household survey on injury and, at the time, the largest ever accomplished in Asia. The government initially balked at accepting the results because they were more serious than expected but would later use evidence from the report, such as accident rates, to underpin action.

A tipping point: 2002

By the beginning of 2002, it was clear that both the Vietnamese government and their international partners were determined to develop mandatory helmet use regulations that could be successfully implemented. Along with the fact that in 2002 Vietnam recorded the most traffic accident deaths and injuries ever, several events made this year a tipping point: the government passed Resolution No. 13, strong legislation to check the rise in and gradually reduce traffic accidents and congestion, and a few months later, the Communist Party of Vietnam became actively involved, issuing a directive to strengthen leadership countrywide on this issue. Bui Huynh Long – who had served on the National Traffic Safety Committee in different positions since 1997, emerging as a helmet use champion – assumed leadership of the NTSC, giving international groups working on helmet use programmes a passionate, committed government partner. Finally, AIPF began to develop a high profile for non-profit helmet manufacturing and mandatory helmet use with the opening of a Protec helmet factory for the production of appropriate, affordable tropical helmets for both adults and children.

2002–2007: An intensive push for success

If the period between 1997 and 2001 had seemed full of new helmet use projects and players, it was nothing like the crowded field that developed over the next five years. The number of people and organizations involved exploded, resulting in many major projects that directly contributed to or had some bearing on the Helmet Day story. Every government ministry was made aware of the helmet initiative, and the Party strongly signalled the problem as a priority. The media was taking up the cause, and celebrities became involved. There would continue to be starts and stops on the road to success, but all the actors believed the effort toward compulsory helmet usage was firmly on track.

Political will and government action: workable laws and serious implementation

In 2002, the government agreed that helmets would be worn on national highways that posted signs stating that helmets were required, and this became the 'law'. Signs began to be posted, and fines were imposed on some highways. However, the regulated national highways and provincial roads covered only 18 per cent of Vietnam's road system, missing the cities where motorcycle use was highest. Local leadership varied, so action and enforcement were not consistent from one locale to another. Helmet usage was growing, but the lack of universality in what was required on which roads and the unevenness of sanctions and their enforcement made it the exception, not the rule, especially in urban areas. Social conformity is strong in Vietnam, which hindered the emergence of significant 'early adopters' for voluntary behavioural change; thus, having everyone don their helmets at once would facilitate acceptance of and compliance with the structural intervention.

Mr Long, now the Secretary of the NTSC, and the Minister of Transport leveraged Vietnam's strong support for APEC, a regional economic forum, to engage the prime minister's backing for aggressive road safety strategies (Long 2008),[3] and in mid-2007, the government unanimously agreed helmet wearing would be compulsory from 15

September on all national highways and from 15 December on all roads. The national universal helmet policy was issued at the end of June in Government Resolution No. 32, which also included a number of urgent measures to control traffic accidents and congestion, triggering a chain of related laws and subordinate policies. The sanction law was amended, and fines were significantly raised.

The political will that led to the government's helmet policy included support from the Party, a largely missing element in earlier periods. Provincial people's committee chairs (the highest ranking Party officials in provinces and the equivalent of governors) became the heads of local NTSC branches, thus lodging responsibility for traffic safety, injuries, and mortality squarely with those leaders responsible for implementing national policy at the local level. In August 2007, the Party issued a report that affirmed that road safety is a political task – and a mass task – and stated that all must comply with and implement Resolution No. 32. This provided the prime minister with the needed authority to issue a formal directive to branches, agencies, offices, and political-social organizations at every level to mobilize them to make sure everyone knew about the rules and fines and would be wearing their helmets on 15 December.

Funding, passion, vision, and leadership: expanding networks, evidence, and education

The policy shift supporting helmet usage was greatly enabled by a significant increase in the number of players involved in the helmet use movement. The international, national, and local synergy electrified participants. While not always well coordinated, planning and organization increased significantly as cooperation and momentum built. One of the most important leaders to join the effort in this period was the prime minister, who lent his personal prestige and moral suasion to the movement and, through his personal involvement, set a positive example for government officials.

Significant donors joined Atlantic in funding the work in Vietnam after the United Nations (UN) adopted the 2005 General Assembly Resolution on Improving Global Road Safety, which prescribed helmet use, among other important measures. The network of organizations that supported the UN resolution began to look at Vietnam as an initial site for its application and saw AIPF as an able facilitator. This led to the World Bank's Global Road Safety Facility and the Bloomberg Family Foundation becoming two key new donors.

There was much collaboration and cooperation among funders and advocates on communications and education work. SIDA continued to fund the Ministry of Health to carry out the Swedish-Vietnam Safe Community collaboration through 2007, and all affiliate Safe Community Network members provided helmet use training and education. At the beginning of 2006, the programme produced national guidelines on criteria for awarding safe family, safe community, and safe school certificates that included helmet wearing.

As in previous periods, AIPF was a linchpin. The organization provided free helmets and a safety demonstration to one of the Safe Community schools. It was also a member of a Make Roads Safe campaign coordinated by the FIA Foundation, a UK charity that supports an international programme of activities promoting road safety, the environment, and sustainable mobility. That coalition had lobbied hard for the government resolutions and – guided by AIPF – brought spokesperson Michelle Yeoh to Vietnam to promote helmet use.

The nascent network joined forces at two pivotal moments during this period. The first was a National Helmet Action Plan Workshop in December 2006. Co-chaired by the Global Road Safety Partnership and the French Red Cross, the workshop was organized by AIPF and the NTSC. The 2006 WHO publication *Helmets: A Road Safety Manual for Decision-makers and Practitioners*, available in Vietnamese, provided a framework for planning Helmet Day. Mr Long was convinced enough of the soundness of the resulting National Helmet Action Plan and the backing of the international players that he proposed December 2008 to the government as the start date for mandatory helmet use.

The second key moment was a national helmet-wearing campaign held in March and April 2007. Greig Craft, AIPF president, tried a new approach to public education and worked closely with Ogilvy and Mather (Vietnam) – an advertising, marketing, and public relations agency – on an extraordinary campaign with the messages 'Enough is enough' and 'No excuses … Wear a helmet'. Launched during the first UN Road Safety Week, the campaign was made possible by funding from the National Helmet Wearing Coalition, which was made up of international groups, embassies, and others that Mr Craft had asked Klaus Rohland at the World Bank to pull together to raise money. The NTSC credits the campaign for influencing the government to move up the date for mandatory helmet use to 15 December 2007.

An initial endpoint: 15 December 2007

Compliance with the new mandate was immediate and nearly complete. On Helmet Day, Da Nang's helmet use went from about 4 per cent to 98 per cent overnight (Scott 2008). Compliance in Ha Noi and Ho Chi Minh City was closer to 99 per cent (Long 2008). The next day, *Saigon Giai Phong* newspaper (2007) reported, 'A new cultural characteristic has been established'.

The positive effect on health outcomes was apparent. The Ministry of Health – with WHO's technical assistance – carried out monitoring at twenty provincial and central hospitals over three months before and after Helmet Day. Results showed a decrease of 24 per cent in patients admitted with head injuries and 14 per cent in road traffic deaths (MOH/WHO 2008). Other government monitoring reports from the first six months of mandatory helmet use supported these findings.

The entire exercise in behaviour change was an enormous accomplishment, a victory over the many obstacles to mandatory helmet use. The government, people, and partners of Vietnam had achieved results that most developing countries could only dream of.

Epilogue: sustaining and fine-tuning success

After the initial success of Helmet Day, the coalition of domestic and international players remained committed and was able to forge ahead to sustain and enhance the behaviour change already in place, focusing attention on both unexpected complications and what had been considered second-order issues, such as helmets for children, helmet quality, and proper wearing of helmets.

While almost all children wore helmets on 15 December, within 10 days, children's helmet use fell to no more than 20 per cent after a media report erroneously cited the opinion of a medical practitioner that helmet use might increase the risk of neck injuries in children. Parents and young teenagers also quickly found out that there were no fines for children under age 16. The coalition decided to accelerate work in two areas: public education targeted to parents and remedying the fines loophole in the law that essentially allowed children to go without helmets. Public education targeted at parents included public service announcements made by AIPF to deliver accurate medical evidence. And the government approved a new schedule of fines in Decree No. 34, effective 20 May 2010, which holds adult drivers accountable for the helmet use compliance of their child passengers and makes it easier for authorities to enforce child helmet usage through schools and parent associations.

Issues with helmet quality were addressed in November 2008 with the revision of the existing adult and child helmet standards into a single consolidated, government-approved National Standards for Helmets. Because the safety standards applied only to motorbike helmets, however, producers of low-quality helmets avoided fines by labelling them as other products, such as 'sport hats'. So in May 2011, the Department of Standards, Measures, and Quality submitted a proposal to the government aimed at listing helmets as goods that require certain production standards and banning all fake helmets.

It was clear that some helmet wearing was done to avoid fines and not for safety. By the end of August 2008, many people were riding around the streets of Ha Noi with their helmet straps unbuckled. In response, in November 2008, the Ministry of Public Security released a circular equating unfastened helmets to no helmet at all and stipulating hefty fines for drivers and passengers who do not use helmet straps. This new regulation can be credited with a noticeable increase in the number of properly fastened helmets.

Most important, the initial success of the helmet intervention was sustained. Two years later, the sudden behaviour change seen on 15 December 2007 had become the norm. According to a Ministry of Health/WHO road observation study in Yen Bai, Da Nang, and Binh Duong, helmet usage had not significantly diminished as one might have expected. By the end of May 2009, the figures for drivers wearing helmets in each city were 91.7 per cent, 86.3 per cent, and 98.5 per cent, respectively. The percentages of passengers wearing helmets were somewhat lower at 81.1 per cent, 86.3 per cent, and 91.6 per cent, but overall the observed usage changes were positive (MOH/WHO 2009). These rates were representative of those in other provinces, some of which had even higher compliance. By November 2009, the helmet use rate for adults was still around 90 per cent (Passmore and Nam 2009).

Looking back: the case of helmet use in Vietnam

What made Helmet Day possible? For over 10 years, multiple actors contributed in a variety of ways. Certain conditions were created, some of which were necessary but not sufficient. Change happened only when the necessary and the sufficient coalesced.

In the lead up to Helmet Day, the government's strong desire to pass helmet use legislation and their ability to develop and implement a logical legal framework had finally come together. At the same time, sufficient resources were available – including passionate and knowledgeable leaders and funders, both Vietnamese and international – to provide the underpinnings that would enable behaviour change. In a departure from the dualism that too often undermines effective collaboration, international participants played positive roles both externally, bringing pressure and funding to bear on the problem, and internally, engaging fully on the ground to create and support coalitions that could drive achievable solutions.

Everyone interviewed for the evaluation agreed on most of the reasons for the success of Helmet Day. Grounded in an overall increased intensity and momentum, those reasons were:

1   An enhanced legal, administrative, and social environment and a rule for changing behaviour that was:
    • Based on sound data supporting the need for urgent action
    • Issued by the highest political authorities
    • Communicated as an effective, urgent solution
    • Clear to understand, communicate, and enforce verbally, visually, and in writing
    • Universal
    • Backed by a mix of coercive and social sanctions, deterrents, and incentives
    • Modelled by leaders and persons of authority
    • Enforced by all, with determination to catch any and all violators
    • Strategically timed and phased in
    • Publicized and disseminated by mass media and every other means.

2   The means for individuals to comply with the helmet law through:
    • The availability of appropriate helmets
    • Verifiable helmet quality and prices
    • Subsidies and employee benefits
    • Programmes offering free helmets.

3   Strong education and awareness efforts, with a clear message that was:
    • Communicated by creative and prolonged campaigns
    • Funded by donors and the government
    • Intended to reach everyone.

4   Effective planning and coordination, from the top to the grassroots:
    • Direction of the campaign by the prime minister to its success and beyond
    • Careful planning on the part of the NTSC
    • Zealous mobilization of influential organizations.

Thus, the Helmet Day case study reveals the gradual evolution of a well-thought-out plan to institute and enable widespread behavioural change through structural interventions in the policy and legal arenas. Once the initial behaviour was established, remaining barriers could be addressed and emerging challenges identified and ameliorated.

Looking forward: potential applications to other public health behaviour change programmes

There are many lessons from Vietnam's helmet story that can be applied to other public health issues that involve programming to change embedded socio-cultural norms and individual behaviour.

The primary lesson of the Helmet Day story is that policy change can be an important element in behavioural change, especially in an environment, such as Vietnam, where the government is a major player. It is more complex though than simply making a law and providing for its implementation. In Vietnam, the government set the policy target, became thoroughly committed to the cause, acquired knowledge of implementation strategies, and mobilized all the other parts of the state to achieve the goal. At the same time, there were additional people involved who – driven by a passion for the work – brought money, knowledge, and leverage to the mix. They knew how to make things happen, were risk-takers when they needed to be, and had the experience to step back and imagine the results. These people were, in this context, a mixture of Vietnamese and international actors whose skills and knowledge were complementary. Planning and coordination among these players was critical so that essential factors could come together powerfully. Without that eventual synchronization, failure was likely.

The second critical lesson drawn from our experience in Vietnam is that initial change must be sustained and supplemented. The initial change will always be imperfect, and there will always be the need to sustain and fine-tune policies and behaviours after the initial change takes hold. It is important to plan for this from the outset and not attempt more than is doable. The initial focus of attention in Vietnam was on getting appropriate helmets on most heads. This was seen as the first step, with secondary attention to issues such as helmet quality, proper use, and sustainability of the effort. Whether handled in phases or thought through all at once, a behaviour change strategy that aims for mass adoption must be coupled with a strategy and action plan for sustaining change and enhancing health outcomes in the longer term.

Additional lessons learned that could potentially be applied to other behaviour change programmes, particularly structural interventions, include the following:

- There must be a credible, understandable knowledge base.
- Cultural context is critical.
- A compulsory element is often essential to changing risky behaviours.
- Any regulation must be clear, easy to understand, and well communicated.
- All essential pieces of legislation must be in place at the same time – the legal authority, the rule, and the sanction, as well as the instructions for implementation and enforcement.
- Education and communications must be appropriate to the audience and cultural context, creative, clear, repeated, truthful, and linked to evidence.
- Education and communications efforts must be simultaneous and constant.
- Capacity-building among key players is essential.
- Local–international partnerships can both develop new and adapt older best practices.
- Global–local interaction can amplify messaging.
- Public–private partnerships can be built to fund and implement injury prevention and other public health programmes.

Conclusion

The Helmet Day case offers lessons on how to initiate and sustain behaviour change in a developing-country setting with respect to a complicated public health issue. It also presents clues to two kinds of roles that strategic learning and assessment can play in nurturing an intervention's intermediate and ongoing success: concurrent process evaluation that identifies areas for adjustment as the intervention unfolds and retrospective outcome evaluation that provides broader insights based on identified trends and patterns.

The complexity and longevity of a major structural intervention prohibit any one actor from fully controlling the process or outcome. Multiple actors must cooperate over extended periods of time. Thus, evaluation and learning on the part of each separate component, while desirable, is insufficient. To grasp the full picture, a cluster evaluation that involves both continuous, real-time assessment and post-investigation of all components is necessary. The cluster evaluation should be thorough and ideally interdisciplinary, integrating findings from desk research, multiple rounds of interviews, and *in situ* observation with measurement of change. Meaningful evaluation therefore takes time and perspective, both of which come more readily to an external team that can focus objectively on all elements – individually and as a whole, systematically and analytically – and synthesize results.

These evaluation constraints and considerations can make it difficult to integrate a thorough strategic learning and assessment component into the initial design of a comprehensive behaviour change intervention. However, the return on this investment can be huge. If an external cluster evaluation team with such goals had been in place for all the years it took the helmet use intervention in Vietnam to come to fruition, positive results might have been achieved faster, more efficiently, and with fewer missteps.

Notes

1   The SSRC Strategic Learning and Evaluation Research Team comprised chief investigator Mary Byrne McDonnell, executive director of the SSRC and director of the Council's Vietnam Programme; project coordinator Van Bich Thi Tran, assistant director of the Vietnam Programme; and Nina R. McCoy, a population health expert and the SSRC's representative in Vietnam.
2   The story told here is based on the original *Helmet Day!* report by Mary Byrne McDonnell, Van Bich Thi Tran, and Nina R. McCoy (2010). Please see that report for a comprehensive listing of key local and international actors in Vietnam's helmet intervention over the years.
3   See the priority action areas of APEC's Transportation Working Group, http://www.apec. org/Home/Groups/SOM-Steering-Committee-on-Economic-and-Technical-Cooperation/ Working-Groups/Transportation.

References

ADB/ASEAN (Asian Development Bank/Association of Southeast Asian Nations) (2003) *Regional Road Safety Program Accident Costing Report: The Cost of Road Traffic Accidents in Vietnam*, Manila: ADB/ASEAN.

Linnan, M., Pham, C.V., Le, L.C., Le, P.N., and Le, A.V. (eds) (2003) *Report to UNICEF on the Vietnam Multi-center Injury Survey*, Hanoi: Hanoi School of Public Health. Online, available at: http://www.tasc-gcipf.org/downloads/Vietnam%20-%20UNICEFfinalVMISreportfinal.pdf (accessed 20 January 2012).

Long, Bui Huynh (National Traffic Safety Committee) (2008) Interview with SSRC Strategic Learning and Evaluation Research Team, 25 August.

McDonnell, M.B., Tran, V.B.T., and McCoy, N.R. (2010) *Helmet Day! Lessons Learned on Vietnam's Road to Healthy Behavior,* New York: Social Science Research Council. Online, available at: http://www.ssrc.org/publications/view/5DBB6A15–2E6F-DF11–9D32–001CC477EC84/ (accessed 20 January 2012).

MOH/WHO (Vietnam Ministry of Health and World Health Organization) (2008) 'Effect of mandatory motorcycle wearing on head injuries in Vietnam', August, unpublished report.

MOH/WHO (2009) *Report: Helmet Observation in Yen Bai, Da Nang and Binh Duong,* May 2009, Ha Noi: MOH/WHO.

Passmore, J. and Nam, N.P. (WHO) (2009) Interview with SSRC Strategic Learning and Evaluation Research Team, 28 October.

Saigon Giai Phong (2007) 'From people throughout the country wearing a helmet, a new cultural characteristic was established', *Saigon Giai Phong,* 16 December.

Scott, I. (Alliance for Safe Children) (2008) Interview with SSRC Strategic Learning and Evaluation Research Team, 20 June.

17

ENDING THE TOBACCO EPIDEMIC

From the genetic to the global level

Jonathan M. Samet and Heather L. Wipfli

Introduction

The epidemic of cigarette smoking and the epidemics of disease that it has caused have now been in progress for more than a century. In the prosperous Western countries where cigarette smoking became highly prevalent at the start of the twentieth century, rates of smoking have been declining for about 40 years and incidence and mortality rates for signature diseases caused by smoking, like lung cancer, have now been falling for several decades, particularly among males. Unfortunately, tobacco use, primarily cigarettes, remains high in many low- and middle-income countries and multinational tobacco companies continue to aggressively target these nations to expand their markets (WHO 2011).

The history of tobacco control activities provides a rich resource for explicating the rationale for structural approaches to disease control and public health. Approaches to tobacco control have evolved over more than half a century, beginning with one centred on individual smokers following the identification of smoking as a cause of disease in the early 1950s and culminating now with implementation of a global strategy, the World Health Organization's (WHO) Framework Convention on Tobacco Control (FCTC). This evolution has been driven by a growing understanding of nicotine addiction and substantial evidence on the efficacy and effectiveness of tobacco control measures.

In this chapter, we offer a structured framework for tobacco control, extending from the genomic to the global level, and chart the recognition of the need over time for structural approaches and their implementation and evaluation. We offer 'lessons learned' for disease control in general, and comment on future directions in global tobacco control, post-FCTC implementation. We begin by offering a general multi-level model for tobacco control, and within this structure, we trace the origin of approaches to tobacco control.

Of necessity, we have greatly oversimplified a complex topic with a long and rich history, although surprisingly little has been written about the conceptual evolution of tobacco control. While this discussion focuses on the United States, the 'lessons learned' have global import. We also examine nations where understanding of structure is critical to any effort to control tobacco use; China is the exemplar in this regard. There are many additional outstanding historical accounts of the tobacco epidemic, though most emphasize the United States (see Brandt 2007; Kluger 1996; Proctor 2011). Accounts specific to the United States are provided in the first monograph in the National Cancer Institute series, *Strategies to Control Tobacco Use in the United States* (National Cancer Institute 1991) and in the 2000 report of the Surgeon General (US Department of Health and Human Services 2000). For a broad and recent international perspective on tobacco control, we recommend the second edition of *Tobacco and Public Health: Science, Policy, and Public Health* (Boyle *et al.* 2010).

A structured framework for tobacco control

In this new era of genomics and advanced understanding of the mechanisms of disease causation, there is much discussion of disease paradigms that extend 'from cells to society'. At one extreme, so-called 'personalized medicine' promises approaches to diagnostics and therapeutics that are tailored to individuals, based on genomic and other data; at the other, frameworks for global health give emphasis to factors operating across borders, whether vectors for infectious diseases, multinational food corporations, or greenhouse gases causing climate change. Such layered frameworks have now become implicit to tobacco control.

We offer a hierarchical structural model for tobacco control that follows a general framework set out by Glass and McAtee (2006) (Figure 17.1). Glass and McAtee offered a model for factors affecting health that begins at its lowest level with the genome and extends across multiple levels, with the global level at its highest. Intermediate levels include the family and the neighbourhood. The model incorporates a life-course element that extends from conception or even pre-conception for some diseases to late life.

Figure 17.1 offers an adaptation of this model for tobacco smoking. All of its elements are relevant. At the lowest level, we are learning that genetic factors figure in determining liability to addiction and risk for disease in smokers. Intermediate levels are also relevant: the roles of family and peers in tobacco initiation are well established. The broader neighbourhood, municipal, state, and national levels are also critical in establishing both positive and negative pressures for tobacco use; the balance between these pressures integrated across these levels sets the 'cultural norm' around smoking. Cultural norms may make smoking acceptable as in present-day China, where cigarettes have well-established roles in social interactions, or unacceptable as in much of the United States today. Advertising bans, pack warnings, and taxation rates – potentially determined at multiple governmental levels of organization – also affect the environment for smoking and tobacco control. In recent decades, the global level has become ever more relevant as the tobacco industry has consolidated into a limited number of multinational companies, including Philip Morris International, British American Tobacco, Japan Tobacco International, Imperial Tobacco/Altadis, and a few others (Shafey *et al.* 2009). The largest producer is China National Tobacco Corporation, a state monopoly that manufactures more than 90 per cent of cigarettes consumed by China's 300 million smokers.

The life-course perspective also fits well with understanding how tobacco smoking damages health and causes addiction. For women who smoke, fertility is reduced and increasingly strong evidence suggests that smoking during pregnancy increases risk for congenital abnormalities and may introduce changes in the epigenome (the noncoding factors that control gene expression) with lasting consequences (US Department of Health and Human Services 2010). The developing brain of the foetus may also be

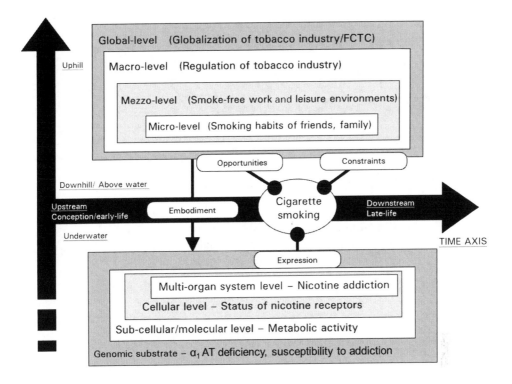

Figure 17.1 Axis of nested hierarchies for tobacco control

Source: Adapted from Glass and McAtee 2006

affected by *in utero* nicotine exposure. Health consequences of involuntary smoking begin during gestation and extend across the lifespan. Experimentation and initiation of smoking typically begin during adolescence, and addiction may extend across the lifespan. For smokers, the adverse consequences of smoking begin immediately after starting and lead to an ever-increasing risk of smoking-caused diseases with ageing (US Department of Health and Human Services 2004).

We introduce a second model for this chapter – the conventional epidemiological triangle of agent, vector, and host – with adaptation to cigarette smoking (Figure 17.2). Used conventionally for infectious diseases (e.g. malaria, mosquito, humans, a wet environment, and no mosquito nets), it is also relevant to the causation of non-communicable diseases, including those caused by smoking. For smoking, the components are cigarettes as agent, non-smokers and smokers as hosts, and the industry as vector; the environment has structure and multiple components. People, as host, include groups with possibly different genetically determined liabilities to become nicotine-addicted and to end addiction by quitting successfully. Notably, the industry is an 'adaptive' vector that dynamically changes strategies to target by host characteristics (age, gender, and race) and to counter efforts toward tobacco control.

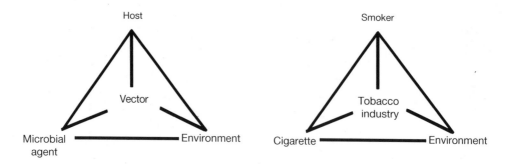

Figure 17.2 The epidemiologic triangle and the tobacco epidemic

Elements of the tobacco control framework

The individual and genetics

Serious efforts to curb tobacco use date to the identification of smoking as a cause of disease, beginning with the seminal reports in 1950 on smoking and lung cancer. In the 1950s, the public learned about the adverse effects of smoking through the media, and individuals were left to weigh the evidence and decide whether to start or to continue to smoke, even as the tobacco industry initiated aggressive efforts to undermine the research findings. The initial scientific reports had impact on smokers, who quit in large numbers, but only transiently as the tobacco industry countered with filter-tip cigarettes. At this time, the tobacco industry's credibility was undiminished, the social environment was supportive of smoking, and cigarette consumption continued to increase (Figure 17.3). Reviewers of this phase of tobacco control have concluded that early informational campaigns failed because efforts to provide information alone to individuals had insufficient impact (National Cancer Institute 1991). However, some groups with first-hand understanding of the health consequences of smoking began to quit for the long term, physicians in particular.

Since the 1950s, emphasis on the individual has continued, particularly around promotion of cessation. For example, interactions of individuals with health care providers are a critical opportunity to promote cessation. Therapies have been developed that increase the likelihood of successful cessation and health care providers are trained to intervene. Media campaigns target individual smokers and in many countries, quit lines (telephone-based counselling services) or other resources are in place to help them quit smoking. In the United States, the prevalence of current smoking continued to decline over the next few decades (Figure 17.4).

Fortunately, not all people who smoke develop one of the many diseases caused by smoking; in fact, most smoking-caused diseases are multifactorial in aetiology, and smoking is neither a necessary nor sufficient causal agent for many, except for nicotine addiction. When the link between smoking and lung cancer was first identified, R.A. Fisher offered a 'constitutional hypothesis' that inherent characteristics led some people to smoke and to have increased risk for lung cancer (Fisher 1959). This alternative hypothesis to direct causation received serious discussion in the 1964 Surgeon General's report (US Department of Health Education and Welfare 1964). Now, research is

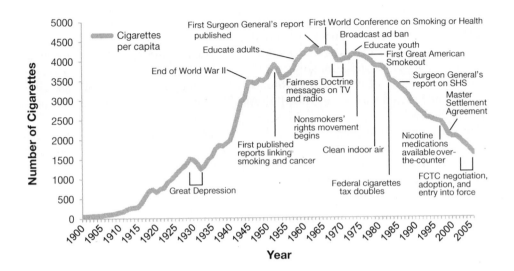

Figure 17.3 Annual cigarette consumption per capita among adults* and major smoking and health events in the United States, 1900–2006

Source: CDC Office on Smoking and Health 2010

Notes: FCTC=Framework Convention on Tobacco Control; SHS=secondhand smoke

*Adults aged 18 and over. US military forces overseas are included in the estimated consumption for the periods 1917–1919 and 1940–2006 and in the estimated per capita consumption for 1930–2006.

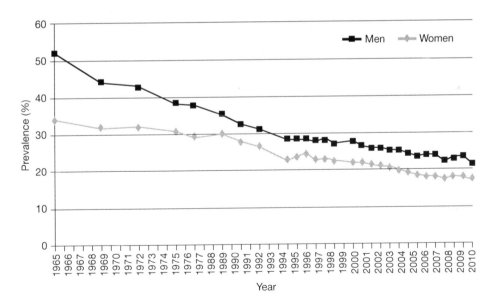

Figure 17.4 Prevalence of current smoking among adults in the USA 1965–2010

Source: Centers for Disease Control and Prevention, Office on Smoking and Health, US National Health Interview Survey, 2012

exploring the genetic basis for nicotine addiction and risk for smoking-caused disease (US Department of Health and Human Services 2010). We are learning that genetic factors may affect the phenotype of nicotine addiction, including the pace at which addiction develops following initiation and the likelihood of successful cessation. Genes affecting metabolism of nicotine and tobacco smoke components may influence risks both for addiction and smoking-caused diseases, findings anticipated by the constitutional hypothesis.

Understanding at the genetic level has little relevance to population-level interventions intended to remove the disease-causing agent – the cigarette. However, individually directed therapeutic interventions may be developed in the future that incorporate genotype. Additionally, mechanistic insights gained from investigating the genetic basis of tobacco-caused disease may prove useful for evaluating claims for reduced-risk products.

The family

The 'microenvironment' of the household has implications for the initiation of smoking by children and the likelihood of cessation by adults. Children of smokers are more likely to become smokers themselves than children of non-smokers. Additionally, smokers tend to partner with smokers, thus creating an accepting environment for smoking that diminishes the likelihood of successful cessation. In some countries, cigarettes or other tobacco products are engrained in behaviour within families. Cigarettes are commonly offered as part of social discourse and may be a component of social events, such as offering gift cigarettes at weddings in China.

The home is also a critical venue for exposure to secondhand smoke (SHS), as people in most societies spend the majority of their time indoors at home. Consequently, the microenvironment of the home is a dominant locale for SHS exposure, particularly for women and children. Wipfli et al. (2008) carried out a study including 31 countries of the exposure of women and children to SHS at home. Using air nicotine monitoring and an exposure biomarker, hair nicotine, they documented the strong contribution of smoking by men to the SHS exposure of women and children.

Socioeconomic status of the household is a key determinant of smoking and disease outcomes (US Department of Health and Human Services 1994). In nearly all countries, tobacco use is higher among poorer, less educated individuals. In very poor families, tobacco use can account for a significant amount of household income, redirecting funds away from essential foods and schooling.

Neighbourhood and local levels

Many aspects of the neighbourhood determine the environment for tobacco control, including the presence and extent of advertising and promotions, displays at point of purchase, the density of neighbourhood stores selling cigarettes and other tobacco products, and the extent of tobacco control counter-advertising. Over time, the environment at this level of organization has changed substantially, moving from widespread billboard advertising to far more confined approaches, such as point of purchase displays. Social norms around smoking are also set at the neighbourhood level.

The actions of the tobacco industry and governments are key in determining the strength of tobacco control laws and their implementation. In some countries, such as the United States, local efforts have been essential to progress in tobacco control. This is partly because of the disadvantage the tobacco industry has at this level, where their activities are more easily revealed and their influence on local policymakers is reduced. The sheer number of localities makes it difficult for the industry to have influence across all of them. Public health policy action at the local level can include smoking bans in public places, provision of nicotine replacement therapy (NRT), and more recently, prohibiting smoking in buildings with multiple residential units. The challenge for the industry to respond to local action does not mean, however, that the industry neglects all local markets. Low-income communities in the United States, for example, are often targeted by the tobacco industry. For example, the density of tobacco advertising in a low-income, minority community in Boston, Massachusetts has been found to be greater than in a neighbouring higher-income community (Seidenberg *et al.* 2010).

State level

In many countries, activities at the state or provincial level have proved pivotal in determining the strength of tobacco control and its outcomes. In many countries, particularly high-income countries, states have taken critical policy steps, including implementation of smoking bans, allocation of funds for tobacco control, tax increases, and implementation of quit lines and counter-marketing. The actions of states have also retarded progress in tobacco control; in the United States, tobacco-growing states have long lagged behind others in implementing effective tobacco control measures, and consequently, the prevalence rates of smoking have remained higher in these states. In other countries, states that benefit from tobacco production may also be resistant to tobacco control, as in the tobacco-growing provinces of China. The steps taken for over two decades by the State of California in the United States illustrate the potential for state-level action to have strong impact (Rogers 2010; see also California Department of Public Health 2010).

One critical illustration of the potential for state-level influence was provided by the American Stop Smoking Intervention Study for Cancer Prevention (ASSIST), a quasi-experimental study that implemented evidence-based interventions in 17 states, leaving the remainder as controls (National Cancer Institute 2006). The study was initiated in 1991 and the intervention extended over six years (Stillman *et al.* 2003). In the intervention states, funding was provided to implement three types of interventions: policy, media, and programme service. A multi-level analysis, reflecting the structure of tobacco control in the United States, showed a small, albeit statistically significant, effect of the intervention (National Cancer Institute 2006).

National level

Even before it was identified as a cause of disease, there were efforts to eliminate smoking by crusaders (US Department of Health and Human Services 2000). In the 1960s, evidence-based actions at the national level began with the release of government and other expert reports on the consequences of smoking, including the two landmarks: the 1962 report of the Royal College of Physicians in the United Kingdom (Royal College of Physicians of London 1962) and the 1964 Surgeon General's Report in the United

States (US Department of Health Education and Welfare 1964). The latter report was an impetus to action at the national level in the United States. It was followed by the placement of the Surgeon General's warnings on tobacco packaging and the testing and labelling of cigarettes for tar and nicotine yields. Legal action also led to the banning of television advertisements for tobacco.

Activities at the national level have had varying influence, depending on how they intersect with those at lower levels of organization. National-level actions can have substantial impact. Some of the most critical outcomes include achieving appropriate taxation, implementing smoke-free policies, controlling smuggling, and addressing issues around tobacco agriculture. In the example of the United States and other Western, high-income countries, the tobacco industry has held policy influence at the national level, in part by securing support from politicians. The Tobacco Institute was long a powerful lobbying force in the United States, until closed down consequent to litigation. In some countries, the tobacco industry remains a part of the government and as a result maintains power over the tobacco control landscape. For example, China National Tobacco Corporation is a national monopoly, and Japan Tobacco is still majority owned by the government.

Global level

Tobacco has long been a globalized industry, dating to the export of tobacco from the English colonies. The cigarette industry is among the first multinational industries, reflecting the dominance of James B. Duke and his global tobacco monopoly. By the early twentieth century, he controlled much of the global cigarette market and most of the United States market, until his empire was broken up under the Sherman Anti-Trust Act of 1890. The struggle between Duke's American Tobacco Company and Imperial Tobacco for global dominance led to the formation of British American Tobacco, which included countries outside the United States and English territories in its market. Today, a small number of companies still account for most cigarettes sold.

The multinational nature of the tobacco industry has resulted in challenges to tobacco control that require multinational solutions; one of the most critical challenges is smuggling in order to avoid taxation and to take advantages of price differentials across borders. Additionally, there has been wide variation in the strength of tobacco control worldwide, giving the industry opportunities to find new markets in low- and middle-income countries where tobacco control has been weak or even non-existent.

Until recently, there was little explicit structure defining activities in tobacco control at the global level. For the most part, tobacco control was not an issue of intense international concern during the twentieth century. Only in the final years of the century did a truly global discourse regarding the health and economic impact of tobacco use emerge including both developed and developing countries. While the World Conferences for Tobacco or Health provided a key venue for international networking beginning in the 1960s, it was the Internet that transformed international communication for tobacco control. Initial and haphazard tobacco control networking over the Internet received a major boost in 1992 when the American Cancer Society turned over control of GLOBALink (then mainly a domestic US online tobacco control network) to the International Cancer Control Union (UICC) (GLOBALink 2011). Membership in GLOBALink rapidly increased during the late 1990s to include individuals from low- and middle-income countries, and online tobacco control networking has continued to expand in recent years to multiple platforms (including Facebook).

A second revolution in global tobacco control was the negotiation, adoption and entry into force of the WHO FCTC (WHO 2003). First endorsed by the World Health Assembly in 1996, the formal FCTC negotiations took place between 2000 and 2003. The initiation of the FCTC process in 1998 marked the first time that member states of the WHO enacted the Organization's power under Article 19 of its constitution to negotiate and sign a binding treaty aimed at protecting and promoting public health. It also represented the first time that member states cooperated worldwide to form a collective response to the causation of avoidable chronic disease.

Over 170 states participated in at least one of the six negotiating sessions held in Geneva between 2000 and 2003. The World Bank's 1999 publication of *Curbing the Epidemic* provided perhaps the single most important tool in support of the FCTC negotiations. The report identified cost-effective interventions that enhance revenues and promote health (Jha and Chaloupka 1999). In doing so, it provided a credible evidence base for global regulation and helped to reverse the longstanding perception that the tobacco industry was economically too beneficial to developing countries to allow for effective regulation, including for tobacco producers. The impact of civil society on the FCTC was greatly enhanced by the development of the Framework Convention Alliance (FCA). The FCA served to increase communication between non-governmental organizations (NGO) that were already engaged, and sought to systematically reach out to and support new and small NGOs, particularly in low-income countries. By the end of the negotiations, the FCA comprised more than 200 NGOs from over 90 countries, and had established itself as an important lobbying alliance for the FCTC (Collin 2004; White 2004).

The WHO member states unanimously adopted the final text of the FCTC in May 2003. Many universal elements of national tobacco control policy became core provisions of the FCTC final text. The key provisions include a comprehensive ban on tobacco advertising, promotion, and sponsorship (with an exception for countries, such as the United States, which deem it unconstitutional); a ban on misleading descriptors that convince smokers that certain products are safer than standard cigarettes (for example, the term 'lights' in Marlboro Lights); and a mandate to place rotating warnings that cover at least 30 per cent of tobacco packaging, with encouragement for even larger, graphic warnings (Table 17.1). The FCTC also encourages countries to implement smoke-free workplace laws, address tobacco smuggling, and increase tobacco taxes.

The FCTC entered into force in February 2005 after 40 countries had ratified the treaty. Within five years, over 170 countries had ratified the treaty, including all major countries with the exception of the United States and Indonesia. FCTC implementation received a major boost with the launch of the Bloomberg Initiative to Reduce Tobacco Use in 2006. The initiative has supported the establishment of tobacco control programmes in a number of priority countries and provided grants to many low- and middle-income countries. The initiative, in collaboration with the United States Centers for Disease Control and Prevention (CDC) and the WHO, has also supported the implementation of the Global Adult Tobacco Survey, providing the first systematic adult survey of tobacco use worldwide. To help countries fulfil their WHO FCTC obligations, in 2008 the WHO introduced the MPOWER package of six evidence-based tobacco control measures that are proven to reduce tobacco use and save lives (WHO

Table 17.1 Key demand reduction provisions of the Framework Convention for Tobacco Control (FCTC)

Article 6: Price and tax measures to reduce the demand for tobacco	Recognizes that price and tax measures are an effective and important means of reducing tobacco consumption, especially among young people
Article 8: Protection from exposure to tobacco smoke	Requires Parties to adopt and implement effective measures 'providing for protection from exposure to tobacco smoke in indoor workplaces, public transport, indoor public places and, as appropriate, other public places'. (p. 8)
Article 9: Regulation of the contents of tobacco products	Obligates countries to require that manufacturers and importers of tobacco products disclose to governmental authorities information about product contents and emissions. Measures for public disclosure must be adopted.
Article 10: Regulation of tobacco product disclosures	Conference of the Parties is to develop guidelines that can be used by countries for the testing, measurement, and regulation of contents and emissions. Parties must adopt pertinent measures at the national level.
Article 11: Packaging and labelling of tobacco products	Requires Parties to adopt and implement effective measures requiring large, clear health warnings, using rotating messages approved by a designated national authority. Provides that these warnings should cover 50% or more of the principal display areas and must occupy at least 30% of the area. Requires the Parties adopt and implement effective measures to ensure tobacco product packaging and labelling do not promote a tobacco product by any means that are false, misleading, deceptive, or likely to create an erroneous impression about its characteristics, health effects, hazards, or emissions.
Article 12: Education, communication, training, and public awareness	Requires the adoption of legislative, executive, administrative, or other measures that promote public awareness and access to information on the addictiveness of tobacco, the health risks of tobacco use and exposure to smoke, the benefits of cessation, and the actions of the tobacco industry.
Article 13: Tobacco advertising, promotion, and sponsorship	Requires, in accordance with constitutional limitations, a comprehensive ban on all tobacco advertising, promotion, and sponsorship.
Article 14: Demand reduction measures concerning tobacco dependence and cessation	Requires creation of cessation programmes in a range of settings, includes diagnosis and treatment of nicotine dependence in national health programmes, establish programmes for diagnosis, counselling, and treatment in health care facilities and rehabilitation centres.

Source: World Health Organization 2003

2008). The MPOWER measures provide practical assistance with country-level implementation of effective policies to reduce the demand for tobacco.

In the years since the FCTC came into force, governments around the world have taken measures to better align themselves with the treaty's goals. The WHO Report on the Global Tobacco Epidemic found in 2011 that roughly 3.8 billion people (55 per cent of the world's population) are covered by at least one measure at the highest level of achievement, including 1.1 billion people covered by a new policy since 2008 (WHO 2011). However, implementation of the FCTC and MPOWER remains a large challenge, with only a small percentage of the world's population covered by all six effective tobacco control policies.

Lessons learned

This brief review documents the underlying structure that is relevant to tobacco control. While individuals smoke, their addiction results from the interplay of factors that act at levels ranging from genetic to global. We show that the understanding of this structure has evolved over time and led to changes in approaches to tobacco control, leading to the present situation of a global treaty. We conclude with several general 'lessons learned' from tobacco control.

Perhaps the most basic lesson was the evolution of understanding how structural approaches are relevant to tobacco control. From the 1950s to the present, we have moved from public education campaigns and cessation initiatives to a global treaty. The tobacco industry has responded aggressively and dynamically to essentially all tobacco control measures, acting at various levels within the framework structure. The industry documents provide the industry's 'playbook', which involved actions extending to the global level. For example, the industry's concern about the implications of the evidence on SHS and disease risk led to global initiatives to discredit the research. At present, industry strategies are clearly in play to diminish the effectiveness of the FCTC.

Given the reach of the implicit framework to the global level, surveillance is needed that reaches from the local to the global level. At the state and local levels, particularly in high-income countries, smoking prevalence is increasingly heterogeneous, necessitating the collection of relatively fine-grained data to target control. At the same time, information is needed at the global level, not only on smoking prevalence but also on policy initiatives by nations, their follow-through with FCTC commitments, and on the actions of the multinational tobacco companies. These needs have been recognized and the WHO is tracking policy through its Report on Global Tobacco Epidemic and is partnering with the US CDC to monitor smoking through the Global Tobacco Surveillance System (GTSS).

The record also makes clear that interventions need to reflect underlying structure and to acknowledge the potential for cross-level interactions, some synergistic and others antagonistic. Over time, the mix of tobacco control interventions has expanded to include programmes directed at most levels. The optimal mix reflects this breadth of coverage. The WHO's MPOWER strategy, which is grounded in the FCTC, includes a set of strategies that have multi-level impact: warnings, tax and price, cessation, enforcement, and protection from SHS (WHO 2008). The multinational corporations have also learned to act across levels: for example, luring young urban adults with promotion in entertainment venues at one end, and diminishing the FCTC at the other.

We now have tools to model tobacco control activities across the various levels of this structured framework. Substantial effort has been directed at developing models for tobacco control (Luke and Stamatakis 2011; National Cancer Institute 2007). These tools can be used to simulate the dynamics of tobacco control and to select the optimum package of interventions.

In closing, much has been learned from tobacco control about the need for structural approaches to control the epidemic of tobacco use. This knowledge has been critical in successes achieved to date. It has guided us to a global strategy, the FCTC, and led to a global campaign against a global threat to public health. We have tools to optimize tobacco control strategies in this effort to end one of the world's deadliest epidemics.

References

Boyle, P., Gray, N., Henningfield, J., Seffrin, J., and Zatonski, W. (2010) *Tobacco and Public Health: Science, Policy, and Public Health*, Oxford: Oxford University Press.

Brandt, A.M. (2007) *The Cigarette Century: The Rise, Fall, and Deadly Persistence of the Product that Defined America*, New York: Basic Books.

California Department of Health (2010) *California Tobacco Control Program*. Online, available at: http://www.cdph.ca.gov/programs/tobacco (accessed 22 May 2012).

Centers for Disease Control and Prevention (CDC), Office on Smoking and Health (2010) *Smoking and Tobacco Use – Consumption Data*. Available at: http://www.cdc.gov/tobacco/data_statistics/tables/economics/consumption/ (accessed 20 May 2012).

Centers for Disease Control and Prevention (CDC), Office on Smoking and Health (2012) Data from the National Health Interview Survey, Hyattsville, MD: National Center for Health Statistics.

Collin, J. (2004) 'Tobacco politics', *Development*, 47: 91–6.

Fisher, R.A. (1959) *Smoking. The Cancer Controversy. Some Attempts to Assess the Evidence*, Edinburgh, Scotland: Oliver & Boyd.

Glass, T.A. and McAtee, M.J. (2006) 'Behavioral science at the crossroads in public health: extending horizons, envisioning the future', *Social Science & Medicine*, 62 (7): 1650–71.

GLOBALink (2011) *GLOBALink Tobacco Control, The International Tobacco Control Community*. Online, available at: http://www.globalink.org/ (accessed 10 Jan 2012).

Jha, P. and Chaloupka, F.J. (1999) *Curbing the Epidemic: Governments and the Economics of Tobacco Control*, Washington, D.C.: World Bank.

Kluger, R. (1996) *Ashes to Ashes: America's Hundred-year Cigarette War, the Public Health, and the Unabashed Triumph of Philip Morris*, New York, Alfred A. Knopf.

Luke, D.A. and Stamatakis, K.A. (2011) 'Systems science methods in public health: dynamics, networks, and agents', *Annual Reviews of Public Health*, 33: 357–76.

National Cancer Institute (1991) *Strategies to Control Tobacco Use in the United States. A Blueprint for Public Health Action in the 1990s.* Smoking and Tobacco Control Monograph 1, Rockville, MD: US Department of Health and Human Services.

National Cancer Institute (2006) *Evaluating ASSIST: A Blueprint for Understanding State-level Tobacco Control. Monograph 17*, Bethesda, MD: US Department of Health and Human Services, National Institutes of Health.

National Cancer Institute (2007) *Greater than the Sum: Systems Thinking in Tobacco Control. Monograph 18*. Bethesda, MD: National Cancer Institute, US Department of Health and Human Services, Public Health Service, National Institutes of Health.

Proctor, R. (2011) *Golden Holocaust: Origins of the Cigarette Catastrophe and the Case for Abolition*, Berkeley, CA: University of California Press.

Rogers, T. (2010) 'The California tobacco control program: introduction to the 20-year retrospective', *Tobacco Control*, 19 Suppl. 1: i1–2.

Royal College of Physicians of London (1962) *Smoking and Health*, Summary of a report of the Royal College of Physicians of London on smoking in relation to cancer of the lung and other diseases, London: Pitman Medical Publishing.

Seidenberg, A.B., Caughey, R.W., Rees, V.W., and Connolly, G.N. (2010) 'Storefront cigarette advertising differs by community demographic profile', *American Journal of Health Promotion*, 24 (6): e26–31.

Shafey, O., Eriksen, M., Ross, H., and Mackay, J. (2009) *The Tobacco Atlas*, 3rd edition, Atlanta, GA: American Cancer Society.

Stillman, F.A., Hartman, A.M., Graubard, B.I., Gilpin, E.A., Murray, D.M., and Gibson, J.T. (2003) 'Evaluation of the American stop smoking intervention study (ASSIST): a report of outcomes', *Journal of the National Cancer Institute*, 95 (22): 1681–91.

US Department of Health and Human Services (1994) *Preventing Tobacco Use Among Young People: A Report of the Surgeon General*, Atlanta, GA: Department of Health and Human Services, Public Health Service, Centers for Disease Control and Prevention, National Center for Chronic Disease Prevention and Health Promotion, Office of Smoking and Health.

US Department of Health and Human Services (2000) *Reducing Tobacco Use: A Report of the Surgeon General*, Atlanta, GA: US Department of Health and Human Services, Centers for Disease Control and Prevention, National Center for Chronic Disease Prevention and Health Promotion, Office on Smoking and Health.

US Department of Health and Human Services (2004) *The Health Consequences of Smoking. A Report of the Surgeon General*, Atlanta, GA: US Department of Health and Human Services, Centers for Disease Control and Prevention, National Center for Chronic Disease Prevention and Health Promotion, Office on Smoking and Health.

US Department of Health and Human Services (2010) *How Tobacco Smoke Causes Disease: The Biology and Behavioral Basis for Smoking-attributable Disease. A Report of the Surgeon General*, Atlanta, GA: US Department of Health and Human Services, Centers for Disease Control and Prevention, National Center for Chronic Disease Prevention and Health Promotion, Office on Smoking and Health.

US Department of Health Education and Welfare (1964) 'Smoking and health', Report of the Advisory Committee to the Surgeon General, Washington, D.C.: US Government Printing Office.

White, A. (2004) 'Controlling big tobacco – the winning campaign for a global tobacco control treaty', *Multinational Monitor*, 25 (1).

Wipfli, H., Avila-Tang, E., Navas-Acien, A., Kim, S., Onicescu, G., Yuan, J., Breysse, P., Samet, J.M., and FAMRI Homes Study Investigators (2008) 'Secondhand smoke exposure among women and children: evidence from 31 countries', *American Journal of Public Health*, 98 (4): 672–9.

World Health Organization (WHO) (2003) *World Health Assembly Resolution 56.1, WHO Framework Convention on Tobacco Control*, Geneva: WHO.

World Health Organization (WHO) (2008) *WHO Report on the Global Tobacco Epidemic, 2008: The MPOWER Package*, Geneva: WHO.

World Health Organization (WHO) (2011) *WHO Report on the Global Tobacco Epidemic, 2011: Warning about the Dangers of Tobacco*, Geneva: WHO.

18

SOCIAL POLICY INTERVENTIONS AND HEALTH

Celina Su and Peter Muennig

Among the poorest nations, economic development is critically important for health (Preston 1976). In these nations, income provides a means to purchase food, cleaner water, and basic medicines. By overcoming hunger and infectious disease, a nation can greatly reduce mortality, especially among children. This probably explains why small changes in national per capita gross domestic product are associated with large increases in life expectancy in the poorest nations. However, once a nation's gross national income exceeds about US $5,000 per capita (adjusting for purchasing power parity), the relationship between income and life expectancy becomes less straightforward. In richer nations, social services – such as schools, health, transit, and safety net programmes – probably matter more for health (Schoeni *et al.* 2008). These services provide buffers that allow people to live in safer homes, be on safer roads, live with less stress, exercise more, and eat more healthfully.

In middle- and high-income nations, many of the social policy interventions that make the greatest impact on health lie outside the health care system (Muennig *et al.* 2010). Because middle-income nations are generally faced with the challenge of conquering chronic diseases rather than infectious diseases and hunger, many experts believe that we should again turn to structural, non-medical policies in the hope that we can realize similar success (Marmot and Wilkinson 2006; Schoeni *et al.* 2008).

These policies include enhancements to schooling or other social welfare programmes. One idea that has gained traction is to couple welfare payments to classroom attendance and receiving regular medical care, a concept known as conditional cash transfers (Adato *et al.* 2011; Cueto 2009; Fernald *et al.* 2008; Paes-Sousa *et al.* 2011). At first glance, social policies such as payments for primary school attendance may not seem as closely linked to health as clean water, but they may provide the next major boost to life expectancy among many nations tackling chronic diseases.

Such social policies can take very broad forms. Even democracy itself is thought to be lifesaving. The Nobel Prize-winning economist Amartya Sen declared that famine is rare in a functioning democracy because mass starvation is not good for anyone's political career (Sen 1999). Likewise, democracy provides a means for people to demand lifesaving programmes, such as better schools, roads, and access to medical care.

In this chapter, we discuss several prominent cases of social policy interventions at least partly aimed at improving health outcomes. We focus on conditional cash transfers, participatory budgeting, and governance and administrative innovations in Brazil, comprehensive early childhood development services in the United Kingdom (UK), and changes to the built environment in New York and San Francisco. We weigh the evidence on the impact of these interventions and the conditions in which they work best, and we conclude with some potential lessons for practice and research.

A rise in targeted social policy interventions

Innovative social policy reforms have proliferated and gained prominence in public policy debates since the 1990s. Latin American cases have dominated many of these debates for several reasons. First, many of the largest economies in the region – Brazil, Argentina, and Chile, for example – returned to democratic governance after military dictatorships (Shifter 2009: 55). Second, the structural adjustment crises of the 1980s that ravaged South America highlighted the importance of sustainable social programmes to policymakers. Third, some economists had previously conceptualized social programmes as arising from economic growth rather than contributors to economic growth, but prevailing opinions began to recognize the importance of both pathways (Bloom et al. 2004; Sachs 2002; Waitzkin 2003). Fourth, there was growing awareness that steep wealth inequalities could lead to civil unrest (Blattman and Miguel 2010; Collier et al. 2003). Finally, the rise of China led to a demand-driven commodity boom that benefited Latin America economically, opening the door to more expensive, innovative social programmes (Nelson 2011).

Of course, this is not to say that innovative policy interventions are not happening elsewhere. Indeed, we reference cases from other low- and middle-income countries, such as India, and from industrialized nations such as the UK.

Conditional cash transfers

Child-centred conditional cash transfers (CCTs) attempt to simultaneously promote poverty alleviation and civic responsibility in the short term and investment in human capital in the longer term. In CCT programmes, families receive monthly cash payments if they meet certain behavioural criteria, such as sending their primary school-age children to school on more than 85 per cent of school days, complying with prenatal visits to clinics, and having their children receive recommended vaccinations.

For instance, Brazil's Bolsa Família began in rural areas, when local governments simultaneously extended after-school programmes and paid families with 5- to 16-year-old children to keep them in school all day, rather than have them work in degrading or hazardous conditions. Other components of Bolsa Família ask that pregnant women attend prenatal medical check-ups, complete immunizations for their children, and breastfeed. In Mexico, additional food cash transfers are given after families attend nutrition seminars.

Mexico's Oportunidades programme (formerly known as Progresa, and the first nation-wide programme of this kind) and Brazil's Bolsa Família are among the largest and most well-known CCT programmes. Bolsa Família alone reached 11 million families, or 46 million people, in 2006 (Lindert et al. 2006; Soares et al. 2010), affecting 100 per cent of Brazil's poor and 25 per cent of the entire population at the time. Other countries with CCTs include Bolivia, Colombia, Jamaica, and Nicaragua (Lund et al. 2010; Soares et al. 2009).

Currently, in Bolsa Família, poor families receive monthly benefits of 140 reals (US $88.60), plus 32 reals per child aged 15 or younger for up to three children. For teenagers aged 16 to 17, families receive 32 reals (US $21) a month for up to two teenagers. Families with incomes below the extreme poverty line receive additional cash transfers of 70 reals (US $44.30). Thus, a very poor family with three children and two teenagers would receive 242 reals (US $153) (Soares 2011). As a point of comparison, the current minimum wage is 545 reals a month (US $344).

These programmes have yielded some impressive outcomes. After the implementation of Bolsa Família, Brazil's poverty rate fell from 39 per cent in 2001 to 25 per cent in 2009 – the lowest rate in decades – and overall income inequalities also fell (ECLAC 2010). Secondary school enrolment increased by 13 per cent, from 69 per cent in 2000 to 82 per cent in 2008 (Loyka 2011). A growing number of Asian, African, and North American governments have followed suit (Schubert and Slater 2006). The CCT programmes' key features appear to be their eligibility rules, coordination with supply-side increases in funding of public services, and administrative structures and transparency.

Eligibility and conditionalities

The programmes' eligibility rules are tied to certain conditions. First, all eligible families must be poor. Brazil's Bolsa Família considers only household income in determining eligibility. This is challenging because many beneficiaries work in the informal sector, so they do not report their income to the government. In Mexico and Chile, social workers use an index to determine eligibility (Soares et al. 2009). Chile's Solidario programme is aimed at the indigent, the poorest 225,000 families in the nation.

Solidario builds upon the premise that many indigent families do not access public services partly because they face discrimination, lack information, and lack a sense of agency; social workers can help to remedy this by relying more on judgement than workers in Mexico. However, eligibility requirements, including possession of birth certificates, proof of citizenship, marriage certificates and divorce decrees, employment-related requirements, and unemployment affidavits, can increase barriers to access. These barriers to entry often come with high opportunity costs and have been more common in more recent programmes, such as one in the Western Cape in South Africa (Lund et al. 2010).

In 2009, Bolsa Família revised its coverage target from 11.1 million to 12.9 million families, despite the fact that poverty rates had fallen. In doing so, it expanded the programme's eligibility criteria and working definition of poverty: a family was poor even if its income exceeded thresholds as long as its income was volatile and risked falling below the poverty threshold in a two-year period (Soares 2011).

Access to social services

In Brazil, if families do not meet conditionalities – the things they are required to do to receive benefits – they go through five stages of warnings and suspensions before benefits cease. Even then, under-16-year-old children are not affected, and the warnings trigger a social worker visit to such families. For example, if a 16-year-old has partly missed school because he/she was caring for a younger sibling after their mother got a new job, the social worker helps the family attain alternate childcare. The programme emphasizes opportunities for greater well-being, rather than punitive measures for poor performance.

Mexico's CCTs operate similarly to Brazil's and Chile's, though they give more generous conditional scholarships to upper secondary school students. As a point of comparison, the CCT ceiling for a very poor family with two teenagers was US $239 in Mexico in 2007, US $91 (adjusting for purchasing power parity) in Brazil in 2003, and just US $33 in Chile in 2003 (Soares *et al.* 2009).

Chile's Solidario programme may seem stingy at first glance. However, it combines CCTs with unconditional family subsidies for the very poor, potable water subsidies (in a country where water provision is privatized in many areas), disability and pension subsidies, and greater access to social services. Chile's Solidario attempts to tackle social exclusion by mandating that social workers collaborate with families to develop action plans for access to employment and domestic violence programmes that may fall outside the parameters of bigger CCT programmes. The amount of the CCT is calculated to ensure that the families can afford a certain basket of goods, amenities, and services below which they would be considered socially excluded. The CCT amount decreases and then ceases over a two-year period. Families are then given a graduation bonus and preferential treatment in accessing social services for another three years.

Transparent administration

Brazil's Bolsa Família was able to achieve notable outcomes because it learned from its mistakes. For instance, its 2003 food subsidy programme quickly lost support because it was seen as too bureaucratic; beneficiaries had to provide proof of their purchases to local managers, leading to barriers to access and heavy administrative costs. As a result, the Brazilian government unified all welfare programmes under Bolsa Família and encouraged civil society to participate (De Janvry *et al.* 2006). The government also coordinated the programme with the Departments of Education and Health (Lindert *et al.* 2006).

The central government now bypasses the country's 27 governors and the legislative branch, working with executive branch agencies and municipal agencies instead. Municipal governments must register families and transfer data to individual ministries (such as that of education). A fully updated and accurate registry earns the town a high 'decentralized management index' score, which then translates into more funds from the central government each month. The local government has general guidelines but considerable discretion on how to spend this money. This way, the national government ensures cooperation by simultaneously mandating responsibilities and providing incentives and funding to municipal governments.

In many traditional welfare programmes, street-level bureaucrats and social workers perform surveillance over beneficiaries, but there is little bottom–up or peer accountability. In contrast, the money in Bolsa Família is given directly to the households via 'Citizen Cards' mailed to each residence. Families use the Citizen Card as they would any debit card, withdrawing money at any ATM belonging to Caixa Econômica Federal, a government-owned savings bank. Further, an online portal publishes names of all persons enrolled in the programme and their CCT amounts. The federal government also launched a single household database to combine all beneficiary databases for all social programmes, including gas, electricity, and food subsidies, Bolsa Família, and youth employment (De la Brière and Lindert 2003).

Outcomes

The amounts transferred to each family are quite modest, totalling extremely small amounts of the GDP in Chile to roughly 0.5 per cent of total GDP in Brazil and Mexico. Nevertheless, these programmes have reduced income inequalities in all three countries (Soares *et al.* 2009). This suggests that when CCT programmes achieve both good targeting and scale, they can be cost-effective poverty eradication policies.

While Brazil's Bolsa Família lowered child labour rates, it *raised* adult labour force participation rates, especially among women (Soares *et al.* 2010). This counters arguments by some critics, including the Brazilian Catholic Church, that the subsidies act as handouts that 'disincentivize' work. It remains unclear the extent to which adults are partly making up for the pay their children no longer earn.

As discussed above, better education translates into greater abilities to earn a living, make choices that yield longer-term benefits, and be informed citizens. Bolsa Família made the greatest difference for students in north-eastern Brazil (the country's poorest region), older students aged between 15 and 17, and girls. Female beneficiary students aged 15 to 17 in north-eastern Brazil were 28 per cent more likely to stay in school (Soares 2011).

In Mexico, Oportunidades increased school enrolment and lowered dropout rates, but it also lowered academic performance because low-achieving students became more likely to stay in school (Soares *et al.* 2010). It is hoped that these students still accrue many of the labour market benefits of having a high school degree, but it remains unclear whether the poorer performers are impacting the performance of the other students.

Hopefully, these changes improve health outcomes in the longer term, promote greater social cohesion and socioeconomic security, and reduce material deprivation. In terms of more immediate health outcomes, newborns of beneficiary pregnant women in Oportunidates were 14 per cent more likely to experience longer gestations (fewer premature births), and beneficiary children were 39 per cent more likely to avoid malnutrition and achieve normal body mass index scores (Soares 2011). Nutritional supplements are sometimes shared by everyone in the household, possibly diminishing returns to children under five (Lund *et al.* 2010). This contrasts with the experiences of Mexico and Colombia, where all beneficiaries under the age of two became significantly less likely to suffer from stunting (Soares *et al.* 2010). It is unclear exactly what local circumstances – advice on preventing malnutrition, monitoring by health clinicians, governance, culture, and so on – made the difference.

There were also some notable failures. For instance, Bolsa Família's cash payments for vaccinations among children did not seem to improve immunization rates, possibly because vaccination services were not available in some localities. In contrast, immunizations rose dramatically in Colombia and Mexico, where payments were only made within localities that actually offered such services. In Ecuador, the first few years of CCTs were actually unconditional in municipalities where adequate services provision and monitoring had not yet been set up (Soares *et al.* 2010).

Remaining problems

These promising but mixed results hint at several important issues. First, payments only work when quality services are available. For example, payments for school attendance, the cornerstone of Latin American CCT programmes, would not make a difference in educational achievement in South Africa, where 8-year-olds achieve an astounding 98 per cent average attendance rate (Lund *et al.* 2010). However, in Kenya, where attendance is low, covering the cost of a school uniform increased attendance by 6.4 per cent and reduced dropout rates and teenage pregnancy rates among girls (Glennerster and Kremer 2011; Kremer *et al.* 2004).

Opportunity NYC, the New York City programme that ran from 2007 to 2010, focused on education, health, and work CCTs. In the randomized control trial, beneficiary families received an average of US $3,000 a year, and CCTs decreased poverty by 8 per cent and extreme poverty by almost half. Programmes that linked poor families to existing institutions and provided intensive guidance were quite successful. The most dramatic health outcome lay in a 10 per cent increase in dental visits to two per year. Still, other outcomes were small; beneficiaries were 2 per cent more likely to hold health insurance (from unusually high baseline rates) and 3 per cent more likely to have been treated for a medical condition (Riccio 2010). This is probably related to the higher baseline rate of health insurance in both groups.

Second, governments recognize that the poverty lines do not accurately differentiate the poor from the non-poor. This is a problem that led to public scrutiny of Brazil's Bolsa Família. In 2011, President Dilma Rousseff announced a new 'Brazil without Misery' programme aimed at eliminating indigent poverty by 2014. This will resemble Chile's Solidario programme, developing more comprehensive action plans for the poorest. Ideally, this would expand the pool of beneficiaries to further move Brazil toward a society with a guaranteed basic income.

Third, policymakers are uncertain about the full range of desirable habits that can or should be shaped via conditionalities. Newer proposed conditionalities to tie cash payments to school achievement scores have been controversial. Mandatory 'volunteering' in the community has also been attempted; however, not only is mandatory volunteering oxymoronic, it risks stigmatizing welfare beneficiaries and real volunteers alike.

Such political questions plagued Opportunity NYC as well, which was criticized by conservatives for 'bribing' poor people to do what they should do anyway. Liberals also criticized it for attempting to correct individuals' 'poor values' in a 'culture of poverty' without adequately addressing larger structural inequalities. Student beneficiaries were 15 per cent more likely to have attendance rates of 95 per cent or better, but conditionalities tied to outcomes (such as high achievement scores), rather than participation in activities, yielded few results. In one case, thousands of students protested a dearth of college preparatory and Advanced Placement (AP) classes even as programmes offered US $1,000 bonuses to Latino or Black students who scored perfectly on AP exams (Su 2010). Few single mothers in the programme were able to maintain a job and attend a skills-building course, despite the US $3,000 bonus. Childcare problems, the Great Recession, high unemployment, and the lack of suitable courses were all notable problems. In other cases, full-time workers who met all conditionalities were still unable to raise themselves out of poverty, for their jobs did not pay living wages (Goldstein 2009; Riccio 2010).

Finally, political and social context also matters. Conditionalities that help adolescents stay in school rather than work full-time in hazardous conditions might be more appropriate in Brazil than in the United States (US), where students are more likely to drop out for different reasons. A programme that gave mothers in Rajasthan, India a kilogram of lentils each time their children received vaccines raised immunization rates from 5 per cent to 38 per cent (Glennerster and Kremer 2011), but these conditional lentil transfers would hardly work in other middle-income countries. (For one, in our humble opinion, American lentil soup is much less tasty than Indian daal.)

South African welfare programmes have a history of using so-called 'conditions' that are not easily monitored and act as normative injunctions, i.e. that the child must be 'properly' clothed. At the same time, these welfare benefits are often meagre, so that parents struggle to meet conditions. Further, past conditionalities demanded that families participated in 'livelihood activities' in neighbourhoods where such projects did not exist (Lund et al. 2010).

Getting at education early

Sizeable income-related gaps in cognitive development are often present in children even before they attend school (Hart and Risley 1992). Children from poorer families tend to enter kindergarten far behind their peers with respect to vocabulary and math skills, making it much more difficult to catch up. This gap appears to be primarily attributable to changeable factors, such as maternal health and parenting styles (Waldfogel and Washbrook 2011). One idea, then, is for governments to enhance these skills for the very poorest children, and to help parents (for instance, those with two jobs) cope with the demands of parenting.

There is evidence that such programmes not only improve earnings once the children grow up, but also reduce criminal behaviour, improve health, and reduce the use of social services (Belfield et al. 2006; Muennig et al. 2009; Muennig et al. 2011). In fact, in the US, one programme was shown in a small randomized trial to produce a net benefit of US $1 million dollars over the lifetime of every child in the experimental group.

Sure Start Children's Centres in the UK attempt to address health disparities by offering services aimed at young children and their families. It has some similarities to Ontario's Early Years Plan in Canada and Head Start in the US. However, Sure Start is more comprehensive than Head Start. In addition to creating children's centres, the British government more generally revamped social service programmes to (1) make work pay; (2) raise incomes for families with children; and (3) invest in children's services (Waldfogel 2010).

The first component of the UK programmes, making work pay, consisted of establishing a national minimum wage and rendering tax rates more progressive by lower payroll tax rates for low-income earners. It also established a Working Families Tax Credit. This is similar to the Earned Income Tax Credit in the US, which provides income supplementation for workers in low-wage jobs. The second component of the anti-poverty strategy expands on this family-based supplemental income approach by increasing New Child Tax Credits, grants to children under ten years, and other child benefits. There were also reductions in primary school class sizes, increases in education spending, and an increase in the minimum school-leaving age from 16 to 18. The most prominent aspect of the campaign probably lay in the Sure Start Children's Centres (Waldfogel 2010).

Between 2002 and 2004, the UK opened 500 Children's Centres serving around 800 children each. These centres ran independently of local governments and received funds so rapidly that only 9 per cent of 1999 moneys were spent that year. In 2005, control of the Centres was transferred from central to local governments (Melhuish *et al.* 2010).

Between 1999 and 2008, the UK experienced a 50 per cent drop in children's poverty. Health outcomes associated with the programmes included improved mental health and school performance among adolescents in single-parent households, a dramatic increase in the consumption of fresh fruits, and decreased spending on tobacco and alcohol by parents (Waldfogel 2010). The implementation of these social programmes was also associated with increased numeracy and literacy among children. Interestingly, outcomes for parenting behaviour, especially in dealing with children's noncompliance, violence, and aggression, were positive and statistically significant in more strictly implemented settings, such as randomized control trials in Wales (Hutchings *et al.* 2007). Outcomes overall were modest or negligible in 2005 but more pronounced in 2008, suggesting that Sure Start programmes improved over time (Mackenbach 2010; Melhuish *et al.* 2010). Though they appeared to be largely successful, the British government announced an end to many of these programmes and reductions in others due to massive deficits from the Great Recession (Ramesh and Gentleman 2011).

Innovations in the built environment

Health insurance status appears to play little role in explaining the massive health disparities according to race, education, income, and region within non-poor societies (Muennig *et al.* 2010). For example, Asian-American women in Bergen County, New Jersey in the US live to an average of 91 years, while Native American men in the Dakotas live to an average of 58 years – a 33-year gap in life expectancy. These differences largely persist after holding constant health insurance status and excluding HIV and homicide. Further, the ten leading risk factors for poor health outcomes in the US (smoking, obesity, high blood pressure, illicit drug use, unsafe sex, etc.) cumulatively only account for 30 per cent of disease among men in the US (Murray *et al.* 2006), and do not appear to explain international changes in life expectancy over time (Muennig and Glied 2010). In response, an increasing number of city planners see that public transit, housing, economic development legislation, zoning, and other aspects of the built environment help to determine how, and how long, residents live.

For instance, New York City embarked upon a multi-pronged approach of giving away free bicycling gear (lights, helmets, and maps), promoting bicycling through advertising, and building (or painting green) 390 miles of new bicycle lanes between 2002 and 2010. By 2011, the number of commuter bicyclists in New York City had risen by 62 per cent since 2008 and 262 per cent since 2000 (O'Grady 2011). While progress was sometimes slowed by a lack of community input, resulting in backlash, the overwhelming majority of new bicycle lanes have been implemented without incident and widely adopted by local residents.

Nevertheless, New York remains behind cities such as Barcelona, Spain; Paris, France; London, England; and for that matter, Curitiba, Brazil; and Hangzhou, China, in promoting transportation alternatives to cars. In those cities, individuals who cannot afford to buy a bicycle (or worry about it getting stolen) can still cheaply rent bicycles at stations conveniently located at public transit stations. Congestion pricing also heavily taxes cars. Both citywide changes, especially in zoning and the promotion of mixed-use and dense areas, and individual-based incentive programmes appear to be essential in encouraging population-wide lifestyle changes (Appleyard *et al.* 2007; Goldman and Gorham 2006).

San Francisco has attempted to tackle health disparities by changing the built environment in other ways (City and County of San Francisco 2010). In the mid to late 1990s, the Bay Area experienced a housing boom because of Silicon Valley and Internet-related industry. The housing pressures persisted even during the economic recession of the 2000s. In response, community organizations struggled to address persistent health disparities (especially in conditions such as asthma and lead poisoning) caused by unsafe housing, proximity to toxic industrial spaces and hazardous land use, and lack of access to public transit, amenities, and good jobs. By 2001, the city had begun to use Health Impact Assessments (HIAs) of proposed built environment developments such as new condominium towers at Rincon Hill, an intra-urban freeway in the Excelsior neighbourhood, and redevelopment of two federal public housing sites. Whenever possible, the Department of Public Health attempted to mandate HIAs alongside the government's or private developer's more typical cost–benefit analyses and environmental impact assessments (Corburn 2009).

In 2004, the city worked to consolidate lessons from different HIAs. It forwarded a Strategic Plan to tackle four priority social determinants: (1) low socioeconomic status; (2) social isolation; (3) institutional racism (including racial disparities regarding the locations of sewage treatment plants, hazardous lots, amenities like public parks and well-funded schools, and well-stocked produce suppliers); and (4) transportation. By 2007, they had developed the Healthy Development Measurement Tool, a comprehensive evaluation metric for all cities and neighbourhoods to use themselves in considering health needs in urban development. The tool includes six key elements, 28 objectives, and 125 indicators. For example, the 'Healthy Economy' key element has four objectives, such as 'Increase high-quality employment opportunities for local residents'. This particular objective has four indicators, including 'jobs paying wages greater than or equal to the self-sufficiency wage'. Each of these indicators then comes with a table on the exact local 'self-sufficiency wages', as well as how they were calculated, so that policymakers in other cities can calculate their own.

Innovations in administration and governance

As the Bolsa Família case suggests, good governance is an integral component of many innovative social policy interventions. Indeed, there has also been a growth in experimental governance structures in the past two decades (De Sousa Santos 2005; Fung *et al.* 2003). Here, we briefly discuss two governance cases: Ceará state in Brazil, where the state government bolstered a preventive care programme by bypassing local governments and strengthening civil society instead; and the city of Porto Alegre, Brazil, where city residents decide annual city budgets themselves, instead of leaving them up to elected city officials.

In 1987, the Ceará state government launched a new health worker programme that managed to lower infant mortality by 36 per cent, triple immunization rates, and almost quadruple the number of municipalities with nurse access – all in just five years, and all with low-paid, unskilled health workers. It managed to do so by coordinating health worker salaries and the recruitment process via the state capital. This way, local mayors could not distribute these funds or jobs via their patronage networks. It also won over local nurses (the main point of resistance because their jobs were threatened by low-wage workers) by giving them considerable training and supervisory powers over these new health workers. Finally, it launched massive publicity campaigns that encouraged the community, including the many applicants who did not receive the jobs, to respect these new health worker public servants, and to hold them accountable via evaluations. All of the public servants felt both pressure to perform well and newfound prestige, despite their low pay. And they succeeded, often performing tasks beyond those formally prescribed. This case runs contrary to what decentralization and privatization proponents would have expected. The state government actually increased its involvement in public programmes, but it was able to reap some of the typical benefits of decentralization, such as knowledge of local contexts, by empowering local communities to hold civil servants accountable (Tendler 1997).

Another approach is to include public participation in developing local budgets. Porto Alegre began its first participatory budgeting process in 1989. Participatory budgeting is a process in which people within a community – rather than elite policymakers – help to determine how government funds are spent. In Porto Alegre, a city of roughly 1.5 million people, a disproportionate percentage of government funds historically went to middle- and upper-class neighbourhoods. This was true even as slums continued to lack access to potable water and other amenities.

The participatory budgeting process forced elected officials and roughly 50,000 residents to meet with one another and justify their budget priorities in public, deliberative assemblies. After hearing residents' concerns, delegates translated these concerns into specific programme and policy proposals. City officials, in turn, worked with these delegates to make the programmes and policies technically and financially feasible. The resulting budgets from this process are binding. After the process, the proportion of the city budget that went to poor districts and to basic public services rose dramatically (Baiocchi 2003).

Many of the middle- and upper-class residents who attended neighbourhood assemblies voted for projects in slum neighbourhoods rather than their own. As a result, sewer and electricity rates rose from 75 to 98 per cent, and the number of schools quadrupled. Health and education budgets increased from 13 to almost 40 per cent (Bhatnagar et al. 2003). An analysis of Brazil's 220 largest cities suggested that participatory budgeting is statistically significantly correlated with lower rates of extreme poverty (Boulding and Wampler 2010). Participatory budgeting has now spread to over 1,000 cities around the world – hundreds in Latin America and dozens in Europe, Africa, Asia, and North America. By building a more equitable distribution of lifesaving resources – such as water, sanitation, education, and public transit – it becomes possible to better tackle the health problems associated with poverty in such nations.

Concluding lessons

Social policy interventions are messy. However, tinkering with policies to make them better – as policymakers did with Bolsa Família, the Health Agent Programme in Ceará, and Sure Start in the UK – should not be viewed as a sign of dysfunction. In fact, the governments' responses to the criticisms ultimately rendered the programmes successful.

It is also important not to attempt to generalize successful programmes from one place across entirely different foreign contexts. Chile, Mexico, and Brazil all launched successful CCT programmes, but in very different ways: Brazil chose administrative decentralization and income as the sole criterion, Mexico chose centralization and a multidimential poverty index, and Chile chose social worker empowerment and a multidimential index (Soares *et al.* 2009). Real estate brokers' mantra of 'location, location, location' matters as much as in social policy as it does in housing markets.

Nevertheless, some themes emerge. In all of the successful cases, civil society and the state were mutually reinforcing rather than mutually exclusive. Decentralization only works if central governments have also worked to bypass corrupt networks in local governments, coordinated programmes, trained workers, and infused resources into the programmes. This increased funding might come about because of newly elected governments or systems of governance (like participatory budgeting), but it must be institutionalized in a transparent manner.

Structural approaches work best when they combine environmental changes and increases in public services with individual and family-based programmes like conditional cash transfers. Poor people's risky behaviours might change, but it takes a long time (and many synergistic policies) to shape health outcomes in sustained ways. Still, these cases ultimately demonstrate that thoughtfully designed social policy interventions are worth a shot; when they do work, they tackle the root causes of health disparities in ways medical approaches cannot.

References

Adato, M., Roopnaraine, T., and Becker, E. (2011) 'Understanding use of health services in conditional cash transfer programs: insights from qualitative research in Latin America and Turkey', *Social Science & Medicine*, 72 (12): 1921–9.

Appleyard, B., Zheng, Y., Watson, R., Bruce, L., Sohmer, R., Li, X., *et al.* (2007) *Smart Cities. Solutions for China's Rapid Urbanization*, New York: National Resources Defense Council.

Baiocchi, G. (2003) 'Participation, activism, and politics: The Porto Alegre experiment', in E.O. Wright and A. Fung (eds) *Deepening Democracy*, New York: Verso Books.

Belfield, C. R., Nores, M., Barnett, W. S., and Schweinhart, L. (2006) 'The High/Scope Perry Preschool Program', *Journal of Human Resources*, 41 (1): 162–90.

Bhatnagar, D., Rathore, A., Torres, M. i. M., and Kanungo, P. (2003) *Empowerment Case Studies: Participatory Budgeting in Brazil*, Washington, D.C.: World Bank.

Blattman, C. and Miguel, E. (2010) 'Civil war', *Journal of Economic Literature*, 48 (1): 3–57.

Bloom, D. E., Canning, D., and Sevilla, J. (2004) 'The effect of health on economic growth: a production function approach', *World Development*, 32 (1): 1–13.

Boulding, C. and Wampler, B. (2010) 'Voice, votes, and resources: evaluating the effect of participatory democracy on well-being', *World Development*, 38 (1): 125–35.

City and County of San Francisco (2010) *Program on Health, Equity and Sustainability*. Online, available at: http://www.sfphes.org/phes_mission.htm (accessed 20 September 2010).

Collier, P., Elliott, V., Hegre, H., Hoeffler, A., Reynal-Querol, M., and Sambanis, N. (2003) *Breaking the Conflict Trap: Civil War and Development Policy*, Washington, D.C.: World Bank and Oxford University Press.

Corburn, J. (2009) *Toward the Healthy City: People, Places, and the Politics of Urban Planning*, Cambridge, MA: MIT Press.

Cueto, S. (2009) 'Conditional cash-transfer programmes in developing countries', *The Lancet*, 374 (9706), 1952–3.

De Janvry, A., Sadoulet, E., Solomon, P., and Vakis, R. (2006) *Evaluating Brazil's Bolsa Escola Program: Impact on Schooling and Municipal Roles*, Berkeley, CA: University of California.

De la Brière, B. and Lindert, K. (2003) *Reforming Brazil's Cadastro Único to Improve the Targeting of the Bolsa Família Program*, Washington, D.C.: World Bank.

De Sousa Santos, B. (2005) *Democratizing Democracy: Beyond the Liberal Democratic Canon*, New York: Verso Books.

Economic Commission for Latin America and the Caribbean (ECLAC) (2010) *Social Panorama of Latin America*, Santiago, Chile: United Nations Economic Commission on Latin America and the Caribbean.

Fernald, L.C., Gertler, P.J., and Neufeld, L.M. (2008) 'Role of cash in conditional cash transfer programmes for child health, growth, and development: an analysis of Mexico's Oportunidades', *The Lancet*, 371 (9615): 828–37.

Fung, A., Wright, E. O., and Abers, R. (2003) *Deepening Democracy: Institutional Innovations in Empowered Participatory Governance*, New York: Verso Books.

Glennerster, R. and Kremer, M. (2011) 'Small changes, big results: behavioral economics at work in poor countries', *Boston Review*, March/April, 36. Online, available at: http://bostonreview.net/BR36.32/glennerster_kremer_behavioral_economics_global_development.php

Goldman, T. and Gorham, R. (2006) 'Sustainable urban transport: four innovative directions', *Technology in Society*, 28 (1–2): 261–73.

Goldstein, D. (2009) 'Behavioral theory: can Mayor Bloomberg pay poor people to do the "right" thing?', *American Prospect*, 24 August.

Hart, B. and Risley, T. R. (1992) 'American parenting of language-learning children: persisting differences in family-child interactions observed in natural home environments', *Developmental Psychology*, 28 (6): 1096–105.

Hutchings, J., Bywater, T., Daley, D., Gardner, F., Whitaker, C., Jones, K. *et al.* (2007) 'Parenting intervention in Sure Start services for children at risk of developing conduct disorder: pragmatic randomised controlled trial', *British Medical Journal*, 334 (7595): 678.

Kremer, M., Miguel, E., and Thornton, R. (2004) *Incentives to Learn*, Cambridge, MA: National Bureau of Economic Research.

Lindert, K., Linder, A., Hobbs, J., and De la Brière, B. (2006) *The Nuts and Bolts of Brazil's Bolsa Família Program: Implementing Conditional Cash Transfers in a Decentralized Context*, Washington D.C.: World Bank.

Loyka, M. (2011) *Inequality and Poverty in Latin America: Can the Decline Continue?*, Washington, D.C.: Council on Hemispheric Affairs.

Lund, F., Noble, M., Barnes, H., and Wright, G. (2010) 'Is there a rationale for conditional cash transfers for children in South Africa?', *Transformation: Critical Perspectives on Southern Africa*, 70: 70–91.

Mackenbach, J.P. (2010) 'The English strategy to reduce health inequalities', *The Lancet*, 377 (9782): 1986–8.

Marmot, M.G. and Wilkinson, R.G. (2006) *Social Determinants of Health*, 2nd edition, New York: Oxford University Press.

Melhuish, E., Belsky, J., and Barnes, J. (2010) 'Evaluation and value of Sure Start', *Archives of Disease in Childhood*, 95 (3): 159–61.

Muennig, P. and Glied, S.A. (2010) 'What changes in survival rates tell us about US health care', *Health Affairs (Millwood)*, 29 (11): 2105–13.

Muennig, P., Fiscella, K., Tancredi, D., and Franks, P. (2010) 'The relative health burden of selected social and behavioral risk factors in the United States: implications for policy', *American Journal of Public Health*, 100 (9): 1758–64.

Muennig, P., Robertson, D., Johnson, G., Campbell, F., Pungello, E.P., and Neidell, M. (2011) 'The effect of an early education program on adult health: the Carolina Abecedarian Project randomized controlled trial', *American Journal of Public Health*, 101 (3): 512–16.

Muennig, P., Schweinhart, L., Montie, J., and Neidell, M. (2009) 'Effects of a prekindergarten educational intervention on adult health: 37-year follow-up results of a randomized controlled trial', *American Journal of Public Health*, 99 (8): 1431–7.

Murray, C., Kulkarni, S., Michaud, C., Tomijima, N., Bulzacchelli, M., Iandiorio, T. *et al.* (2006) 'Eight Americas: investigating mortality disparities across races, counties, and race-counties in the United States', *PLoS Medicine*, 3 (9): 1513–24.

Nelson, J.M. (2011) 'Social policy reforms in Latin America: urgent but frustrating', *Latin American Research Review*, 46 (1): 226–39.

O'Grady, J. (2011) 'Biking on the rise in the city, DOT says', *National Public Radio*, 29 April. Online, available at: http://www.wnyc.org/articles/wnyc-news/2011/apr/29/department-transportation-says-streets-aresafer-biking/.

Paes-Sousa, R., Santos, L.M., and Miazaki, E.S. (2011) 'Effects of a conditional cash transfer programme on child nutrition in Brazil', *Bulletin of the World Health Organization*, 89 (7): 496–503.

Preston, S.H. (1976) *Mortality Patterns in National Populations with Special Reference to Recorded Causes of Death*, New York: Academic Press.

Ramesh, R. and Gentleman, A. (2011) 'Cuts will force 250 Sure Start centres to close, say charities: 60,000 families could lose local centre despite "family-friendly" coalition agenda', *Guardian*, 28 January.

Riccio, J. (2010) *Sharing Lessons from the First Conditional Cash Transfer Program in the United States*, Ann Arbor, MI: National Poverty Center.

Sachs, J.D. (2002) 'Macroeconomics and health: investing in health for economic development', *Revista Panamericana de Salud Pública*, 12 (2): 143–4.

Schoeni, R.F., House, J.S., Kaplan, G.A., and Pollack, H. (eds) (2008) *Making Americans Healthier: Social and Economic Policy as Health Policy*, New York: Russell Sage Foundation.

Schubert, B. and Slater, R. (2006) 'Social cash transfers in low-income African countries: conditional or unconditional?', *Development Policy Review*, 24 (5): 571–8.

Sen, A. (1999) *Development as Freedom*, New York: Knopf.

Shifter, M. (2009) 'Managing disarray: the search for a new consensus', in A.F. Cooper and J. Heine (eds) *Which Way Latin America? Hemispheric Politics Meets Globalization*, Tokyo: United Nations University Press.

Soares, F.V. (2011) 'Brazil's Bolsa Família: a review', *Economic and Political Weekly*, 46 (21): 55–60.

Soares, F.V., Ribas, R.P., and Osório, R.G. (2010) 'Evaluating the impact of Brazil's Bolsa Família: cash transfer programs in comparative perspective', *Latin American Research Review*, 45 (2): 173–90.

Soares, S., Osório, R.G., Veras Soares, F., Medeiros, M., and Zepeda, E. (2009) 'Conditional cash transfers in Brazil, Chile and Mexico: impacts upon inequality', *Estudios Económicos*, 1: 207–24.

Su, C. (2010) 'Marginalized stakeholders and performative politics: dueling discourses in education policymaking', *Critical Policy Studies*, 4 (4): 362–83.

Tendler, J. (1997) *Good Government in the Tropics*, Baltimore, NJ: Johns Hopkins University Press.

Waitzkin, H. (2003) 'Report of the WHO Commission on Macroeconomics and Health: a summary and critique', *The Lancet*, 361 (9356): 523–6.

Waldfogel, J. (2010) *Britain's War on Poverty*, New York: Russell Sage Foundation.

Waldfogel, J. and Washbrook, E. (2011) 'Early years policy', *Child Development Research*, Article 343016: 1–12.

INDEX